Advances in Pediatric Thoracic Imaging

Guest Editor

EDWARD Y. LEE, MD, MPH

RADIOLOGIC CLINICS OF NORTH AMERICA

www.radiologic.theclinics.com

Consulting Editor
FRANK H. MILLER, MD

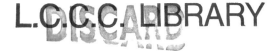
September 2011 • Volume 49 • Number 5

SAUNDERS an imprint of ELSEVIER, Inc.

W.B. SAUNDERS COMPANY
A Division of Elsevier Inc.

1600 John F. Kennedy Boulevard • Suite 1800 • Philadelphia, Pennsylvania 19103-2899

http://www.theclinics.com

RADIOLOGIC CLINICS OF NORTH AMERICA Volume 49, Number 5
September 2011 ISSN 0033-8389, ISBN 13: 978-1-4557-1151-2

Editor: Barton Dudlick
Developmental Editor: Donald E. Mumford

Radiologic Clinics of North America (ISSN 0033-8389) is published bimonthly by Elsevier Inc., 360 Park Avenue South, New York, NY 10010-1710. Months of issue are January, March, May, July, September, and November. Periodicals postage paid at New York, NY and additional mailing offices. Subscription prices are USD 386 per year for US individuals, USD 610 per year for US institutions, USD 185 per year for US students and residents, USD 450 per year for Canadian individuals, USD 766 per year for Canadian institutions, USD 556 per year for international individuals, USD 766 per year for international institutions, and USD 266 per year for Canadian and foreign students/residents. To receive student and resident rate, orders must be accompanied by name of affiliated institution, date of term and the signature of program/residency coordinatior on institution letterhead. Orders will be billed at individual rate until proof of status is received. Foreign air speed delivery is included in all *Clinics* subscription prices. All prices are subject to change without notice. **POSTMASTER:** Send address changes to *Radiologic Clinics of North America*, Elsevier Health Sciences Division, Subscription Customer Service, 3251 Riverport Lane, Maryland Heights, MO63043. **Customer Service: Telephone: 1-800-654-2452** (U.S. and Canada); **1-314-447-8871** (outside U.S. and Canada). **Fax: 1-314-447-8029. E-mail: journalscustomerservice-usa@ elsevier.com** (for print support); **journalsonlinesupport-usa@elsevier.com** (for online support).

Reprints. For copies of 100 or more of articles in this publication, please contact the Commercial Reprints Department, Elsevier Inc., 360 Park Avenue South, New York, New York 10010-1710. Tel.: (+1) 212-633-3812; Fax: (+1) 212-462-1935; E-mail: reprints@elsevier.com.

Radiologic Clinics of North America also published in Greek Paschalidis Medical Publications, Athens, Greece.

Radiologic Clinics of North America is covered in *MEDLINE/PubMed (Index Medicus), EMBASE/Excerpta Medica, Current Contents/Life Sciences, Current Contents/Clinical Medicine, RSNA Index to Imaging Literature, BIOSIS, Science Citation Index,* and *ISI/BIOMED.*

Printed in the United States of America.

Contributors

CONSULTING EDITOR

FRANK H. MILLER, MD
Professor of Radiology; Chief, Body Imaging
Section and Fellowship Program and GI
Radiology, Medical Director MRI, Department
of Radiology, Northwestern University
Feinberg School of Medicine, Chicago, Illinois

GUEST EDITOR

EDWARD Y. LEE, MD, MPH
Assistant Professor of Radiology; Chief,
Division of Thoracic Imaging, Departments of
Radiology and Medicine, Pulmonary Division,
Children's Hospital Boston and Harvard
Medical School, Boston, Massachusetts

AUTHORS

PHILLIP M. BOISELLE, MD
Professor of Radiology, Department of
Radiology, Beth Israel Deaconess Medical
Center and Harvard Medical School, Boston,
Massachusetts

ALAN S. BRODY, MD
Professor of Radiology, Department of
Radiology, Cincinnati Children's Hospital
Medical Center, Cincinnati, Ohio

L.P. BROWNE, MD
Assistant Professor, Edward B. Singleton
Department of Pediatric Radiology, Texas
Children's Hospital, Houston, Texas

DOROTHY BULAS, MD
Professor of Radiology and Pediatrics,
Department of Diagnostic Imaging and
Radiology, Children's National Medical Center,
The George Washington University School of
Medicine and Health Sciences, Washington, DC

T. CHUNG, MD
Department of Pediatric Radiology, Children's
Hospital & Research Center Oakland, Oakland,
California

BRIAN D. COLEY, MD
Clinical Professor of Radiology and Pediatrics;
Chief, Section of Ultrasound, Columbus
Children's Hospital, The Ohio State University
School of Medicine and Public Health,
Columbus, Ohio

MELISSA DAUBERT, MD
Cardiology Fellow, Stony Brook University
School of Medicine, Stony Brook, New York

HENRY DORKIN, MD
Associate Professor of Pediatrics, Director,
Associate Chief, Division of Respiratory
Diseases, Department of Medicine, Children's
Hospital Boston and Harvard Medical School,
Boston, Massachusetts

ALEXIA M. EGLOFF, MD
Clinical Instructor, Department of Diagnostic
Imaging and Radiology, Children's National
Medical Center, Washington, DC

MONICA EPELMAN, MD
Assistant Professor of Radiology; Director,
Neonatal Imaging, The Children's Hospital of
Philadelphia, University of Pennsylvania
School of Medicine, Philadelphia, Pennsylvania

HEDIEH K. ESLAMY, MD
Clinical Instructor, Department of Radiology, Lucile Packard Children's Hospital, Stanford University School of Medicine, Stanford, California

DONALD P. FRUSH, MD, FACR, FAAP
Professor of Radiology and Pediatrics; Chief, Pediatric Radiology, Department of Radiology, Children's Health Center, Duke University Medical Center, Durham, North Carolina

HYUN WOO GOO, MD
Associate Professor, Department of Radiology and Research Institute of Radiology, Asan Medical Center, University of Ulsan College of Medicine, Songpa-gu, Seoul, South Korea

FREDERICK D. GRANT, MD
Division of Nuclear Medicine and Molecular Imaging, Department of Radiology, Children's Hospital Boston; Associate Training Program Director, Joint Program in Nuclear Medicine; Assistant Professor in Radiology, Harvard Medical School, Boston, Massachusetts

S. BRUCE GREENBERG, MD
Professor of Radiology and Pediatrics, University of Arkansas for Medical Sciences, Arkansas Children's Hospital, Little Rock, Arkansas

R. PAUL GUILLERMAN, MD
Associate Professor of Radiology, Department of Pediatric Radiology, Texas Children's Hospital, Baylor College of Medicine, Houston, Texas

JEFFREY C. HELLINGER, MD
Associate Professor of Radiology and Pediatrics; Associate Director, Advanced Cardiovascular Imaging; Director, Advanced Imaging and Informatics Laboratory, Stony Brook Long Island Children's Hospital, Stony Brook University School of Medicine, Stony Brook, New York

R. KRISHNAMURTHY, MD
Assistant Professor, Edward B. Singleton Department of Pediatric Radiology, Texas Children's Hospital, Houston, Texas

EDWARD Y. LEE, MD, MPH
Assistant Professor of Radiology; Chief, Division of Thoracic Imaging, Departments of Radiology and Medicine, Pulmonary Division, Children's Hospital Boston and Harvard Medical School, Boston, Massachusetts

MICHAEL A. MOORE, MB BCh
Department of Radiology, Cork University Hospital, Wilton, Cork, Ireland

BEVERLEY NEWMAN, MD
Professor of Radiology, Department of Radiology, Lucile Packard Children's Hospital, Stanford University School of Medicine, Stanford, California

S. TED TREVES, MD
Chief, Division of Nuclear Medicine and Molecular Imaging, Department of Radiology, Children's Hospital Boston; Director, Joint Program in Nuclear Medicine; Professor in Radiology, Harvard Medical School, Boston, Massachusetts

SARA O. VARGAS, MD
Associate Professor of Radiology, Department of Pathology, Children's Hospital Boston and Harvard Medical School, Boston, Massachusetts

E. CHRISTINE WALLACE, MB BCh
Assistant Professor of Radiology; Pediatric Radiologist, Department of Radiology, UMass Memorial Medical Center, University of Massachusetts Medical School, Worcester, Massachusetts

SJIRK J. WESTRA, MD
Associate Professor of Radiology; Pediatric Radiologist, Division of Pediatric Radiology, Department of Radiology, Massachusetts General Hospital, Harvard Medical School, Boston, Massachusetts

Contents

> Advances in high-resolution prenatal ultrasound and fetal magnetic resonance (MR) imaging have changed the practice of obstetrics by allowing better visualization of intrathoracic and neck structures and better estimation of lung volumes. More accurate prenatal diagnosis has increased options for pregnancy management and treatment, delivery planning, and postnatal care. Anyone who is interested in the fascinating field of fetology should become familiar with the current state of fetal imaging of the chest as well as potential advances in technology and research.

> Ultrasound of the thorax is particularly rewarding in children, because their unique thoracic anatomy provides many available acoustic windows into the chest. Newer ultrasound techniques can allow better understanding of lung disease. With minimum effort and creativity, chest ultrasound can provide important clinical information without radiation exposure or sedation sometimes required for computed tomography and magnetic resonance imaging.

> It is much more challenging in children than in adults to obtain computed tomography images of the lung parenchyma at optimal lung volumes without motion artifact. Some of the more common forms of diffuse lung disease in adults rarely occur in children, and several forms of diffuse lung disease are unique to children. Recognition of these differences has led to the development of a new classification scheme for pediatric diffuse lung disease. Knowledge of this classification and recognition of characteristic imaging findings of specific disorders will lead to accurate diagnosis and guide appropriate treatment of children with diffuse lung disease.

> Advances in multidetector computed tomography (MDCT) technology have given rise to improvements in the noninvasive and comprehensive assessment of the large airways in pediatric patients. Superb two-dimensional and three-dimensional reconstruction MDCT images have revolutionized the display of large airways and enhanced the ability to diagnose large airway diseases in children. The 320-MDCT scanner, which provides combined detailed anatomic and dynamic functional information assessment of the large airways, is promising for the assessment of dynamic

large airway disease such as tracheobronchomalacia. This article discusses imaging techniques and clinical applications of MDCT for assessing large airway diseases in pediatric patients.

Pneumonia is an infection of the lung parenchyma caused by a wide variety of organisms in pediatric patients. The role of imaging is to detect the presence of pneumonia, and determine its location and extent, exclude other thoracic causes of respiratory symptoms, and show complications such as effusion/empyema and suppurative lung changes. The overarching goal of this article is to review cause, role of imaging, imaging techniques, and the spectrum of acute and chronic pneumonias in children. Pneumonia in the neonate and immunocompromised host is also discussed.

Congenital pulmonary malformations represent a heterogeneous group of developmental disorders affecting the lung parenchyma, the arterial supply to the lung, and the lung's venous drainage. In both asymptomatic and symptomatic pediatric patients with congenital pulmonary malformations, the diagnosis of such malformations usually requires imaging evaluation, particularly in cases of surgical lesions for preoperative assessment. The goal of this article is to review the current imaging techniques for evaluating congenital pulmonary malformations and their characteristic imaging findings, which can allow differentiation among various congenital pulmonary malformations in pediatric patients.

Given the heterogeneous nature of pediatric chest trauma, the optimal imaging approach is tailored to the specific patient. Chest radiography remains the most important imaging modality for initial triage. The decision to perform a chest computed tomography scan should be based on the nature of the trauma, the child's clinical condition, and the initial radiographic findings, taking the age-related pretest probabilities of serious injury into account. The principles of as low as reasonably achievable and *Image Gently* should be followed. The epidemiology and pathophysiology, imaging techniques, characteristic findings, and evidence-based algorithms for pediatric chest trauma are discussed.

Congenital thoracic vascular anomalies include embryologic developmental disorders of the thoracic aorta, aortic arch branch arteries, pulmonary arteries, thoracic systemic veins, and pulmonary veins. Diagnostic evaluation of these anomalies in pediatric patients has evolved with innovations in diagnostic imaging technology. State-of-the-art magnetic resonance (MR) imaging, MR angiography multidetector-row computed tomographic (MDCT) angiography, and advanced postprocessing visualization techniques offer accurate and reliable high-resolution two-dimensional and three-dimensional noninvasive anatomic displays for interpretation and clinical management of congenital thoracic vascular anomalies. This article reviews vascular MR imaging, MR angiography, MDCT angiography, and advanced visualization techniques and applications for the assessment of congenital thoracic vascular anomalies, emphasizing clinical embryology and the characteristic imaging findings.

Cardiac multidetector computed tomography (MDCT) for congenital heart disease is a useful, rapid, and noninvasive imaging technique bridging the gaps between echocardiography, cardiac catheterization, and cardiac MRI. Fast scan speed and greater anatomic coverage, combined with flexible ECG-synchronized scans and a low radiation dose, are critical for improving the image quality of cardiac MDCT and minimizing patient risk. Current MDCT techniques can accurately evaluate extracardiac great vessels, lungs, and airways, as well as coronary arteries and intracardiac structures. Radiologists who perform cardiac MDCT in children should be familiarized with optimal cardiac computed tomography (CT) scan techniques and characteristic cardiac CT scan imaging findings.

Cardiovascular magnetic resonance imaging (CMR) plays an important role in the preoperative and postoperative evaluation of congenital heart disease with newer techniques enabling faster and more comprehensive evaluation of the pediatric patient. This article reviews the clinical applications of CMR before and after surgery in the most common congenital heart anomalies in pediatric patients.

In the chest, the indications for nuclear medicine studies are broader and more varied in children than in adults. In children, nuclear medicine studies are used to evaluate congenital and developmental disorders of the chest, as well as diseases more typical of adults. In the chest, pediatric nuclear medicine uses the same radiopharmaceuticals and imaging techniques as used in adults to evaluate cardiac and pulmonary disease, aerodigestive disorders, and pediatric malignancies. The introduction of PET (mostly using ^{18}F-FDG) has transformed pediatric nuclear oncology, particular for imaging malignancies in the chest.

The chest is the most frequently evaluated region of the body in children. The majority of thoracic diagnostic imaging, namely "conventional" radiography (film screen, computed radiography and direct/digital radiography), fluoroscopy and angiography, and computed tomography, depends on ionizing radiation. Since errors, oversights, and inattention to radiation exposure continue to be extremely visible issue for radiology in the public eye it is incumbent on the imaging community to maximize the yield and minimize both the real and potential radiation risks with diagnostic imaging. Technical (e.g. equipment and technique) strategies can reduce exposure risk and improve study quality, but these must be matched with efforts to optimize appropriate utilization for safe and effective healthcare in thoracic imaging in children. To these ends, material in this chapter will review practice patterns, dose measures and modality doses, radiation biology and risks, and radiation risk reduction strategies for thoracic imaging in children.

GOAL STATEMENT

The goal of the *Radiologic Clinics of North America* is to keep practicing radiologists and radiology residents up to date with current clinical practice in radiology by providing timely articles reviewing the state of the art in patient care.

ACCREDITATION

The *Radiologic Clinics of North America* is planned and implemented in accordance with the Essential Areas and Policies of the Accreditation Council for Continuing Medical Education (ACCME) through the joint sponsorship of the University of Virginia School of Medicine and Elsevier. The University of Virginia School of Medicine is accredited by the ACCME to provide continuing medical education for physicians.

The University of Virginia School of Medicine designates this enduring material activity for a maximum of 15 *AMA PRA Category 1 Credit*(s)™ for each issue, 90 credits per year. Physicians should only claim credit commensurate with the extent of their participation in the activity.

The American Medical Association has determined that physicians not licensed in the US who participate in this CME enduring material activity are eligible for a maximum of 15 *AMA PRA Category 1 Credit*(s)™ for each issue, 90 credits per year.

Credit can be earned by reading the text material, taking the CME examination online at http://www.theclinics.com/home/cme, and completing the evaluation. After taking the test, you will be required to review any and all incorrect answers. Following completion of the test and evaluation, your credit will be awarded and you may print your certificate.

FACULTY DISCLOSURE/CONFLICT OF INTEREST

The University of Virginia School of Medicine, as an ACCME accredited provider, endorses and strives to comply with the Accreditation Council for Continuing Medical Education (ACCME) Standards of Commercial Support, Commonwealth of Virginia statutes, University of Virginia policies and procedures, and associated federal and private regulations and guidelines on the need for disclosure and monitoring of proprietary and financial interests that may affect the scientific integrity and balance of content delivered in continuing medical education activities under our auspices.

The University of Virginia School of Medicine requires that all CME activities accredited through this institution be developed independently and be scientifically rigorous, balanced and objective in the presentation/discussion of its content, theories and practices.

All authors/editors participating in an accredited CME activity are expected to disclose to the readers relevant financial relationships with commercial entities occurring within the past 12 months (such as grants or research support, employee, consultant, stock holder, member of speakers bureau, etc.). The University of Virginia School of Medicine will employ appropriate mechanisms to resolve potential conflicts of interest to maintain the standards of fair and balanced education to the reader. Questions about specific strategies can be directed to the Office of Continuing Medical Education, University of Virginia School of Medicine, Charlottesville, Virginia.

The faculty and staff of the University of Virginia Office of Continuing Medical Education have no financial affiliations to disclose.

The authors/editors listed below have identified no financial or professional relationships for themselves or their spouse/partner:
Phillip M. Boiselle, MD; Alan S. Brody, MD; L.P. Browne, MD; Dorothy Bulas, MD; T. Chung, MD; Brian D. Coley, MD; Melissa Daubert, MD; Barton Dudlick (Acquisitions Editor); Alexia M. Egloff, MD; Monica Epelman, MD; Hedieh K. Eslamy, MD; Hyun Woo Goo, MD; Frederick D. Grant, MD; Jeffrey C. Hellinger, MD; Edward Y. Lee, MD, MPH (Guest Editor); Frank H. Miller, MD (Consulting Editor); Michael Moore, MB, BCh; Beverley Newman, MD; S. Ted Treves, MD; Sara O. Vargas, MD; E. Christine Wallace, MB, BCh; Sjirk J. Westra, MD.

The authors/editors listed below have identified the following financial or professional relationships for themselves or their spouse/partner:
Henry Dorkin, MD is an industry funded research/investigator, is a consultant, and is on the Advisory Board for Novartis, Bayer, Gilead, and Vertex.
Donald P. Frush, MD is an industry funded research/investigator for GE Healthcare.
S. Bruce Greenberg, MD is on the Speakers' Bureau for Toshiba, and is a consultant for Vital Images.
R. Paul Guillerman, MD is a consultant for PTC Therapeutics.
Klaus D. Hagspiel, MD (Test Author) is an industry funded research/investigator for Siemens Medical Solutions.
R. Krishnamurthy, MD is on the Speakers' Bureau for Vital Images, and is an industry funded research/investigator for Eisai Pharmaceuticals.

Disclosure of Discussion of Non-FDA Approved Uses for Pharmaceutical Products and/or Medical Devices
The University of Virginia School of Medicine, as an ACCME provider, requires that all faculty presenters identify and disclose any off-label uses for pharmaceutical and medical device products. The University of Virginia School of Medicine recommends that each physician fully review all the available data on new products or procedures prior to clinical use.

TO ENROLL

To enroll in the Radiologic Clinics of North America Continuing Medical Education program, call customer service at 1-800-654-2452 or sign up online at http://www.theclinics.com/home/cme. The CME program is available to subscribers for an additional annual fee USD 245.

Radiologic Clinics of North America

THE CLINICS ARE NOW AVAILABLE ONLINE!

Access your subscription at:
www.theclinics.com

Preface
Pediatric Thoracic Imaging

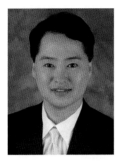

Edward Y. Lee, MD, MPH
Guest Editor

Among the numerous technological advances that have occurred in medicine over the past decade, none has created a greater change in clinical practice than those that employ state-of-the-art imaging modalities and imaging processing techniques. The increased capability to detect and diagnose various congenital and acquired thoracic diseases in infants and children is an especially compelling example of the paradigm shift created by these advances. With these technological developments, however, there are also new challenges for radiologists who must clearly understand these advances in technology in order to implement new applications and protocols in the field of pediatric thoracic imaging. The overarching goal of this issue of *Radiologic Clinics of North America* is to address these challenges by providing the readers with an up-to-date review of what is new and also currently relevant to the practice of pediatric thoracic radiology.

As the guest editor for this issue, I have selected topics that are considered to be helpful not only for understanding recent and innovative technological advances of imaging studies but also for providing optimal management of pediatric patients with various thoracic disorders. The major aim of this issue is to facilitate the reader's ability to successfully employ these imaging studies for evaluating thoracic diseases in infants and children in daily clinical practice. An additional goal of this review is to close the gap that presently exists between knowledge and practice with a view toward creating a uniform standard of care for major thoracic diseases of childhood.

I had the great privilege and pleasure of working with highly experienced and talented contributing authors—all of whom are experts in the field of pediatric thoracic imaging. Their invaluable efforts and extraordinary expertise have helped create a resource of information that should facilitate the understanding of pediatric thoracic imaging. I would also like to thank Phillip Boiselle, MD, of the Beth Israel Deaconess Medical Center, for his guidance with this project; Richard Robertson, MD, my department chair, and Caroline Robson, MD and Kirsten Ecklund, MD, my department vice chairs, for their support; my colleagues at Children's Hospital Boston, for their encouragement; Barton Dudlick and his colleagues at Elsevier for their administrative and editorial assistance; and my family for their constant encouragement and support.

Edward Y. Lee, MD, MPH
Division of Thoracic Imaging
Departments of Radiology and Medicine
Pulmonary Division
Children's Hospital Boston and
Harvard Medical School
300 Longwood Avenue
Boston, MA 02115, USA

E-mail address:
Edward.Lee@childrens.harvard.edu

Radiol Clin N Am 49 (2011) xi
doi:10.1016/j.rcl.2011.06.011

Fetal Chest Ultrasound and Magnetic Resonance Imaging: Recent Advances and Current Clinical Applications

Dorothy Bulas, MD[a],*, Alexia M. Egloff, MD[b]

KEYWORDS
• Fetal • Chest • Ultrasound • Magnetic resonance imaging

Nearly every pregnant woman in the United States today is offered fetal screening ultrasonography (US) during the second trimester. Advances in prenatal US, including three-dimensional (3D)/four-dimensional (4D) imaging, have increased the rate of fetal chest anomaly detection. As the diagnosis of fetal anomalies increase, more aggressive options for pregnancy management and treatment have been developed. Magnetic resonance (MR) imaging has become a complementary tool in the assessment of fetal chest anomalies because of its exquisite delineation of the airway and lung parenchyma. Accurate prenatal diagnosis is fundamental to assess prognosis, perform appropriate counseling, and plan prenatal management and delivery as well as postnatal therapy.

Various anomalies are now identified within the fetal chest, the prognosis of which can be variable. This article reviews current fetal US and MR imaging techniques as well as imaging findings of commonly encountered fetal thoracic anomalies. Anomalies that are discussed in this article include congenital bronchopulmonary malformations (BPMs), pleural effusions, congenital diaphragmatic hernia (CDH), congenital high airway obstruction (CHAOS), and pulmonary hypoplasia.

IMAGING TECHNIQUES
US

US is the screening imaging modality of choice and can provide accurate visualization of the anatomy of the fetus and uterus. It is widely available, inexpensive, and easy to perform. Limitations of US can be secondary to maternal obesity, oligohydramnios, fetal position, and overlying osseous structures, which decrease the ability to visualize fetal structures and the diagnostic accuracy of the study. Another limitation is the wide range of sensitivities in abnormality detection, dependent on the type of anomaly, gestational age at time of the study, and the skill of the sonographer. Detection rates of fetal chest lesions with US vary widely from as low as 22% to as high as 90%.[1]

In recent years, advances in US technology have improved the sensitivity and specificity of identifying fetal lung anomalies. High-resolution transducers with advanced pulsed, color, and power

Disclaimer: This article includes a discussion of fetal MRI technology, which has not received FDA approval. The authors have nothing to disclose.

[a] Department of Diagnostic Imaging and Radiology, Children's National Medical Center, The George Washington University School of Medicine and Health Sciences, 111 Michigan Avenue, NW, Washington, DC 20010, USA
[b] Department of Diagnostic Imaging and Radiology, Children's National Medical Center, 111 Michigan Avenue, NW, Washington, DC 20010, USA
* Corresponding author.
E-mail address: dbulas@cnmc.org

Radiol Clin N Am 49 (2011) 805–823
doi:10.1016/j.rcl.2011.06.005
0033-8389/11/$ – see front matter © 2011 Elsevier Inc. All rights reserved.

Doppler imaging, and 3D/4D postprocessing software have revolutionized fetal US assessment and advanced guided therapeutic procedures.

US is considered safe to perform at any gestation. However, there are theoretic safety risks from US energy, including thermal damage or cavitation. A gray-scale US examination produces energies ranging between 10 and 20 mW/cm^2, markedly less than the safety threshold of 100 mW/cm^2.[2] The use of power Doppler increases energy output. Therefore, conservative use of Doppler, particularly in the first trimester, should be emphasized.

MR Imaging

Fetal MR imaging has been used clinically for more than 20 years and its role in fetal evaluation has increased with time. It is considered an adjunct to fetal US evaluation and is typically not used as a screening tool. Fast scanners using ultrafast sequences have been fundamental in the increasing use in fetal imaging by substantially reducing motion artifact and limiting the need for sedation. MR imaging has multiple major advantages in the assessment of fetal lung disorders. It provides multiplanar capability, large fields of view, and excellent contrast between bowel, lung, and lung masses. Unlike US, MR imaging is not operator dependent, and is not limited by fetal position, overlying bowel gas, or osseous structures. Limitations in the use of MR imaging include cost and availability. Studies can be limited because of large maternal size, claustrophobia, maternal discomfort, and fetal motion. Currently available wide-bore magnets and faster sequences can decrease some of these limitations.

A fast, multiplanar, spoiled gradient-echo sequence or large-field-of-view coronal single-slice fast spin echo (ssFSE) localizer can first be performed to evaluate fetal position. Each subsequent plane is placed orthogonal to the previous sequence to account for fetal movement. Axial, sagittal, and coronal T2-weighted (T2W) images angled to the fetal chest are obtained at 3-mm to 5-mm thickness without gap. For complete assessment of the fetus, planes angled to the brain and abdomen should also be obtained. A fetal study may take 20 to 40 minutes depending on fetal movement, which is especially problematic when polyhydramnios is present or when the fetus is small and young.

Sequences useful in evaluating the fetal lung include ssFSE (GE, Milwaukee, WI, USA), and half-Fourier acquisition single-shot turbo spin echo (HASTE) (Siemens, Erlangen, Germany).[3,4] These T2W images can provide good contrast and spatial resolution as well as high signal/noise

ratios. Slices are acquired individually with each slice obtained by a single excitation pulse taking less than 400 milliseconds. A series can be obtained in less than 30 to 40 seconds with slices as thin as 2 to 3 mm.

Heavy T2W hydrography, fast T1-weighted (T1W) sequences including fast multiplanar spoiled gradient-echo, diffusion-weighted sequences, and 2-dimensional (2D) fast low-angle shot can also be used to evaluate the fetal chest. However, these sequences typically take longer, may require breath holding, and require thicker slices for sufficient signal/noise ratios.

Documentation of long-term safety of MR imaging exposure to the fetus is paramount. No definite harmful effects have been shown using 1.5 T magnets.[5,6] There continues to be research as to whether higher strength magnets and prolonged MR imaging studies can cause injury to the developing fetus.[7,8] To date, no definite growth abnormalities or genetic defects have been identified in animal studies and embryos.[9,10] A maximum specific absorption rate (SAR) of 10 g is recommended to be in compliance with the Medical Device Agency (MDA) guidelines to limit fetal exposure to potential heating risks.[11] Currently, MR imaging studies in the first trimester are typically avoided. Gadolinium can cross the placenta and reach the fetal circulation. Animal studies have reported growth retardation after administration of high doses of gadolinium and, thus, administration is contraindicated for fetal MR imaging studies.[12]

Fetal Lung Volume Assessment

Anatomic evaluation of the lung combined with an assessment of the fetal lung volume is important in fetal imaging. Accurate assessment of lung hypoplasia is paramount in the planning of perinatal management. Normative data of fetal lung volume are currently available but limited for different gestational ages, with high variability dependent on the methodology used.[13]

US measurements of lung volume have been used to assess pulmonary hypoplasia. Ratios such as thoracic circumference/abdominal circumference ratio, lung length/thoracic circumference ratio, and lung length/head circumference ratio, have been described with mixed reliability.[14] Use of 3D US has resulted in improved volumetric measurements of fetal lungs. 2D equations have been validated and can be used to obtain fetal lung volumes when 3D technology is not available.

Lung volume measurements using 2D US include:

1. 4.24+{1.53 × [(area of base of both lungs) × 1/3 height of right lung)]}. Moeglin and colleagues[15]

considered the lung as a regular pyramid and, using a transverse plane of the thorax at the level of the 4-chamber view, the area of the base of the lung is obtained. Height is measured on a sagittal image, between the apex of the lung and the apex of the diaphragm.

2. [Anteroposterior diameter × transverse diameter × cranial-caudal diameter of the right lung] × 0.152 + [anteroposterior diameter × transverse diameter × cranial-caudal diameter of the left lung] × 0.167, as described by Araujo Jr and colleagues,[16] who considered the lung as an ellipsoid. The anteroposterior and transverse diameters are obtained from the axial image at the level of the 4 chambers of the heart, and the craniocaudal dimension is obtained on a sagittal view using the clavicles and the diaphragms as limits.

Lung volume measurement techniques using 3D US include:

1. Lung volume = thoracic volume−heart volume. Thoracic volume is obtained by measuring and adding areas of serial transverse slices from the apex of the diaphragm to the clavicle. Heart volume is obtained by measuring and adding areas of serial transverse slices of the heart.[17] Limitations of this method are caused by overestimation of the lung volume because of the presence of mediastinal structures such as trachea, esophagus, great vessels, and thymus.
2. Lung volume equals consecutive axial slices of lung parenchyma added together. Mediastinal structures are not included in the lung volume.[18]
3. Lung volume using rotational technique. Each lung volume is obtained by serial contouring of the pulmonary area after rotating the volumetric image. This method allows finer contouring of the lung, and thus is better at estimating volumes when lungs are irregular and small, such as in fetuses with CDH.
4. Lung volume using a computer-aided volumetric calculation analysis method (virtual organ computer-aided analysis [VOCAL]). Measurement calipers demarcate upper and lower margin of fetal lung, software calculates volume of each lung, and volumes of each lung are added to obtain the total lung volume.[14]

2D measurements have been statistically lower than 3D measurements.[14] Low agreement between lung volumes obtained by 3D US and 2D US suggests that 2D equations probably should not be used despite convenience and low cost.[14] 3D US allows assessment and correction of uneven surfaces, and thus is more accurate. Use of 2D equation revalidated by 3D US represents a promising method for predicting pulmonary hypoplasia in prenatal phase in places where 3D technology is not available.[14] Advantages of 3D US compared with MR imaging are lower cost and availability as well as assessment of volume growth over time. However, US measurements of fetal lung volume have many limitations, including poor visualization of lung parenchyma in cases of oligohydramnios and obesity, time-consuming technique, and poor reliability.[19] Therefore, many have turned to MR for fetal lung volume measurements.

Lung volume measurements using MR include:

1. Total lung volume by planimetric analysis measuring the lung area on each MR imaging section, multiplying by slice thickness to obtain the volume and summing all section volumes.[20]
2. Counting number of pixels in the region of interest, multiplying by area corresponding to the pixel, and multiplying by slice thickness.[21]
3. Volume calculation from 3D reconstructed images. Images reconstructed at a workstation and automatically measured using postprocessing by cutting, erosion, dilatation, thresholding, and segmentation.[22,23]

When using MR, measurements can be performed in any plane. Axial plane measurements have been shown to be more accurate in some series,[24] but validity may be independent of plane of imaging.[25] High variability in absolute lung volumes is described, with volumes ranging from 20 to 35 mL at 25 weeks of gestation and 58 to 95 mL at 35 weeks of gestation.[13] The right lung (56% of the total lung volume) has a slightly larger volume compared with the left.

NORMAL ANATOMY
US of the Normal Fetal Chest

US is a particularly useful imaging modality in the evaluation of the fetal chest. It has high sensitivity in identifying fetal lung lesions because of their abnormal echogenicity and mass effect on adjacent structures. However, many of these lesions appear similarly echogenic on US, and thus there is low specificity. When a pulmonary abnormality is identified, a thorough evaluation of the fetus should be performed to identify other concomitant malformations.

The normal fetal chest is round or oval with ribs surrounding more than half of the circumference. A proportional growth of the fetal chest, lungs, and heart is seen with preservation of the cardiothoracic ratio throughout gestation. The heart is positioned in the anterior half of the chest, with the apex pointing toward the left. This position and axis should not change throughout the pregnancy and, when altered, can suggest the presence of an abnormal lung mass.

The fetal lung parenchyma is homogeneous on US. In early pregnancy, fetal lungs appear hypoechoic compared with the liver parenchyma. With advancing gestational age, the fetal lungs become more fluid filled, which results in increasing its echogenicity. At times, echogenic bowel, liver, and lung masses are difficult to differentiate from adjacent echogenic lung parenchyma. The thymus is a homogeneous, echogenic structure, usually not identified because of overlying rib shadowing. The diaphragms are dome shaped and hypoechoic compared with the adjacent lung parenchyma.

When evaluating the fetal lung, the fetal airway should also be assessed. However, the larynx, pharynx, and trachea are usually difficult to visualize directly by US. At times, a fluid-filled larynx can be seen in the later weeks of gestation, but the trachea is rarely seen when normal.

MR Imaging of the Normal Fetal Chest

Fetal lungs are homogeneous and hyperintense compared with muscle on MR imaging. They show an increase in signal after the 24th week of gestation (Fig. 1). This increase in signal results from the increased amount of fluid present in the lung parenchyma as the alveoli develop. Use of both T1W images (T1WI) and T2W images (T2WI) aids in the differentiation of normal lung parenchyma from adjacent structures such as mediastinum, liver, and bowel. Lungs are hyperintense compared with liver and spleen on T2WI. Conversely, liver, spleen, and meconium in bowel are hyperintense compared with lung on T1WI. The thymus is hyperintense compared with the heart, and well visualized in the third trimester. The heart shows flow void on ssFSE T2WI, and is high in signal on bright blood sequences.

MR imaging is superior to US in the evaluation of the fluid-filled fetal airway (Fig. 2). The larynx, pharynx, and trachea are typically visualized as high-signal, fluid-filled structures. Anomalies that cause airway compression can be evaluated in all 3 planes with high spatial resolution with MR imaging. Advanced techniques such as virtual bronchoscopy can now also be applied to fetal MR imaging.[26]

SPECTRUM OF FETAL THORACIC ANOMALIES
Fetal Lung Anomalies

Congenital BPMs represent a group of lung anomalies that include congenital pulmonary airway malformation (CPAM), bronchopulmonary sequestration (BPS), and congenital lobar overinflation (CLO). BPMs are now believed to represent a spectrum of anomalies that result from airway obstruction and subsequent malformation dependent on the timing, level in the tracheobronchial tree, and severity of airway obstruction.[27–29] There is considerable overlap in imaging findings of BPMs. In recent years, prenatal diagnosis of BPMs has improved the understanding of the natural progression of these lung masses and has become critical in the perinatal management and counseling of these anomalies.

Congenital Pulmonary Airway Malformation

CPAM, previously known as congenital cystic adenomatoid malformation (CCAM), is the most common congenital lung abnormality, representing 30% to 47% of fetal thoracic lung lesions.[27,28] CPAM is a hamartomatous malformation of the lung characterized by abnormal branching of immature bronchioles that communicate with the normal tracheobronchial tree.[27–29] It has arterial blood supply originating from the normal pulmonary circulation and venous drainage into normal pulmonary veins.[27,29] CPAM is most commonly located within only 1 lung (95%).[30] However, it can rarely be seen bilaterally.[30,31] Both lungs are affected with equal frequency. CPAM is usually unilobar (85%–95%), with the lower lobes most commonly affected.[31]

Stocker[32] recently expanded the classification of CPAM into 5 different types from the previous 3 different types. This new classification of CPAM is mainly based on the cyst size and underlying histologic resemblance to segments of the developing bronchial tree and airspaces. Regarding the management implications of CPAM, Adzick[33] described a classification of CPAM into 2 types based on fetal imaging appearance and gross anatomy:

1. Macrocystic CPAM: multiple large cysts measuring more than 5 mm, characterized by a slower growth rate and favorable prognosis
2. Microcystic CPAM: cysts measuring less than 5 mm and thus having a solid appearance.

Depending on the type of CPAM, US and MR imaging appearance may vary. Cystic components of CPAM are anechoic by US and bright on T2WI with MR imaging (Fig. 3). Solid components of CPAM are homogeneously echogenic by US and hyperintense on T2WI with MR imaging (Fig. 4). Large lesions can cause mediastinal shift to the contralateral side and rotation of the heart axis, hindering development of the normal lung, which can result in pulmonary hypoplasia.[34] The lung mass can compress the vena cava and heart

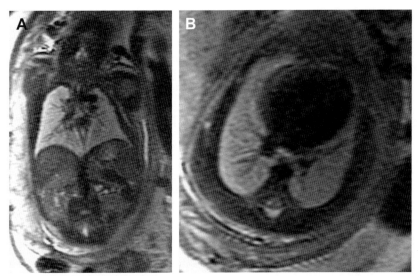

Fig. 1. Normal fetal chest at 37 weeks' gestation. (*A*) Coronal and (*B*) axial ssFSE T2W MR images of the fetal chest show homogeneous high-signal lung parenchyma caused by increased fluid content. Branching pulmonary vessels are of low signal because of flow void.

with impairment of venous return resulting in hydrops with pleural effusion, pericardial effusion, skin thickening, and/or ascites. Compression of the esophagus can also occur and result in proximal esophageal dilatation, small or absent stomach, and polyhydramnios.

As the fetus grows, lung lesions become more difficult to delineate because echogenicity of normal surrounding lung increases and blends in with the echogenic lung lesion.[35] Color Doppler imaging is useful in the evaluation of a possible systemic feeding vessel in hybrid lesions.[30] Although most lesions can be identified by US, MR imaging is useful in assessing residual normal lung volume, differentiating CPAM from other abnormalities such as CDH, and identifying associated congenital anomalies, which is critical for prognosis and counseling.[28,30,31,35]

A ratio between the CPAM volume and the head circumference was developed in an attempt to predict occurrence of hydrops and prognosis before birth.[36] The CPAM volume ratio (CVR) is obtained by calculating the volume of the lung mass and dividing it by the head circumference to normalize it by gestational age.[36] When the ratio measures less than 1.6, the risk of hydrops has been reported to be 14% in macrocystic CPAM,

and 3% in microcystic CPAM. In fetuses with CVR at presentation measuring greater than 1.6, there is a high risk, with 75% developing hydrops in a series reported by Crombleholme.[36,37]

Prognostic indicators besides the CVR include the type of lesion, amount of mediastinal shift, and fetal hemodynamic alterations including the presence of polyhydramnios and hydrops.[32–34,38] The rate of growth, particularly when associated with macrocysts, also increases the risk for developing hydrops.[36] The most important prognostic factor is hydrops. If there is no hydrops, outcome is excellent with more than 95% survival.[39] If hydrops develops, the fetus is at risk for perinatal death,[36,39] with a risk of demise approaching 100% if untreated. In these cases, fetal intervention should be considered.[30] Different interventions have been attempted, including maternal steroids, intrauterine cyst aspiration, fetal thoracentesis and thoracoamniotic shunt, laser therapy, sclerotherapy, and in utero surgical resection.[34,39–42]

Maximum growth of a CPAM lesion typically occurs between 20 and 26 weeks' gestation. Between 26 and 28 weeks, growth of CPAM plateaus.[43] In the late second trimester, the mass often decreases in size.[43] The mass may seem to disappear in up to 50% of cases.[38] When no lesion

$$CVR = \frac{\text{height} \times \text{anteroposterior diameter} \times \text{transverse diameter} \times 0.52 \text{ (constant)}}{\text{Head circumference}}$$

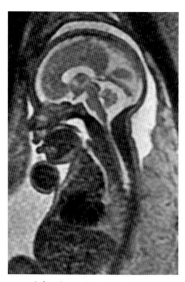

Fig. 2. Normal fetal trachea. Sagittal ssFSE T2W MR image of the fetal head, neck, and chest show a well-delineated, fluid-filled oropharynx, larynx, and trachea.

is identified on follow-up prenatal studies, postnatal imaging should still be performed because 40% of them have a residual mass. These residual masses often become difficult to see by US in the third trimester because of the normal increase in echogenicity of the surrounding normal lung parenchyma.[33] Complete resolution does occur with lesions that mimic CPAM, such as transient bronchial obstruction with focal fluid retention that can eventually resolve.[38]

Differential diagnostic considerations of CPAM lesions on prenatal imaging studies include BPS, CLO, bronchogenic cyst, CDH, laryngeal or tracheal atresia, neurenteric/enteric cysts, and mediastinal cystic teratomas (Fig. 5).[28,30,44]

Delivery and postnatal management of fetuses with CPAM depends on the characteristics of the lung mass, the associated fetal findings, and maternal health. Respiratory stability and feeding tolerance of infants with CPAM should be assessed following delivery. Follow-up radiographs and computed tomography (CT) scans can be obtained in the immediate postnatal period if the infant is symptomatic, or months later when asymptomatic to determine whether surgery is indicated.

Bronchopulmonary Sequestration

BPS is the second most common cause of fetal lung mass. These lung lesions are composed of nonfunctioning lung tissue with no communication to the bronchial tree, and are supplied by systemic arteries arising from the lower thoracic or upper abdominal aorta. BPSs are most often

hybrid lesions with components of both sequestration and CPAM. BPSs can be supradiaphragmatic, diaphragmatic, or infradiaphragmatic in location. Infradiaphragmatic lesions should be differentiated from neuroblastomas and adrenal hematomas.[27,45]

By US, BPS is usually a homogeneous echogenic mass most commonly located in the base of the lung, adjacent to the diaphragm. It typically has a triangular shape and is characterized by having a feeding systemic vessel (Fig. 6). Doppler examination is useful in identifying these systemic feeding vessels associated with BPS.[45,46] A hybrid lesion is described as a cystic lesion with a feeding systemic vessel, although the vascular structures are not always identified. Typically, these hybrid lesions have a better prognosis compared with CPAM without systemic feeding vessels.[45–47]

MR imaging is useful in the evaluation of BPS by delineating the mass and providing assessment of the contralateral lung.[28,30] BPS appears as a hyperintense T2W lesion in the lower lobe. Macrocysts are present in hybrid lesions. MR imaging does not always show the feeding systemic vessels associated with BPS (Fig. 7). When the feeding systemic vessels are noted, they usually appear as low-signal linear structures extending from the aorta into BPS.[30]

Prognosis for fetuses with BPS is favorable, with hydrops rarely developing. If hydrops does develop before 32 weeks' gestation, steroids, resection of the lesion, or thoracentesis are currently available therapeutic options. If hydrops develops after the 32nd week, early delivery is recommended.[47,48]

Although intrauterine resolution of BPS has been described, postnatal imaging with CT angiography is still indicated because typically a small residual lesion remains.

Congenital Lobar Emphysema

CLO, also known as congenital lobar emphysema, is a lung anomaly characterized by hyperinflation with normal pulmonary vascular supply and without the presence of macroscopic or microscopic cysts. After birth, it is commonly located in the apical and posterior segments of the left upper lobe but can also occur in other lobes.[27–30] By US, an echogenic, homogeneous, hyperechogenic mass without visible macrocysts can be identified in the second trimester. Normal pulmonary vascularity can be tracked within the mass (Fig. 8). The increased echogenicity of CLO is believed to be secondary to an abnormal accumulation of fluids in the lung.[49] By the third trimester, the mass often becomes isoechoic to adjacent normal lung and can be difficult to visualize.

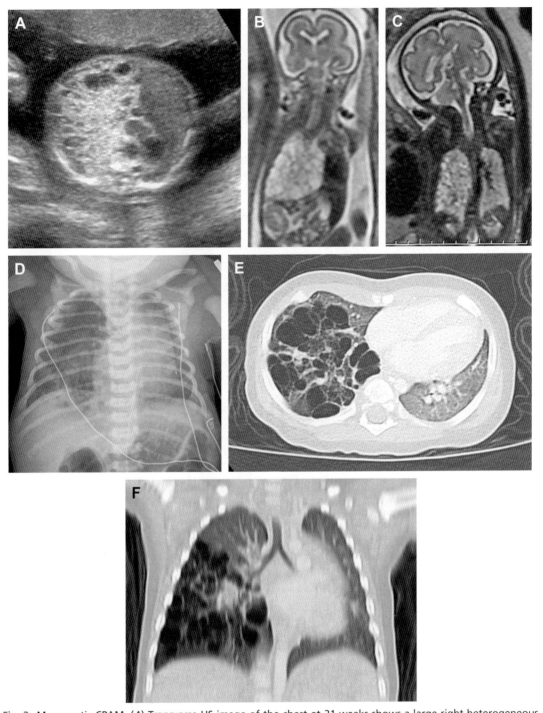

Fig. 3. Macrocystic CPAM. (*A*) Transverse US image of the chest at 21 weeks shows a large right heterogeneous echogenic mass interspersed with hypoechoic cysts. The normal hypoechoic left lung is compressed by the mass. (*B*) Coronal ssFSE T2W MR image at 21 weeks confirms the presence of a large multicystic right lung mass deviating the heart to the left. The CVR measured 2.4 which is high risk for developing hydrops. (*C*) Follow-up coronal ssFSE MR image at 30 weeks' gestation shows an interval decrease in CVR (1.4) with less mediastinal shift and left lung growth. (*D*) Radiograph at 1 day of age shows a heterogeneous right lower lobe in this full-term infant with no respiratory distress. Follow-up computed tomography (CT) scan was performed at 6 months of age. (*E*) Axial and (*F*) coronal reformatted CT images show multiple macrocysts in the right lower lobe with no systemic feeding vessel.

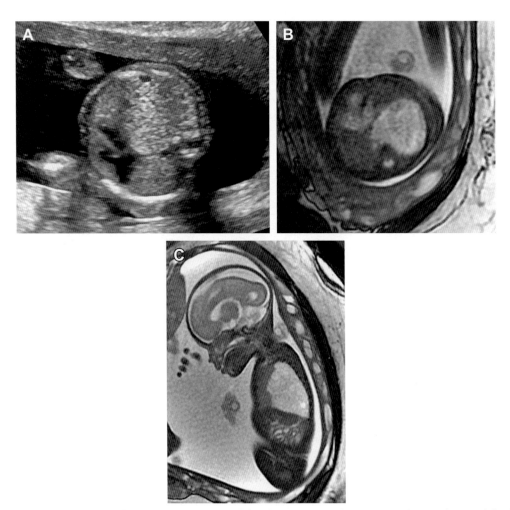

Fig. 4. Microcystic CPAM. (*A*) Transverse US image of the chest at 23 weeks' gestation shows a large solid echogenic mass in the left hemithorax deviating the heart to the right. CVR ratio = 1.8. (*B*) Follow-up MR image at 26 weeks' gestation using steady-state acquisition bright blood sequence in the axial plane shows a large left lower lobe solid mass deviating the heart anteriorly and to the right. (*C*) Sagittal ssFSE MR image shows that the mass is confined to the left lower lobe, flattening the diaphragm.

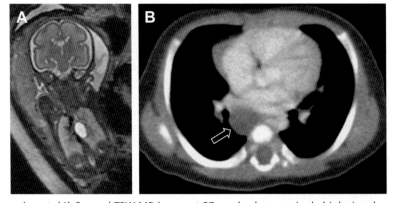

Fig. 5. Bronchogenic cyst. (*A*) Coronal T2W MR image at 27 weeks shows a single high-signal cyst located in the subcarina region and splaying the carina. The lung parenchyma is normal with no obstruction of the bronchi. (*B*) Follow-up postnatal axial CT image obtained at 2 months of age confirms the presence of a bronchogenic cyst (*arrow*).

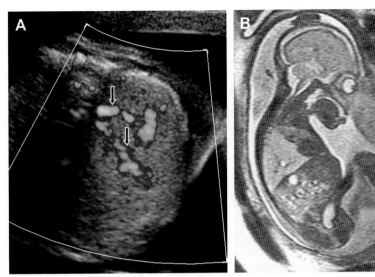

Fig. 6. Hybrid BPS. (*A*) Power Doppler axial US image of the chest at 24 weeks' gestation shows systemic vessels (*arrows*) coursing from the aorta to an echogenic solid mass within the left hemithorax. (*B*) Sagittal ssFSE MR image confirms the presence of a high-signal left lower lobe mass containing a small macrocyst.

Mass effect may be the only clue that a CLO is present on prenatal US. MR imaging shows a hyperintense lesion on T2WI (**Fig. 9**). When large, usually because of lobar bronchial atresia, mediastinal displacement to the contralateral side, polyhydramnios, and hydrops may occur.[49,50]

Differentiation of CLO from a microcystic CPAM or sequestration can be difficult before birth. Hydrops and pulmonary hypoplasia are most often associated with CPAM rather than CLO or BPS. Diagnosis can be confirmed after birth by radiograph and CT imaging.[50,51]

Congenital Diaphragmatic Hernia

Herniated bowel loops into the hemithorax can mimic a multicystic, heterogeneous lung mass by prenatal US. Hernias are more common on the left side (88% vs 10% right sided) but can also be bilateral (2%).[52] When left sided, the stomach can be herniated into the hemithorax, and nonvisualization of the stomach bubble within the abdomen is a helpful clue in the diagnosis.[52–54] When right sided or when the stomach is infradiaphragmatic in position, mediastinal and cardiac deviation may be the first hint that a CDH is present by US. Peristalsis of herniated bowel loops within the thorax can sometimes be seen.[52] Assessment of liver herniation can be difficult by US because of the similarity in echogenicity to fetal lung. When liver herniates, it typically lies anteriorly in the left hemithorax and deviates the stomach posteriorly. Thus, if the herniated stomach is posteriorly positioned, liver herniation is likely present as well. Color Doppler is best in showing kinking of the sinus venosus or bowing of the umbilical portion of the portal vein when liver is herniated into the left hemithorax.[52]

MR imaging is helpful in confirming the diagnosis of CDH. It can also provide specific information on determining size of diaphragmatic defect, assessing amount of liver herniation, delineating small and large meconium-filled bowel in the chest, and measuring volume of ipsilateral and contralateral lung. MR is most helpful in the evaluation of right and bilateral CDH. In these cases, with the stomach often infradiaphragmatic, it may be difficult to differentiate a CPAM from a CDH by US. In such cases, MR imaging can easily distinguish abdominal contents within the chest from cystic pulmonary lesions (**Fig. 10**).

The prognosis of CDH depends on the side of the herniation, the position of the liver, and whether or not there are associated abnormalities. Right-sided CDHs have a better prognosis compared with left-sided hernias (**Fig. 11**). Bilateral CDHs are typically fatal. When the liver is down, survival rate has been reported to be 90%, whereas survival rate decreases to less than 50% when liver is herniated into the thoracic cavity. Presence of other associated fetal abnormalities decreases the survival in fetuses with CDH.[55] Prognosis also depends on the therapy used at individual centers. Variability in treatment options, including the use of nitrous oxide, extracorporeal membrane oxygenation (ECMO), ex utero intrapartum treatment (EXIT) to ECMO, and fetoscopic endotracheal occlusion influence the accuracy of prenatal prognosticators.

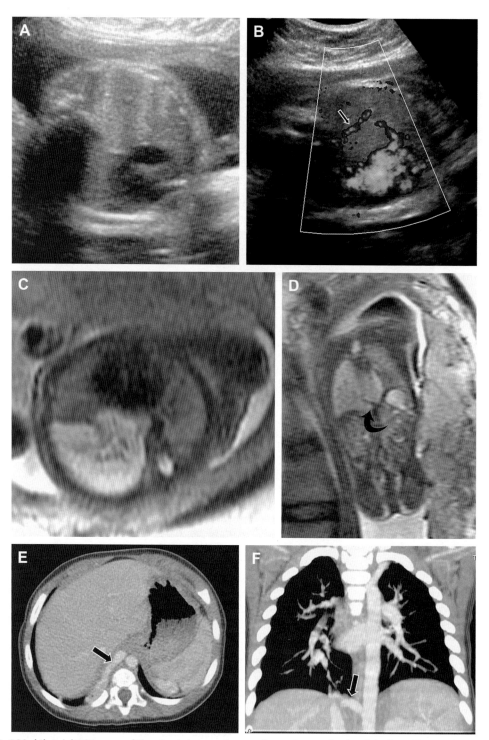

Fig. 7. BPS. (*A*) Axial US image of the chest shows a large echogenic mass in the right hemithorax deviating the heart to the left. (*B*) Power Doppler identifies a systemic vessel (*arrow*) coursing into the solid mass. (*C*) Axial T2W MR image shows the high-signal mass deviating the heart anteriorly and to the left. (*D*) Coronal ssFSE MR image shows a low-signal systemic vessel coursing into the mass (*arrow*). Following delivery, axial CT (*E*) and coronal reformatted CT images (*F*) show a large systemic vessel (*arrow*) arising from the descending aorta with interval involution of the mass.

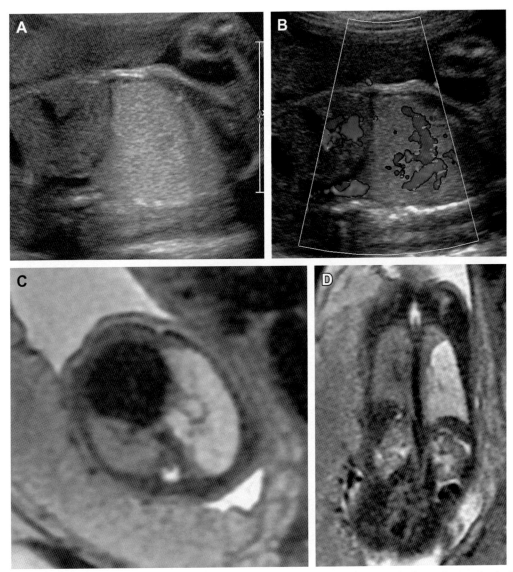

Fig. 8. Congenital lobar emphysema. (*A*) Sagittal US at 27 weeks' gestation shows an echogenic mass in the left lower lobe. (*B*) Color Doppler shows normal pulmonary vessels coursing through the mass. (*C*) Axial and (*D*) coronal ssFSE MR images at 27 weeks confirm the presence of a high-signal mass in the left lower lobe with mediastinal deviation. By 32 weeks' gestation, the mass could no longer be appreciated by US.

Currently, no single measurement has been proved to be an absolute indicator of postnatal outcome in fetuses with CDH. Measurement of the lung/head ratio (LHR) by US has been described as a tool to predict survival and the need for more aggressive treatment such as ECMO. The LHR is a measurement using the orthogonal dimensions of the right lung at the 4-chamber view divided by the head circumference in millimeters to standardize for gestational age. If the LHR is less than 1, outcome is often poor despite aggressive therapy, with a survival rate of approximately 45%.[55,56]

Multiple methods of measuring lung volumes have been attempted by MR to quantify the degree of lung hypoplasia in fetuses with CDH. Absolute total lung volumes can be obtained and compared with expected lung volumes for age.[13] If the lung volume is more than 25 cm³, a favorable prognosis is expected compared with lung volumes less than 18 cm³. A ratio between the observed and the predicted lung volume can also be obtained in an attempt to classify the patients as high or low risk. Several investigators have noted a correlation with this ratio to predict survival in CDH.[13,57,58] Gounicour and colleagues[58] noted low postnatal

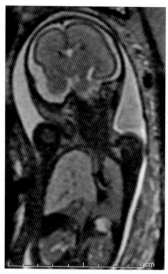

Fig. 9. Congenital lobar emphysema. Coronal ssFSE MR image at 24 weeks' gestation shows a high-signal mass in the right upper lobe with pulmonary vessels coursing from the hilum.

lung volume to obtain a percent predicted lung volume (PPLV).[59] Barnewolt and colleagues[59] noted that a PPLV less than 15% had a 40% survival versus a PPLV of greater than 15% having a 100% survival. Other MR methods that have been suggested to assess fetal pulmonary hypoplasia in CDH have included diffusion-weighted MR imaging. Information regarding peripheral growth and maturation of airways and vessels could be obtained by apparent diffusion coefficient measurement with MR imaging. However, they have not been shown to correlate with lung volume or survival of fetuses with CDH.[60]

Patients with CDHs often have pulmonary hypertension, which can worsen the outcome. The modified McGoon index can be obtained to predict the risk of developing severe pulmonary hypertension. It is obtained by adding the right and left pulmonary artery diameters and dividing it by the aortic diameter either by US or MR imaging. If the result is less than 0.8, the fetus is at high risk of developing pulmonary hypertension, and at low risk if it is more than 1.0.[61]

survival when the observed to expected total fetal lung volume was less than 25%. Another technique to standardize normal lung volume measures fetal thoracic volume then subtracts the mediastinal volume to obtain an estimated expected lung volume. The lung volume in a fetus with CDH is then measured and divided by this expected

All these measurements currently remain controversial with regard to accuracy in predicting outcome.[62,63] Measurement techniques vary between centers, as do therapeutic strategies and outcomes. Each center must define its own method of measuring volumes and correlate them with their center's outcomes. There continues to be an evolution in the evaluation, treatment, and

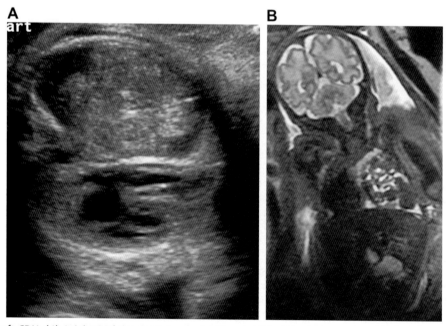

Fig. 10. Left CDH. (A) Axial US of the chest shows significant shift of the heart to the right by a heterogeneous mass. (B) Coronal T2W MR image confirms the presence of herniated small and large bowel within the left hemithorax. The liver and stomach were infradiaphragmatic in location.

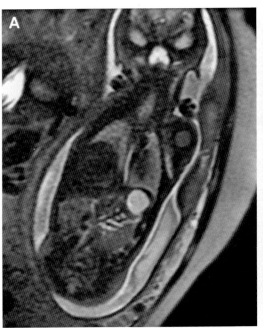 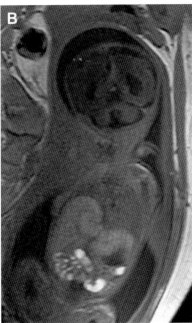

Fig. 11. Right CDH at 31 weeks' gestation. (*A*) Coronal T2W MR shows herniation of the liver into the right hemithorax. (*B*) Coronal T1W MR image confirms liver herniation into the right hemithorax.

outcome of CDH. Prenatal imaging is important for confirming the diagnosis and identifying associated anomalies. Prognostic indicators continue to be refined using US and MR volume measurements as well as Doppler assessment.

Congenital Hydrothorax

Fetal pleural effusion is an abnormal accumulation of fluid in the pleural space at any stage of gestation. It can be unilateral or bilateral. The development of fetal pleural effusion can be primary or secondary. Primary fetal pleural effusions are caused by a chylous leak, which results from thoracic duct anomalies. Secondary fetal pleural effusions can be seen in the presence of pulmonary, cardiac, gastrointestinal, metabolic, infectious, or neoplastic disorders. They can be associated with aneuploidy or other genetic syndromes. Thorough fetal evaluation must be performed to differentiate primary from secondary fetal pleural effusions. A search for other fetal anomalies, fetal echocardiography, and karyotyping is recommended.[64]

By US, an anechoic region surrounding the fetal lung is identified in the fetus with pleural effusions (**Fig. 12**). MR imaging shows high T2 signal in the pleural space. When large, mediastinal shift can occur. Depending on the size of the effusion, the lung can be compressed and subsequently result in pulmonary hypoplasia.

Primary fetal pleural effusions can have spontaneous resolution. When unilateral and without associated mediastinal shift, survival of fetuses with pleural effusions has been reported to be 100%. Thus, small effusions are conservatively managed and followed with imaging. When fetal pleural effusions are bilateral or associated with mediastinal shift and/or diaphragmatic eversion, survival rate decreases to 52%.[53] If pleural effusions progress to hydrops, mortality increases to 75%.

Secondary fetal pleural effusions have a worse outcome than primary fetal pleural effusions. Mortality ranges as high as 95% to 98% depending on the size of the pleural effusion, presence of hydrops, gestational age, and underlying cause. If the pleural effusion is large and the fetus is less than 32 weeks' gestation, fetal thoracentesis and thoracoamniotic shunting are potential prenatal treatment options, although reaccumulation of pleural fluid is frequently described.[65]

Congenital High Airway Obstruction

When bilateral large echogenic lung masses are identified on prenatal imaging studies, CHAOS should be included in the differential diagnosis.[30,66–68] This rare entity can be caused by laryngotracheal atresia, tracheal stenosis, thick tracheal web, laryngeal cyst, subglottic stenosis, and laryngeal or tracheal agenesis, which cause

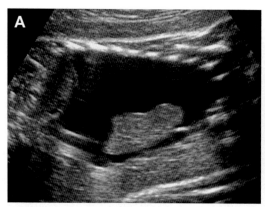
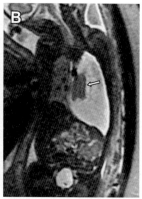

Fig. 12. Pleural effusion. (*A*) Sagittal US of the chest at 30 weeks' gestation shows a large pleural effusion compressing the underlying lung. (*B*) Coronal T2W MR image confirms the presence of a large left pleural effusion with mediastinal shift, diaphragmatic eversion, and underlying hypoplastic left lung (*arrow*).

lung overexpansion with impaired venous return to the heart resulting in hydrops and ascites.[68,69] There may be increased or decreased amniotic fluid, and placentomegaly can also occur.[68,69] Aberrant pulmonary budding off the foregut is present. CHAOS can be part of Fraser syndrome when laryngeal atresia is associated with cryptophthalmos, syndactyly, genital abnormalities, and a positive family history (**Fig. 13**).[67,69]

By US, both lungs are symmetrically enlarged, up to 15 times the normal lung size,[69] and echogenic because of fluid trapping. The heart is centrally located and compressed, whereas the diaphragms are inverted. Doppler imaging can sometimes help identify the level of obstruction by showing absence of flow in the dilated trachea at the site of obstruction.[67,69] MR imaging shows abnormally large lungs with high signal on T2WI with diaphragmatic eversion. Identifying a dilated, fluid-filled trachea and bronchi below the level of obstruction helps localize the level and confirm the diagnosis. When there is a tracheoesophageal fistula or a small laryngotracheal or pharyngotracheal fistula, the airway can be decompressed and accurately making the diagnosis of CHAOS can be difficult.[70]

Recognizing this entity is important to allow proper planning for perinatal interventions and to assess prognosis. Differential diagnosis includes bilateral type III CPAM and extrinsic tracheobronchial obstruction caused by cervical teratoma, lymphatic malformation, or vascular ring.[71]

In the past, CHAOS was considered incompatible with life.[66] However, in recent years, a less severe subtype of CHAOS with a less ominous natural history has been described. This subtype of CHAOS is characterized by the presence of a fistulous connection that allows decompression through a small laryngotracheal or pharyngotracheal fistula.[69] Because of advances in perinatal intervention, EXIT delivery with airway control has been performed before hypoxia, brain injury, or death results.[71] Outcome has improved, although prognosis remains poor. Surviving children have persistent pulmonary abnormalities and often require a long-term tracheostomy.[67,70]

Pulmonary Hypoplasia

Pulmonary hypoplasia is characterized by the presence of underdevelopment and decreased numbers of alveoli and bronchi resulting in a decrease in lung size and weight.[13] When the lung parenchyma and bronchi are absent, it is called lung agenesis. When there is absent lung parenchyma, but rudimentary bronchi are present, it is called lung aplasia. In cases of pulmonary hypoplasia, there is the presence of alveoli and bronchi that are underdeveloped, with a decrease in number of both. These entities can be associated with severe respiratory insufficiency and failure at birth that can potentially lead to death.

Pulmonary hypoplasia can be primary or secondary. Primary pulmonary hypoplasia is less common and can be associated with syndromes such as the VACTERL (vertebral anomalies, anal atresia, cardiac defect, tracheoesophageal fistula, renal abnormalities, and limb abnormalities) sequence (**Fig. 14**). Secondary pulmonary hypoplasia is more common. The underlying causes of secondary pulmonary hypoplasia include premature rupture of membranes, renal malformations with oligohydramnios (**Fig. 15**), lung masses, CDH and skeletal dysplasias, all restricting normal lung expansion and development.[13,72] Severity of pulmonary hypoplasia depends on the gestational

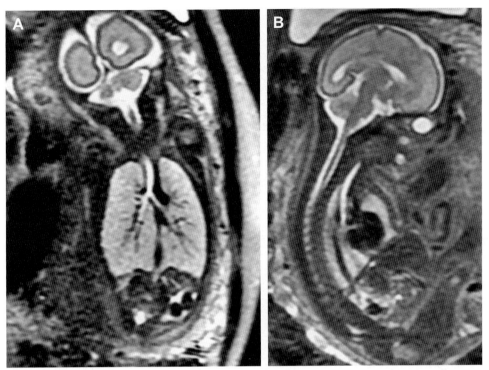

Fig. 13. Fraser syndrome with CHAOS (*A*) Coronal T2W image of a 27-week fetus with oligohydramnios secondary to renal agenesis. Despite the oligohydramnios, the lungs are enlarged and cause flattened diaphragms. (*B*) Sagittal T2W image shows a dilated trachea consistent with fluid trapping within the airway. Note the oval-shaped orbit.

age at onset. Embryologically, alveoli and pulmonary vascularity develop concomitantly, so associated anomalies of pulmonary vessels are common in fetuses with pulmonary hypoplasia.

Fetal ultrasonographic diagnosis of pulmonary hypoplasia is limited, particularly if oligohydramnios is present. Various measurements (eg, areas and ratios of hypoplastic lung to normal lung)

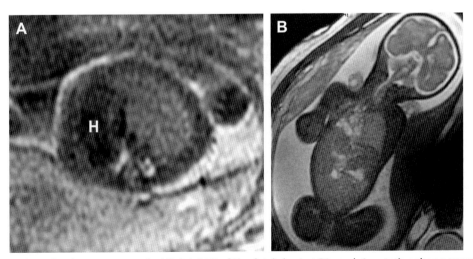

Fig. 14. Unilateral pulmonary agenesis. (*A*) Axial US of the fetal chest at 21 weeks' gestation shows severe deviation of the heart (H) to the right. (*B*) Coronal steady-state acquisition MR at 27 weeks' gestation confirms the absence of the right lung and bronchus.

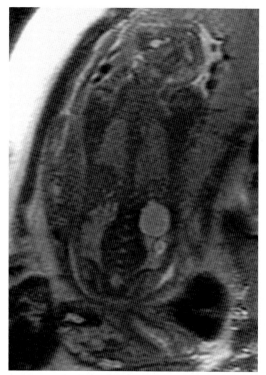

Fig. 15. Pulmonary hypoplasia. A 26-week fetus with cystic dysplastic kidneys resulting in severe oligohydramnios. Coronal T2W MR image shows small lung volumes with low signal in the lung parenchyma.

have been used in an attempt to predict outcome. Doppler imaging can evaluate the high-resistance patterns in peripheral pulmonary arteries that have been reported in fetuses with pulmonary hypoplasia.[73]

A decrease in T2W signal has been described in MR images of hypoplastic lungs compared with the progressive hyperintensity seen in normal developing lungs.[21,74–79] MR imaging, compared with US, allows better evaluation of the fetal anatomy when oligohydramnios is present. MR imaging can provide a better estimation of relative lung volumes based on gestational age and lung volume/body weight ratios. Several studies have suggested that MR spectroscopy may be a method to further assess the severity of hypoplasia in the future.[21,78,79]

Ratios such as the thoracic circumference/abdominal circumference ratio, the lung length/thoracic circumference ratio, and the lung length/head circumference ratio have been used to predict severity of hypoplasia. However, to date, these measurements have not been found to be reliable.[13] Further work on improved accuracy in predicting pulmonary hypoplasia is fundamental for outcome and counseling because a 50%

mortality has been described in fetuses with pulmonary hypoplasia.[13]

SUMMARY

In recent years, earlier and more accurate prenatal diagnosis has become possible with the technological advances that have occurred both in US and MR imaging. With these advances, a better understanding of the underlying pathophysiology and differentiation between the various lung anomalies has become possible, allowing for better prenatal management, delivery planning, and postnatal care. Currently available methods of measurements and volume acquisition of fetal thoracic anomalies can help obtain a more accurate prognosis and facilitate counseling. With the increased use of US screening, lung anomalies are more frequently identified. Fetal MR imaging can further advance the care of fetuses with various thoracic anomalies by helping to confirm the diagnosis, delineating anatomy such as the trachea that is often not well visualized by US, and showing additional associated subtle anomalies. In addition, MR imaging allows experts in fields from otolaryngology, pediatric surgery, and neonatology who are not comfortable interpreting US imaging to provide additional expertise that is useful in the counseling and management of these cases. This multidisciplinary approach becomes particularly crucial for the success of managing fetuses with complex thoracic anomalies.

REFERENCES

1. Bernaschek G, Stuempflen I, Deutinger J. The influence of the experience of the investigator on the rate of sonographic diagnosis of fetal malformations in Vienna. Prenat Diagn 1996;16:807–11.
2. American College of Obstetricians and Gynecologists. Ultrasonography in pregnancy. Washington, DC: American College of Obstetricians and Gynecologists; 2008. Practice Bulletin 98.
3. Coakley FV, Glenn OA, Qayyam A, et al. Fetal MRI: a developing technique for the developing patient. AJR Am J Roentgenol 2004;182:243–52.
4. Prayer D, Brugger PC, Prayer L. Fetal MRI: techniques and protocols. Pediatr Radiol 2004;34: 685–93.
5. Baker PN, Johnson IR, Harvey PR, et al. A three year follow up children imaged in utero with echoplanar magnetic resonance. Am J Obstet Gynecol 1994; 170:32–3.
6. De Wilde JP, Rivers AW, Price DL, et al. A review of the current use of magnetic resonance imaging in pregnancy and safety implications for the fetus. Prog Biophys Mol Biol 2005;87:335.

7. Vadeyar SH, Moore RJ, Strachan BK, et al. Effect of fetal magnetic resonance imaging on fetal heart rate patterns. Am J Obstet Gynecol 2000;182:666–9.

8. Mevissen M, Buntenkotter S, Loscher W. Effect of static and time varying magnetic field on reproduction and fetal development in rats. Teratology 1994; 50:229–37.

9. Yip YP, Capriotti C, Tlagala SL, et al. Effects of MR exposure at 1.5 T on early embryonic development of the chick. J Magn Reson Imaging 1994;4:742–8.

10. Yip YP, Capriotti C, Yip JW. Effects of MR exposure on axonal outgrowth in the sympathetic nervous system of the chick. J Magn Reson Imaging 1995; 5:457–62.

11. Hand JW, Thomas EL, Rutherford MA, et al. Predictions of specific absorption rate in mother and fetus associated with MRI examinations during pregnancy. Magn Reson Med 2006;55(4):883–93.

12. Magnevist official FDA information, side effects and uses. Wayne (NJ): Berlex Labs. Available at: http://www.drugs.com/pro/magnevist.html. Accessed July 8, 2011.

13. Rypens F, Metens T, Rocourt N, et al. Fetal lung volume: estimation at MR imaging – initial results. Radiology 2001;219:236–41.

14. Britto IS, de Silva Bussamra LC, Araujo Junior E, et al. Fetal lung volume: comparison by 2D- and 3D-sonography in normal fetuses. Arch Gynecol Obstet 2009;280:363–8.

15. Moeglin D, Almant C, Duyme M, et al. Fetal lung volumetry using two and three dimensional ultrasound. Ultrasound Obstet Gynecol 2005;25:118–27.

16. Araujo JE, Nardozza LM, Pires CR, et al. Comparison of the two-dimensional and establishment of a new constant for the measurement of fetal lung volume. J Matern Fetal Neonatal Med 2008;21:81–8.

17. Lee A, Kratochwil A, Stümpfelen I, et al. Fetal lung volume determination by three-dimensional ultrasonography. Am J Obstet Gynecol 1996;175:588–92.

18. Pohls UG, Rempen A. Fetal lung volumetry by three dimensional ultrasound. Ultrasound Obstet Gynecol 1998;11:6–12.

19. Deshmukh S, Rubesova E, Barth R. MR assessment of normal fetal lung volumes: a literature review. AJR Am J Roentgenol 2010;194:W212–7.

20. Duncan KR, Gowland PA, Moore RJ, et al. Assessment of fetal lung growth in utero with echo planar MR imaging. Radiology 1999;201:197–200.

21. Keller TM, Rake A, Michel SC, et al. MR assessment of fetal lung development using lung volumes and signal intensities. Eur Radiol 2004;14(6):984–9.

22. Mahieu-Caputo D, Sonigo P, Dommergues M, et al. Fetal lung volume measurement by magnetic resonance imaging in congenital diaphragmatic hernia. BJOG 2001;108:863–8.

23. Jani J, Breysem L, Maes F, et al. Accuracy of magnetic resonance imaging for measuring fetal sheep lungs and other organs. Ultrasound Obstet Gynecol 2005;25:270–6.

24. Büsing KA, Kilian AK, Schaible T, et al. Reliability and validity of MR image lung volume measurement in fetuses with congenital diaphragmatic hernia and in vitro lung models. Radiology 2008;246:553–61.

25. Azizkhan RG, Crombleholme TM. Congenital cystic lung disease: contemporary antenatal and postnatal management. Pediatr Surg Int 2008;24:643–57.

26. Werner H, Dos Santos JR, Fontes R, et al. Virtual bronchoscopy in the fetus. Ultrasound Obstet Gynecol 2011;37:113–5.

27. Langston C. New concepts in the pathology of congenital lung malformations. Semin Pediatr Surg 2003;12:17–37.

28. Epelman M, Kreiger PA, Servas S, et al. Current imaging of prenatally diagnosed congenital lung lesions. Semin Ultrasound CT MR 2010;31:141–57.

29. Correia-Pinto J, Gonzaga S, Huang Y, et al. Congenital lung lesions - underlying molecular mechanisms. Semin Pediatr Surg 2010;19(3):171–9.

30. Daltro P, Werner H, Gasparetto T, et al. Congenital chest malformations: a multimodality approach with emphasis on fetal MR imaging. Radiographics 2010;30(2):385–95.

31. Hubbard AM, Adzick NS, Crombleholme TM, et al. Congenital chest lesions: diagnosis and characterization wit prenatal imaging. Radiology 1999;212: 43–8.

32. Stocker TJ, Manewell JE, Drake RM. Congenital cystic adenomatoid malformation of the lung: classification and morphologic spectrum. Hum Pathol 1977;8:155–71.

33. Adzick NS, Harrison MR, Crombleholme TM, et al. Fetal lung lesions: management and outcome. Am J Obstet Gynecol 1998;179(4):884–9.

34. Kunisaki SM, Fauza DO, Barnewolt CE, et al. Ex utero intrapartum treatment with placement of extracorporeal membrane oxygenation for fetal thoracic masses. J Pediatr Surg 2007;42(2):420–5.

35. Levine D, Barnewolt CE, Mehta TS, et al. Fetal thoracic abnormalities: MR imaging. Radiology 2003;228:379–88.

36. Crombleholme TM, Coleman B, Hedrick H, et al. Cystic adenomatoid malformation volume ration predicts outcome in prenatally diagnosed cystic adenomatoid malformation of the lung. J Pediatr Surg 2002;37(3):331–8.

37. Mann S, Wilson RD, Bebbington MW, et al. Antenatal diagnosis and management of congenital cystic adenomatoid malformation. Semin Fetal Neonatal Med 2007;12:477–81.

38. Cavoretto P, Molina F, Poggi S, et al. Prenatal diagnosis and outcome of echogenic fetal lung lesions. Ultrasound Obstet Gynecol 2008;32:769–83.

39. Morris LM, Lim FY, Livingston JC, et al. High-risk fetal congenital pulmonary airway malformations

have a variable response to steroids. J Pediatr Surg 2009;2004:60–5.

40. Fortunato S, Lombardi SJ, Cantrell J, et al. Intrauterine laser ablation of a fetal cystic adenomatoid malformation with hydrops: the application of minimally invasive surgical techniques to fetal surgery. Am J Obstet Gynecol 1997;177:S84.

41. Adzick NS. Open fetal surgery for life-threatening fetal anomalies. Semin Fetal Neonatal Med 2010; 15(1):1–8.

42. Bermudez C, Pérez-Wulff J, Arcadipane M, et al. Percutaneous fetal sclerotherapy for congenital cystic adenomatoid malformation of the lung. Fetal Diagn Ther 2008;24:237–40.

43. Lecompte B, Hadden H, Coste K, et al. Hyperechoic congenital lung lesions in a non-selected population: from prenatal detection till perinatal management. Prenat Diagn 2009;29:1222–30.

44. Zeidan S, Gorincour G, Potier A, et al. Congenital lung malformation: evaluation of prenatal and postnatal radiologic findings. Respirology 2009;14: 1005–11.

45. Vijayaraghavan SB, Rao PS, Selvarasu CD, et al. Prenatal sonographic features of intralobar bronchopulmonary sequestration. J Ultrasound Med 2003; 22:541–4.

46. Sepulveda W. Perinatal imaging in bronchopulmonary sequestration. J Ultrasound Med 2009;28: 89–94.

47. Witlox RS, Lopriore E, Walther FJ, et al. Single-needle laser treatment with drainage of hydrothorax in fetal bronchopulmonary sequestration with hydrops. Ultrasound Obstet Gynecol 2009;34:355–7.

48. Becmeur F, Horta-Geraud P, Donato L, et al. Pulmonary sequestrations: prenatal ultrasound diagnosis, treatment and outcome. J Pediatr Surg 1998;33: 492–6.

49. Pariente G, Aviram M, Landau D, et al. Prenatal diagnosis of congenital lobar emphysema: case report and review of the literature. J Ultrasound Med 2009;28:1081–4.

50. Seo T, Ando H, Kaneko K, et al. Two cases of prenatally diagnosed congenital lobar emphysema caused by lobar bronchial atresia. J Pediatr Surg 2006;41:E17–20.

51. Bush A, Hogg J, Chitty LS. Cystic lung lesions – prenatal diagnosis and management. Prenat Diagn 2008;28:604–11.

52. Graham G, Devine C. Antenatal diagnosis of congenital diaphragmatic hernia. Semin Perinatol 2005;20:69–76.

53. Claus F, Sandaite I, Dekoninck P, et al. Prenatal anatomical imaging in fetuses with congenital diaphragmatic hernia. Fetal Diagn Ther 2011;29(1): 88–100.

54. Bootstaylor BS, Filly RA, Harrison MR, et al. Prenatal sonographic predictors of liver herniation in congenital diaphragmatic hernia. J Ultrasound Med 1995;14:515–20.

55. Laudy JA, Van Gucht M, VanDooren MF, et al. Congenital diaphragmatic hernia: an evaluation of the prognostic value of the lung-to-head ratio and other prenatal parameters. Prenat Diagn 2003;23: 634–9.

56. Hedrick HL, Danzer E, Merchant A. Liver position and lung to head ratio for prediction of extracorporeal membrane oxygenation and survival in isolated left congenital diaphragmatic hernia. Am J Obstet Gynecol 2007;197:422–32.

57. Jani JC, Peralta CF, Ruano R, et al. Comparison of fetal lung area to head circumference ratio with lung volume in the prediction of postnatal outcome in diaphragmatic hernia. Ultrasound Obstet Gynecol 2007;30:850–4.

58. Gorincour G, Boubenot J, Mourot MG, et al. Prenatal prognosis of congenital diaphragmatic hernia using MRI measurement of fetal lung volume. Ultrasound Obstet Gynecol 2005;26:738–44.

59. Barnewolt CE, Kunisaki SM, Fauza DO, et al. Percent predicted lung volumes as measured on fetal MRI: a useful biometric parameter for risk stratification in congenital diaphragmatic hernia. J Pediatr Surg 2007;42:193–7.

60. Cannie M, Janis J, DeKeyyzer F, et al. Diffusion weighted MRI in lungs of normal fetuses and those with congenital diaphragmatic hernia. Ultrasound Obstet Gynecol 2009;34:678–86.

61. Vuletin JF, Lim FY, Cnota J, et al. Prenatal pulmonary hypertension index: novel prenatal predictor of severe postnatal pulmonary artery hypertension in antenatally diagnosed congenital diaphragmatic hernia. J Pediatr Surg 2010;45(4):703–8.

62. Arkovitz MS, Russo M, Devine P. Fetal lung-head ratio is not related to outcome for antenatal diagnosed congenital diaphragmatic hernia. J Pediatr Surg 2007;42:107–11.

63. Deprest JA, Hyett JA, Flake AS, et al. Current controversies in prenatal diagnosis: should fetal surgery be done in all cases of severe diaphragmatic hernia? Prenat Diagn 2009;29:15–9.

64. Aybard Y, Derouineau I, Aubard V, et al. Primary fetal hydrothorax: a literature review and proposed antenatal clinical strategy. Fetal Diagn Ther 1998;13: 325–33.

65. Longaker MT, Laberge JM, Dansereau J, et al. Primary fetal pneumothorax: natural history and management. J Pediatr Surg 1989;24:573–6.

66. Roybal JL, Liechty KW, Hedrick HL, et al. Predicting the severity of congenital high airway obstruction syndrome. J Pediatr Surg 2010;45:1633–9.

67. Mong A, Johnson AM, Kramer SS, et al. Congenital high airway obstruction syndrome: MR/US findings, effect on management, and outcome. Pediatr Radiol 2008;38:1171–9.

68. Courtier J, Poder L, Wang ZJ, et al. Fetal tracheolaryngeal airway obstruction: prenatal evaluation by sonography and MRI. Pediatr Radiol 2010;40:1800–5.
69. Vidaeff AC, Szmuk P, Mastrobattista JM, et al. More or less CHAOS: case report and literature review suggesting the existence of a distinct subtype of congenital high airway obstruction syndrome. Ultrasound Obstet Gynecol 2007;30:114–7.
70. Kuwashima S, Kazuhiro K, Yasushi K, et al. MR imaging appearance of laryngeal atresia (congenital high airway obstruction syndrome): unique course in a fetus. Pediatr Radiol 2008;38:344–7.
71. Liechty KW, Crombleholme TM. Management of fetal airway obstruction. Semin Perinatol 1999;23:496–506.
72. Ruano R, Joubin L, Aubry MC, et al. A nomogram of fetal lung volumes estimated by 3-dimensional ultrasonography using rotational technique (virtual organ computer-aided analysis). J Ultrasound Med 2006;25:701–9.
73. Chaoui R, Kalache K, Tennsstedt C, et al. Pulmonary arterial Doppler velocimetry in fetuses with lung hypoplasia. Eur J Obstet Gynecol Reprod Biol 1999;84:179–85.
74. Osada H, Kaku K, Masuda K, et al. Quantitative and qualitative evaluations of fetal lung with MR imaging. Radiology 2004;231:887–92.
75. Tanigaki S, Miyakoshi K, Tanaka M, et al. Pulmonary hypoplasia: prediction with use of ratio of MRI measured fetal lung volume to US estimated fetal body weight. Radiology 2004;232:767–72.
76. Ward VL, Nishino M, Hatabu H, et al. Fetal lung volumemeasurements: determination with MR imaging–effect of various factors. Radiology 2006;240(1):187–93.
77. Williams G, Coakley FV, Qayyum A, et al. Fetal relative lung volume: quantification by using prenatal MR imaging lung volumetry. Radiology 2004;233:457–62.
78. Kuwashima S, Nishimura G, Limura F, et al. Low intensity fetal lungs on MRI may suggest the diagnosis of pulmonary hypoplasia. Pediatr Radiol 2001;31:669–72.
79. Zaretsky M, Ramus R, McIntire D, et al. MR calculation of lung volumes to predict outcome in fetuses with genitourinary abnormalities. AJR Am J Roentgenol 2005;185(5):1328–34.

Chest Sonography in Children: Current Indications, Techniques, and Imaging Findings

Brian D. Coley, MD*

KEYWORDS

- Chest sonography • Imaging findings • Thoracic diseases
- Pediatric chest

After plain radiography, CT and MR imaging are the usually preferred modalities for imaging the pediatric chest. With acoustic limitations imposed by bone and air, the thorax at first seems unforgiving place to perform ultrasound (US). Various diseases and pathologic conditions, however, can allow an acoustic window into the chest, and the unique anatomy of the pediatric chest provides other imaging windows for creative sonologists.[1] Advances in thoracic US relying on interpretation of artifacts produced by the interface of air in the lung and pleural space allow important information about the lung itself to be determined by US.[2–9] US will never replace CT and MR imaging, but it can provide important and at times superior information safely and efficiently, particularly in pediatric patients. In this article, current imaging techniques and clinical applications of US for assessing full spectrum of thoracic diseases in children are reviewed.

TECHNIQUE

Although US of the chest may be the first imaging modality used in some acute and critical care settings, in general, pediatric patients undergoing sonographic examination of the chest have a preceding plain radiographic examination.[10–13] This helps focus the US study and the combination of information obtained can improve diagnostic accuracy. As with sonography elsewhere in the body, the appropriate transducers and frequencies vary with the size of the patient and the structure examined. Neonates and small infants are easily examined with high-frequency linear transducers, whereas older children and adolescents require lower-frequency transducers. Smaller footprint sector, vector, or tightly curved array transducers are needed to insonate between ribs, below the diaphragm, or from the suprasternal notch. Linear transducers are valuable for examining chest wall lesions and for examining the lung pleura interface.[2,12,14]

Basic B-mode real-time US is generally all that is required for chest US. The use of M-mode imaging has proved helpful, however, in the evaluation of pneumothorax and quantification of diaphragmatic motion.[15–18] Color Doppler can be useful when evaluating peripheral parenchymal opacities to differentiate vascularized lesions from infarcts.

Useful acoustic windows are shown in **Fig. 1**. The relatively unossified thorax of the neonate and infant, along with the presence of a relatively large thymus allow imaging of the anterior chest and mediastinum through sternal and costochondral cartilages. Suprasternal or supraclavicular approaches may also be useful in examining the anterior mediastinum and thoracic vessels. Intercostal scanning allows imaging of the lung and

Section of Ultrasound, Columbus Children's Hospital, The Ohio State University School of Medicine and Public Health, 700 Children's Drive, Columbus, OH 43205, USA

* Cincinnati Children's Hospital Medical Center, Department of Radiology, ML 5031, 3333 Burnet Avenue, Cincinnati, OH 45229-3039.

E-mail address: brian.coley@nationwidechildrens.org

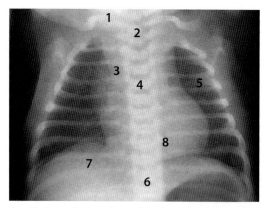

Fig. 1. Acoustic windows for thoracic sonography: 1, supraclavicular; 2, suprasternal; 3, parasternal; 4, transsternal; 5, intercostal; 6, subxyphoid; 7, subdiaphragmatic; and 8, posterior paraspinal. (*Adapted from* Kim OH, Kim WS, Min JK, et al. US in the diagnosis of pediatric chest disease. Radiographics 2000;20: 653–71; with permission.)

pleura throughout the thorax and of the posterior mediastinum.[10,19–24] The inferior thoracic cavity can be examined using the liver, spleen, or fluid-filled stomach as acoustic windows.[25] For evaluation of the lung and pleural space in critically ill patients, a systematic organized approach is required. One suggested approach divides each hemithorax into 4 quadrants: upper anterior, lower anterior, upper lateral, and basal lateral[2]; the anterior axillary line divides the anterior from lateral regions (Fig. 2). If a patient's condition permits, upright posterior imaging should be performed to

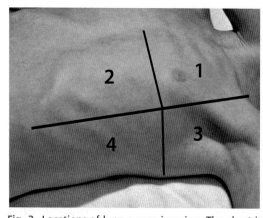

Fig. 2. Locations of lung survey imaging. The chest is divided into anterior and lateral portions by the anterior axillary line: 1, anterior superior; 2, anterior basal; 3, lateral superior; and 4, lateral basal. (*Adapted from* Volpicelli G, Silva F, Radeos M. Real-time lung ultrasound for the diagnosis of alveolar consolidation and interstitial syndrome in the emergency department. Eur J Emerg Med 2011;17:63–72; with permission.)

better evaluate the posterior chest and to improve detection of small pleural effusions.[26,27]

INDICATIONS

The most common indication for chest sonography is to evaluate an opacity detected on a chest radiograph.[10,19,20] In the case of a completely opacified hemithorax, US can differentiate whether parenchymal or pleural disease (or both) is the cause (Fig. 3).[28,29] Such information is often helpful for guiding the appropriate direction of therapy and possible thoracic intervention.[30–34] Focal masses can be imaged to determine location and whether they are solid or cystic. Abnormal mediastinal contours in infants are usually due to an unusually sized or shaped thymus, which can be easily shown by US,[21] obviating CT. Palpable chest wall lesions are best initially imaged with US, because nonpainful pediatric chest wall masses are typically benign and require no further investigation.[35] Although CT and MR angiographic techniques can produce exquisite vascular images, US is often the first and only necessary study for examination of suspected thromboses and other abnormalities of thoracic vasculature.

NORMAL ANATOMY

Unossified costochondral and sternal cartilage appears hypoechoic on US (Fig. 4). The shape of costochondral cartilage is often varied and may produce irregular chest wall "masses."[35] With aging, these cartilages gradually ossify, diminishing acoustic access to the thorax.

The thymus is larger compared with the rest of the thorax during the first year of life. The thymus is physically largest, however, during adolescence.[36] Usually confined to the anterior mediastinum, the thymus may extend into the neck or middle and posterior mediastinum, which may produce concern for pathology.[37] Fortunately, the thymus has a characteristic echotexture, with regular linear and punctate echogenicities that allows its confident recognition and differentiation from mediastinal pathology (Fig. 5).[21,38]

The normal pleural space contains a tiny amount of fluid,[27,39] but fluid is seen with US in only 35% of normal healthy children.[39] The acoustic interface of the chest wall with normal aerated lung provides a strong reflective surface and produces a characteristic reverberation within the US image, often referred to as A lines (Fig. 6). The thinner chest wall of infants and small children, however, may not demonstrate this artifact. Aerated lung is also seen to move along the parietal pleural surface with respiration, termed *the gliding sign*.[22,34,40,41]

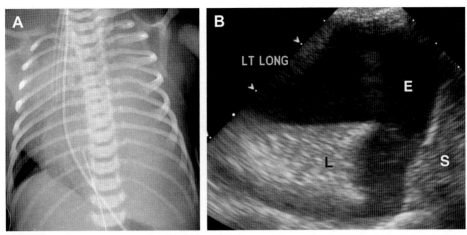

Fig. 3. (A) Newborn with respiratory distress and opaque left hemithorax of unclear etiology. (B) Longitudinal parasternal sonogram shows a large anechoic effusion (E) and consolidated left lung (L). The diaphragm is partially everted, displacing the spleen (S). Aspiration revealed a chylothorax. (*Adapted from* Coley BD. Pediatric chest ultrasound. Radiol Clin North Am 2005;43:405–18; with permission.)

Using M mode, the normal motion of the lung produces a characteristic pattern, termed *the seashore sign* (**Fig. 7**).[16] The recent literature is replete with many other terms, which often are more confusing than clarifying.[7] Recognizing these normal findings, however, is important, because deviations from their appearances provide clues to pleural and parenchymal disease.

THE PLEURAL SPACE
Effusions

Being superficial to normally echogenic aerated lungs, the pleural space is well visualized by US. Although pleural fluid collections are often suspected from chest radiographs, US is more sensitive in detecting pleural fluid than chest radiographs,[42] particularly in critically ill patients in whom upright or decubitus radiographs are not possible. The sonographic appearance of pleural

fluid depends on its composition and may range from completely anechoic, in the case of simple transudative collections, to collections with mobile echogenic debris in cases of infection and hemorrhage, to septated and more solid appearing collections with empyemas and organizing infection (**Fig. 8**).[31,32,43,44] Simple nonloculated collections can be seen to change shape with patient breathing or change in position. The distinction of echogenic

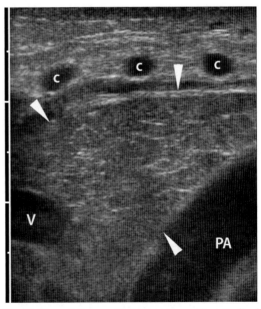

Fig. 5. Normal thymus. Right parasternal longitudinal view shows a normal triangular-shaped right thymic lobe (*arrowheads*) with characteristic linear and punctate echogenicities conforming to the contours of the brachiocephalic vein (V) and main pulmonary artery (PA). Note the hypoechoic costosternal cartilages (C).

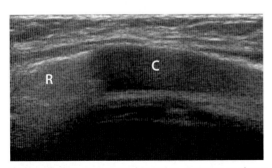

Fig. 4. Normal costosternal junction. Sonogram along the long axis of an anterior rib in a teenager shows the bony portion of the rib (R) with posterior acoustic shadowing and the hypoechoic cartilaginous rib end (C).

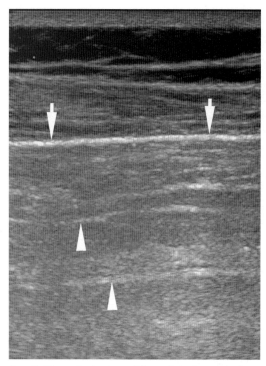

Fig. 6. Normal chest wall/lung interface; A lines. Transverse intercostal sonogram using a linear transducer shows the strong echogenic interface of the aerated lung and pleura (*arrows*) as well as the reverberation artifacts projected within the deeper lung parenchyma (A lines) (*arrowheads*).

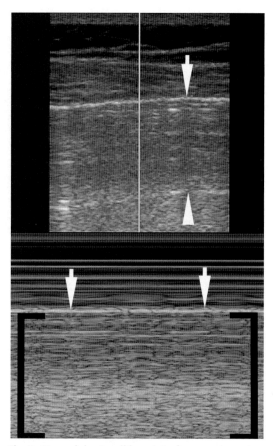

Fig. 7. Normal chest wall/lung interface; seashore sign. Transverse intercostal gray-scale and M-mode image shows a normal lung interface (*arrows*) and a normal A line (*arrowhead*). In the M-mode image, the normal motion of the lung ([ ]) gives a pattern some liken to sand on a beach, thus the term seashore sign.

but still fluid collections from more solid collections can be aided by the fluid color sign, in which mobile debris produces signal with color Doppler whereas nonmobile solid material does not.[45,46]

As infected pleural collections progress and organize, fibrinous strands begin to form. Initially thin and mobile, these fibrin strands thicken and increase, creating multiple loculations in which fluid no longer changes with patient position or respiration. The parietal and visceral pleura may be thickened as well, as often seen with CT. Infected pleural collections may progress to solidify into a homogenous echogenic gelatinous mass encasing the underlying lung, eventually producing a fibrothorax.

US is superior to CT in characterizing the nature of pleural fluid collections[23,47] and can help guide percutaneous drainage.[31,32,34,43,48,49] Simple fluid collections are amenable to percutaneous aspiration and are most safely performed with US guidance (**Fig. 9**). Because up to 50% of pediatric parapneumonic effusions recur after aspiration, however, it is often more prudent to leave a drainage catheter in place, even if only for a short time.[50] The US detection of fibrinous strands and even honeycombing of the pleural space is not

a contraindication to percutaneous drainage, but it does mean that fibrinolytic therapy is required to clear the collections and should be started promptly to achieve proper drainage (**Fig. 10**).[31,32,51–53] In the setting of continued fevers and poor clinical response after pleural drainage, plain radiographs may not adequately assess whether undrained pleural collections or underlying parenchymal infection is the cause, US can adequately assess the pleural space and portions of the underlying lung, although there may be limitations from existing chest tubes, dressings, and patient discomfort. In these complicated and refractory cases, CT may be a better option, especially if surgical intervention is planned.[31,32]

Masses

Malignant disease involving the pleural space is much less common in children than in adults[54]

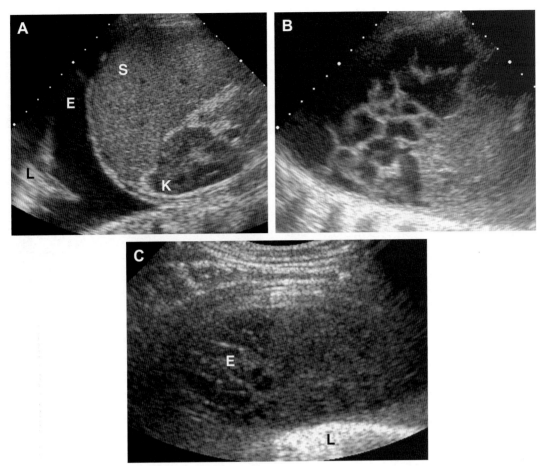

Fig. 8. Sonographic appearances of pleural collections. (*A*) Subdiaphragmatic longitudinal sonogram shows a mostly anechoic left pleural effusion (E) along with consolidated lung (L). The spleen (S) and kidney (K) help to provide acoustic windows into the inferior chest. (*B*) Empyema with the formation of fibrinous septations. (*C*) Well-organized, solid-appearing empyema (E) adjacent to aerated lung (L). (*Adapted from* Coley BD. Pediatric chest ultrasound. Radiol Clin North Am 2005;43:405–18; with permission.)

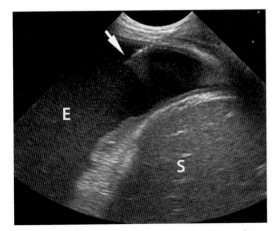

Fig. 9. Pleural effusion aspiration. Transverse intercostal sonogram of the left chest shows a pleural effusion (E) with some echogenic material. The aspirating needle (*arrow*) is seen just entering the pleural space. S, spleen.

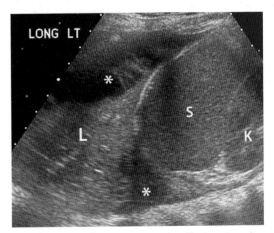

Fig. 10. Septated parapneumonic effusion. Longitudinal sonogram of the left chest shows consolidated lung (L) and complex partially septated fluid (*asterisks*). This collection responded well to interventional drainage and lytic therapy. K, kidney; S, spleen.

but can occur with Wilms tumor, neuroblastoma, leukemia, and sarcomas. Primary chest wall neoplasms and pleural metastases are often accompanied by hemorrhagic pleural effusions, which appear as echogenic debris-filled fluid at sonography. The presence of pleural fluid aids in detection of solid masses adherent to the parietal or visceral pleura (**Fig. 11**). If visible sonographically, pleural masses are readily biopsied with US guidance (**Fig. 12**),[34,48,55–57] allowing confirmatory histologic diagnoses.

Pneumothorax

As discussed previously, the normal strong acoustic interface between pleura and aerated lung produces repeating posterior echogenicities (A lines), and the normal sliding motion of the lung can be seen during respiration (see **Fig. 6**). When air is introduced into the pleural space, the normal tension between the pleural layers is lost, and a gap is created between the parietal and visceral pleura disrupting the normal acoustic interface. The sliding of the underlying lung can no longer be seen, and the normal reverberation is replaced by a static homogeneous posterior acoustic shadowing (**Fig. 13**). Some reports indicate that US is superior to plain radiographs in pneumothorax detection and may be useful in monitoring procedural complications and assessing critically ill and trauma patients.[15–17,58–63] Similarly, the curtain sign has been described in hydropneumothorax where the normal pleural

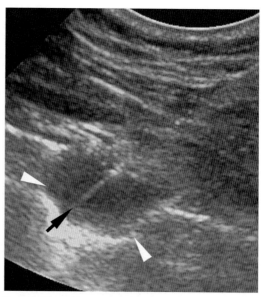

Fig. 12. Pleural biopsy. Intercostal sonogram in a child with Wilms tumor shows a pleural-based solid mass (*arrowheads*). The aspirating needle (*arrow*) is seen within the lesion, and yielded metastatic Wilms tumor.

gliding is lost and mobile air fluid levels are visualized.[40]

LUNG PARENCHYMA
Interstitial Disease

Plain radiography usually suffices for the evaluation of parenchymal lung disease in pediatric patients, but unclear cases may benefit from US or CT examination. The traditional view is that

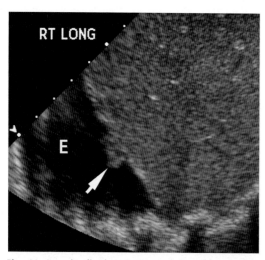

Fig. 11. Longitudinal sonogram of the right chest in a child with Wilms tumor shows a pleural effusion (E) outlining a metastatic deposit on the diaphragmatic parietal pleura (*arrow*). (*Adapted from* Coley BD. Pediatric chest ultrasound. Radiol Clin North Am 2005;43:405–18; with permission.)

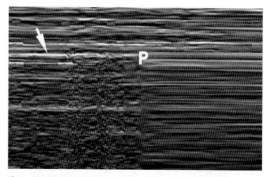

Fig. 13. Pneumothroax. Transverse intercostal sonogram shows a normal pattern of moving lung (seashore sign) deep to the lung pleural interface (*arrow*). On the right hand side of the image, there is loss of this normal pattern with a static series of horizontal echogenicities. Note how this looks different from normal A lines. An absence of normal lung sliding adjacent to normal lung is called the lung point sign (P).

aerated lung must become atelectatic or consolidated before it becomes possible to examine with US. More recent studies have shown that there is significant important clinical information that can be obtained by evaluating the artifacts produced from the surface of aerated lung. The interaction of the sound beam with interlobular septa produces so-called B lines, also referred to as lung rockets or comet tails.[6,9] A few scattered B lines can be normally seen and may be caused by focal subpleural thickening or distortion by parenchymal disease.[64] Multiple B lines can indicate an abnormality with the underlying lung. Anything that thickens the interlobular septa can produce a B line, but the distinction between fibrotic change and interstitial edema can often be made given the clinical context.[65] In adults, this finding has been shown with a variety of disorders, such as pulmonary fibrosis, viral pneumonias, sarcoidosis, lymphangitic carcinomatosis, and bronchiectasis.[64,66] Investigators have subdivided B lines into B7 lines (7 mm apart), indicating thickened interlobular septa, and B3 lines (3 mm apart), indicating the equivalent of the ground glass appearance at CT.[6,41] The presence of B lines is shown to correlate accurately with other imaging, pulmonary artery pressures, and fluid status and seem accurate in diagnosing interstitial and alveolar disease.[2,4,5,8,12,14,67]

Experience in children is more limited, particularly regarding interstitial edema,[68] but my anecdotal experience indicates that similar findings occur in children as well (**Fig. 14**). Surfactant deficiency disease produces variable appearances ranging from multiple B lines to a diffusely echogenic lung, which eliminates visualization of the normal chest wall–pleural interface (**Fig. 15**).[69–71] The sonographic appearance correlates well with the clinical and radiographic findings.[71] Chronic lung disease in the infant produces similar acoustic interfaces as seen in adult parenchymal disease, creating multiple ring-down artifacts (**Fig. 16**). The progression of US findings from surfactant deficiency to bronchopulmonary dysplasia may be useful as a predictor of the development of chronic lung disease and may appear earlier than chest radiographic findings.[70,72] The administration of exogenous surfactant, however, does not seem to improve the sonographic appearance in surfactant deficiency.[73] Interstitial prominence causing B lines persists, indicating that interstitial extravascular fluid clearance remains impaired despite radiographic improvement in aeration and clinical improvement in ventilation.[73]

Consolidation

Airless lung can appear sonographically similar to liver, thus has been termed, *hepatization* (**Fig. 17**). The underlying internal architecture of the lung is preserved, however, allowing differentiation from masses or other processes. Branching linear echogenicities representing air bronchograms are often seen (**Fig. 18**),[74] first described in pediatric patients.[75] Entrapped fluid or mucoid material within bronchi in necrotizing or postobstructive pneumonias produces hypoechoic branching structures, the sonographic fluid bronchogram.[76] Pulmonary vascular flow is preserved in simple

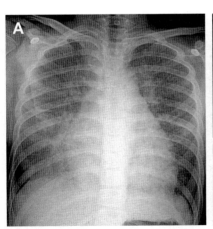
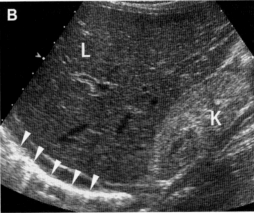

Fig. 14. Interstitial edema. (*A*) Chest radiograph of a teenage girl with dyspnea and new-onset renal failure shows interstitial edema. (*B*) Longitudinal image of the right upper quadrant shows an abnormally echogenic kidney consistent with the subsequent diagnosis of glomerulonephritis. Note the regularly spaced B lines within the right lower lobe (*arrowheads*). These correspond to the thickened interlobular septa seen on the chest radiograph. K, kidney; L, liver.

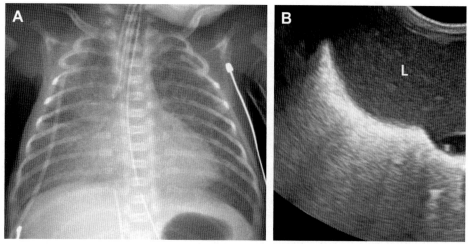

Fig. 15. Surfactant deficiency disease. (*A*) Chest radiograph of a preterm infant shows diffuse granular airspace disease typical of surfactant deficiency, worst in the right lower lobe. (*B*) Transverse sonogram of the right lower chest through the liver (L) shows abnormal increased pulmonary echogenicity of the right lower lobe without visualization of focal B lines.

pneumonic consolidation and is readily demonstrated with color Doppler.[76] With atelectasis, air bronchograms are also present, and blood vessels become crowded together and have a more parallel orientation. Their orderly linear and branching structure is preserved, however, allowing distinction from the more irregular vasculature found in neoplasms.[46]

Distinguishing pneumonic consolidation from simple atelectasis can be difficult radiographically. It has been suggested that US can be more specific in this situation. If there is movement of the air within bronchi, this usually indicates pneumonia,

whereas the air bronchograms in atelectasis are most often static.[2] In a recent study, this dynamic air bronchogram had a sensitivity of 61% and a positive predictive value of 97% in distinguishing pneumonia from atelectasis.[77] Additionally, in adults atelectasis has been reported to transmit cardiac pulsation more readily than pneumonic consolidation, producing the so-called lung pulse sign.[41] I have not found this sign useful in my personal experience, perhaps because of the smaller thoraces of children and closer proximity of the heart producing pulmonary motion regardless of the cause of the underlying lung disease.

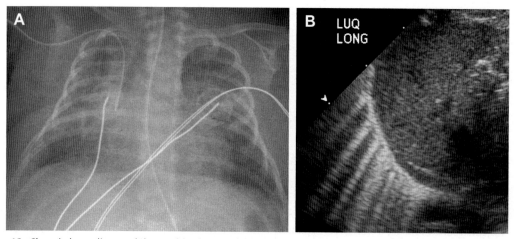

Fig. 16. Chronic lung disease. (*A*) Portable chest radiograph in a former preterm infant with continued oxygen requirements shows increased interstitial markings of chronic lung disease. (*B*) Longitudinal sonogram through the left upper quadrant shows multiple B lines indicating interstitial lung disease. (*Adapted from* Coley BD. Pediatric chest ultrasound. Radiol Clin North Am 2005;43:405–18; with permission.)

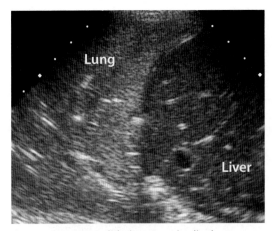

Fig. 17. Lung consolidation. Longitudinal sonogram over the lower right chest shows consolidated lung superior to the liver. Although their echogenicities differ, their internal sonographic appearance is similar. (*Adapted from* Coley BD. Pediatric chest ultrasound. Radiol Clin North Am 2005;43:405–18; with permission.)

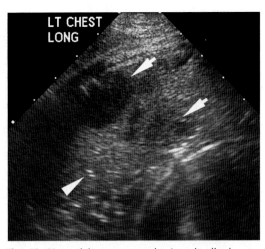

Fig. 19. Necrotizing pneumonia. Longitudinal sonogram shows consolidation of the left lower lobe with air bronchograms (*arrowhead*). There are several areas of decreased echogenicity within the lung (*arrows*) that showed no flow with color Doppler indicating foci of necrosis.

As lung infections progress, areas of parenchymal necrosis may develop. Small areas of lung necrosis appear as areas of decreased echogenicity (**Fig. 19**) that lacks color Doppler flow within a region of pulmonary consolidation.[78] If the area of necrosis progresses and enlarges faster than can be cleared by the body, a lung abscess develops. Larger abscesses may develop a thick wall, and air fluid levels may be seen if there is cavitation or if the abscess communicates with the bronchial tree (**Fig. 20**).[22,32,76] Causative organisms are not always cultured from sputum or peripheral blood. If abutting the pleura, lung abscess are sonographically visible, and US-guided aspiration and drainage can play an important role in diagnosis and treatment.[32,76,79]

Masses

Primary lung neoplasms are fortunately rare in children. Pulmonary blastoma is the most common and usually starts as a peripheral lesion, often attaining large size before becoming clinically apparent.[21] Other less common tumors include mucoepidermoid carcinoma, rhabdomyosarcoma, and bronchogenic tumors. Although US can confirm the presence of a mass, like other imaging modalities US cannot be histologically specific and differentiate among tumor types.[80] As with pleural lesions, if a lung mass is sufficiently peripheral and abuts the lung surface, percutaneous US-guided biopsy is a safe and effective method for obtaining a tissue diagnosis.[57]

Congenital parenchymal masses include congenital pulmonary airway malformation (CPAM) and sequestration. Although often regarded as separate entities, these malformations are part of a spectrum of congenital pulmonary airway malformations and may have overlapping imaging and histologic features.[21,81] These masses may be detected prenatally by US or MR imaging,

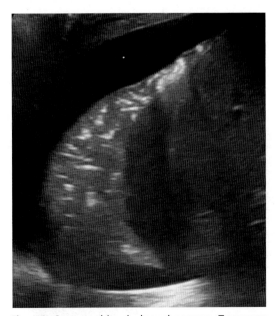

Fig. 18. Sonographic air bronchograms. Transverse sonogram shows pleural effusion and lower lobe consolidation with internal branching bright echogenicities representing air bronchograms. These may move with patient respiratory effort.

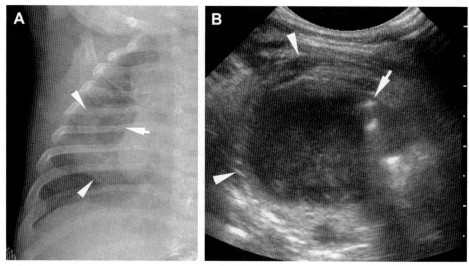

Fig. 20. Lung abscess. (*A*) Chest radiograph in a 4-month-old child with a history of bronchopulmonary dysplasia shows a thick walled cystic mass in the right chest (*arrowheads*) with internal air (*arrow*). (*B*) Transverse sonogram shows the thick-walled abscess (*arrowheads*) with internal air (*arrow*). Percutaneous drainage and antibiotic treatment lead to a complete resolution.

appearing as variably solid or cystic structures.[82] Postnatally, plain radiographs usually show the lesion, often as incidental findings or on images taken for respiratory symptoms. CPAMs have traditionally classified according to their cystic component, although the usefulness of this is questionable. The US appearance follows this histologic typing, demonstrating cysts of varying size amidst echogenic parenchyma (**Fig. 21**).[80] Although spontaneous regression of CPAMs has been reported, and there is controversy as to whether surgery is indicated, most of these lesions are currently surgically resected in the United States.[83] Superimposed infection can pose

difficulties and complications for surgery. Like lung abscesses, US-guided percutaneous drainage can allow successful treatment of infected CPAMs and allow a safer delayed surgical resection.[32]

Intralobar sequestrations are most often found in the lower lobes, presenting with recurrent infections or persistent radiographic opacities.[84] These are typically sonographically solid masses, although there may be cystic components.[19] The key diagnostic feature of sequestration is demonstrating systemic arterial supply, usually from the descending aorta (**Fig. 22**).[46,85,86] Color Doppler sonography is diagnostically reliable in this

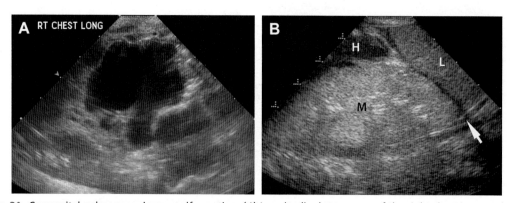

Fig. 21. Congenital pulmonary airway malformation. (*A*) Longitudinal sonogram of the right chest in a newborn with prenatal diagnosis of a lung mass shows a complex mass with a large central cystic component corresponding to a type I CPAM. No normal lung was visualized. (*B*) Longitudinal midline sonogram in another newborn shows a large echogenic mass (M) representing a type III CPAM. This mass displaces the heart (H) anteriorly and to the left, and is inverting the diaphragm (*arrow*) and displacing the liver (L) inferiorly.

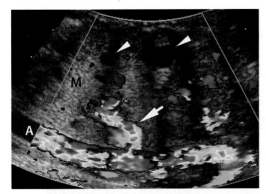

Fig. 22. Congenital pulmonary sequestration with cystic adenomatoid malformation. Coronal sonogram of the inferior left chest shows an echogenic mass (M) representing an intralobar sequestration with a large feeding artery (*arrow*) arising from the thoracic aorta (A). Note the cystic components (*arrowheads*), which were shown histologically to be elements of cystic adenomatoid malformation within the sequestration.

condition in the neonate, infant, and young child, although contrast-enhanced CT and MR imaging are often required in older patients with limited acoustic windows.[87] Extralobar sequestrations have a separate pleural investment and are usually found in the inferior left chest but may even be located below the diaphragm where they may be confused with adrenal pathology. Patients present symptomatically at a younger age than those with intralobar malformation, with cyanosis and dyspnea more common.[80] US features are similar in both conditions, although associated anomalies are more commonly associated with extralobar sequestrations.

MEDIASTINUM

The thymus is the dominant noncardiac mediastinal structure within the pediatric chest. Its appearance on chest radiography is usually clear, although variations in size and position can occasionally be confusing and prompt further imaging for clarification. The characteristic US appearance allows confident diagnosis and obviates the need for further imaging tests (**Fig. 23**).[38] Diminished thymic size is seen in infants and children subject to physiologic stress.[19,88] DiGeorge syndrome is a cellular immunodeficiency disorder related to hypoplasia or aplasia of the thymus. Although the associated anomalies are usually sufficient for diagnosis, failure to visualize the infant thymus by US is strongly confirmatory.[19]

Primary thymic tumors in children are rare.[21] Thymomas usually occur in older children and adolescents, who often present with paraneoplastic syndromes.[89] They can present as aggressive tumors particularly in cases of invasive thymomas.[89] In this age group, mediastinal acoustic windows are more limiting. Therefore, MR imaging and CT are often better imaging choices.[90] Thymomas can be heterogeneous tumors with areas of necrosis and calcification,[91,92] whereas thymolipomas are more homogeneously echogenic due to their fatty content. Secondary neoplastic thymic infiltration is more common, and occurs with leukemia, lymphoma, and Langerhans cell histiocytosis.[93] In these cases, the normal sonographic thymic pattern is replaced with variably echogenic and heterogeneous soft tissue and associated abnormal lobulation of the thymic capsule. Small calcifications have been described with histiocytic infiltration.[21,38] An infiltrated thymus loses its

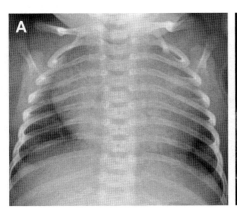

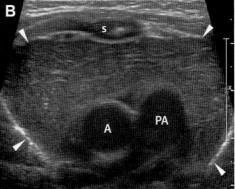

Fig. 23. Prominent thymus. (*A*) Chest radiograph of an infant with respiratory symptoms shows an enlarged cardiomediastinal contour. (*B*) Transverse sonogram of the superior chest shows a normal thymus (*arrowheads*) to be the source of the radiographic findings. The thymus conforms to the contours of the anterior chest wall and drapes around the aorta (A) and pulmonary artery (PA). Note the hypoechoic sternal cartilage with a small ossification center (S).

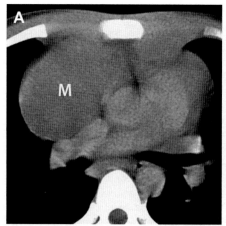
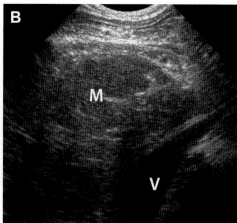

Fig. 24. Lymphoma. (A) Contrast-enhanced chest CT of a 14-year-old girl with fatigue shows an anterior medias-tinal mass (M). (B) Longitudinal sonogram just before percutaneous biopsy shows a predominantly hypoechoic mass (M) anterior to the mediastinal vessels (V). Core biopsies showed nodular sclerosing Hodgkin disease.

normal compliance and may be seen to displace and distort adjacent structures instead of conform-ing to their shape.

The most common benign thymic masses are lymphatic malformations and thymic cysts.[21] Lymphatic malformations are usually comprised of multiple loculated cysts with thin bands of intervening soft tissue. Normally hypovascular, lymphatic malformations may contain hemangiom-atous components that demonstrates flow with color Doppler. Cysts contents are usually anecho-ic, but superimposed hemorrhage or infection produces cyst contents of variable echogenicity or even fluid debris levels. Thymic cysts arise from remnants of the thymopharyngeal ducts,[80] thymic tumors, and cystic degeneration of the thymus itself associated with mediastinal trauma or surgery. Most congenital cases of thymic cysts are diagnosed in childhood, presenting as slowly enlarging masses that may extend into the neck.[94] Thymic cysts typically are unilocular with imperceptible walls and anechoic contents, and sonographic demonstration of their continuity with the thymus allows their diagnosis. Thymic cysts associated with HIV infection are more commonly multiseptated and may cause more diffuse thymic enlargement.[95,96]

The anterior mediastinum is a common site for other neoplasms, in particular lymphoma. The majority of children with lymphoma have anter-ior mediastinal involvement, more frequent with Hodgkin lymphoma than with non-Hodgkin lymphoma.[19,80] Patients may present with con-stitutional symptoms (fever and weight loss), respi-ratory complaints (cough and dyspnea), and occasionally masses are discovered incidentally. Sonographically, lymphomas may appear as discrete masses, nodal enlargement, or with diffuse thymic infiltration. They tend to be hypoe-choic and hypovascular compared with inflamma-tory processes and other neoplasms (Fig. 24).[80] Teratomas and other germ cell tumors may also arise in the anterior mediastinum.[97] The US appearance of germ cell tumors is variable, ranging from purely soft tissue masses to hetero-geneous masses containing fat, bone, and cystic elements (Fig. 25).[19,80,98] A tissue diagnosis is required before chemotherapy, but airway compromise often associated with large masses located within the anterior mediastinum may make surgical biopsy undesirable. US-guided percutaneous biopsy is an excellent alternative in

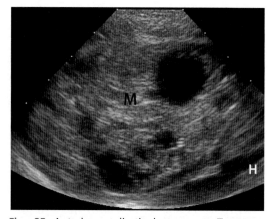

Fig. 25. Anterior mediastinal teratoma. Transverse sonogram of the chest in a newborn shows a complex solid and cystic mass (M) displacing the heart (H). (Adapted from Coley BD. Pediatric chest ultrasound. Radiol Clin North Am 2005;43:405–18; with permission.)

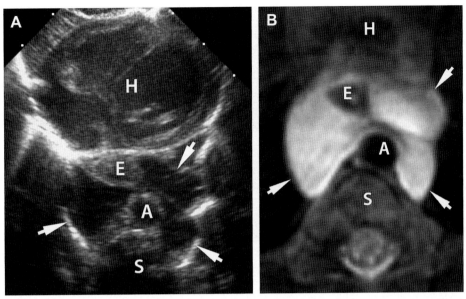

Fig. 26. Middle mediastinal lymphangioma. (A) Transverse sonogram using the heart as an acoustic window in a child with abnormal paraspinal widening on chest radiography shows a septated cystic mass (*arrows*) posterior to the heart (H) and anterior to the spine (S), surrounding the aorta (A) and esophagus (E). (B) Transverse T2-weighted MR imaging at a similar level with the same findings. (*Adapted from* Coley BD. Pediatric chest ultrasound. Radiol Clin North Am 2005;43:405–18; with permission.)

these patients and can be done comfortably and safely, even in critically ill patients.[22,34,48,56]

Middle mediastinal lesions include cystic (bronchogenic, gastrointestinal, pericardial, and lymphatic) and solid (lymphadenopathy) masses. Visualization of these masses with US may become more difficult with increasing age of patients, but the optimal use of acoustic windows can still make US a valuable diagnostic modality.[99]

Lymphadenopathy can arise from underlying neoplasia or infection, appearing abnormally enlarged and hypoechoic, often with color Doppler hyperemia.[100] Bronchogenic cysts are usually thin walled, whereas esophageal duplication cysts may have a hypoechoic muscular rim typical of gastrointestinal duplications elsewhere in the body; this differentiation may, however, be difficult. Pericardial cysts have a typical appearance on plain radiographs, but US can confirm their cystic nature. Lymphatic malformations in the mediastinum appear similar to those elsewhere in the body, as discussed previously (**Fig. 26**).

Posterior mediastinal cystic masses include lymphatic malformations and neurenteric cysts, the latter often associated with vertebral body anomalies.[99] Most pediatric posterior mediastinal masses, however, are solid and arise from neural crest cells within the sympathetic ganglion. In order of decreasing malignancy, these include neuroblastoma, ganglioneuroblastoma, and

ganglioneuroma. Posterior mediastinal masses can often be best visualized via a posterior thoracic or paraspinal approach. Although sometimes containing calcifications, the sonographic appearance of these tumors is nonspecific. Thoracic neuroblastomas commonly extend through neural foramina, causing extradural compression of the

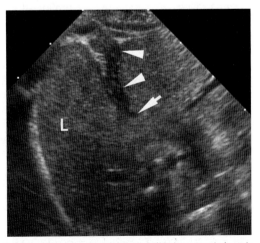

Fig. 27. Right-sided congenital diaphragmatic hernia. Sagittal sonogram through the inferior right chest of an infant with radiographic opacity of unclear etiology shows a defect (*arrow*) in the hypoechoic muscular right hemidiaphragm (*arrowheads*) with herniation of liver (L) into the chest.

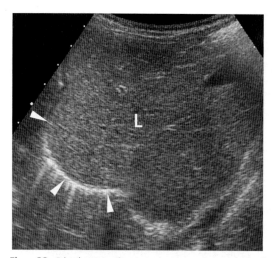

Fig. 28. Diaphragmatic eventration. Longitudinal sonogram of the right upper abdomen in a young child with a diaphragmatic contour abnormality on chest radiographs shows an intact diaphragm with a focal eventration (*arrowheads*) with liver (L) protruding superiorly.

spinal cord that may be symptomatic, and may be demonstrable sonographically. US can also demonstrate neoplastic invasion of the chest wall and bony involvement, although CT and MR imaging are more commonly used and more sensitive than US.

DIAPHRAGM

US is a valuable tool in assessing the diaphragm, allowing delineation of juxtadiaphragmatic masses, contour abnormalities and hernias, and evaluation of diaphragmatic motion.[101–104] Congenital diaphragmatic hernias are typically located on the left and usually pose little diagnostic

confusion on plain radiographs. When radiographic findings are less clear, especially with right-sided hernias, US becomes a useful modality for confirmation and further characterization. Sagittal and coronal scanning allows depiction of the diaphragm and assessment its integrity. Discontinuity of the diaphragm is readily seen, and the herniated viscera can be evaluated (Fig. 27). Eventration of the diaphragm results from a congenital weakness or thinness of the central tendon or muscle.[80] Patients may present with respiratory difficulties, but the radiographic findings are often incidental. Although further imaging may not be required, US can confirm the diagnosis by demonstrating an intact hemidiaphragm, thus helping to exclude contained hernias or masses (Fig. 28).[105]

Elevation of a hemidiaphragm after thoracic surgery raises the question of diaphragmatic paresis or paralysis. US provides a portable method for evaluating diaphragmatic motion without the use of radiation. Sagittal or coronal imaging provides information about that particular hemidiaphragm, whereas transverse imaging allows comparison of both hemidiaphragms and evaluation for paradoxic motion with unilateral paralysis (Fig. 29).[34,54,104,106] With M-mode recording, US can provide quantitative information about diaphragmatic excursion.[102]

CHEST WALL

Abnormalities of the pediatric chest wall are particularly amenable to high-resolution sonography. Nonpainful soft tissue masses are usually benign, and sonography often provides a definitive diagnosis.[35] Cystic and vascular masses are more often benign than solid masses.[80] US can

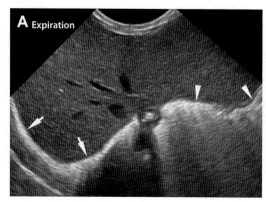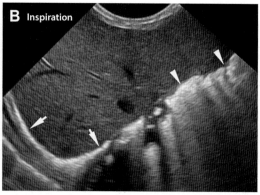

Fig. 29. Diaphragmatic paralysis. Transverse sonogram of the chest in an infant with a persistently elevated right hemidiaphragm after cardiac surgery. (*A*) In expiration the right hemidiaphragm (*arrows*) is higher than the left (*arrowheads*). (*B*) With inspiration there is expected inferior displacement of the left hemidiaphragm (*arrowheads*) but no motion of the right hemidiaphragm (*arrows*).

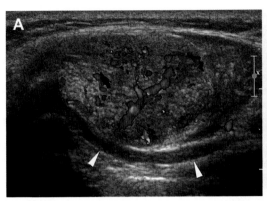
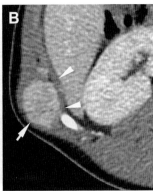

Fig. 30. Chest wall hemangioma. (*A*) Transverse color Doppler sonogram in a 5-year-old child with a soft palpable mass shows heterogeneous ovoid mass with marked vascularity that was arterial on pulsed Doppler interrogation. The mass is superficial to the intercostal musculature (*arrowheads*). (*B*) Contrast-enhanced CT shows intense enhancement within the hemangioma (*arrow*) and redemonstrates its location relative to the intercostal muscles (*arrowheads*). Given the child's age, this represents a noninvoluting congenital hemangioma.

accurately assess the extent and depth of lesions, which are important if surgical resection is considered. Doppler evaluation can help characterize the type of vascular malformation, which can be useful in determining an efficacious treatment.[107,108] Common benign chest wall masses include vascular and lymphatic malformations, lipomas, and lymph nodes.

Hemangiomas and other vascular lesions usually have discoloration of the overlying skin, providing the first clue to diagnosis. On grayscale imaging, hemangiomas are variably echogenic depending on the amount of fatty stroma and are typically well circumscribed. Hemangiomas usually have high Doppler frequency shifts and high color Doppler vessel density, whereas other vascular malformations do not (**Fig. 30**).[107] Venous malformations have a more bluish discoloration of the skin and show multiple serpiginous channels and cystic spaces. Blood flow may be

too slow to produce pulsed or color Doppler signal but with gentle compression and release the slow inflow of blood can be detected. Lymphatic malformations have variably sized cystic components whose echogenicity depends on whether there has been infection or hemorrhage into the normally anechoic cyst fluid. They may be found anywhere in the chest but are most common in the axilla (**Fig. 31**). Extension and infiltration into the mediastinum is common and may necessitate MR imaging for complete evaluation. Treatment may be surgical excision, although less invasive percutaneous sclerotherapies are effective and have less morbidity.[109] Neurofibromas may arise along costal margins within the neurovasvular bundle. Lipomas are generally well-circumscribed masses usually located within the subcutaneous tissues. They are typically echogenic due to their fat content but may be less echogenic than fat elsewhere in the body.[80] Color Doppler flow to lipomas is

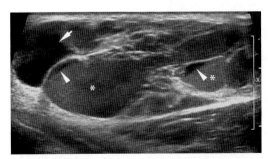

Fig. 31. Lymphatic malformation. Transverse sonogram of the axilla in a teenage girl with swelling and skin discoloration shows a mixed cystic lesion. There are anechoic cysts (*arrow*) along with echogenic cysts (*asterisks*) from internal hemorrhage that demonstrate fluid levels (*arrowheads*).

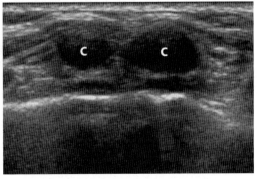

Fig. 32. Bifid rib. Transverse sonogram over an area of painless chest wall asymmetry in a 12-year-old girl shows a bifid anterior rib with two costosternal cartilages (C), a normal variant.

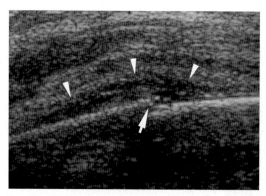

Fig. 33. Rib fracture. Longitudinal sonogram along a painful rib after a football injury shows cortical discontinuity (*arrow*) and a small associated hematoma (*arrowheads*) of a radiographically occult rib fracture.

minimal. Lymph nodes are usually recognizable by their echogenic fatty hila containing the central nodal blood supply, although inflamed and infiltrated nodes may have distorted internal architecture and color Doppler flow.

Firm, nontender masses may be secondary to bony or cartilaginous anomalies.[35,110] Bony abnormalities are often detectable by plain radiographs, but US can clarify and confirm findings. Anomalous rib ends can be diagnosed. Osteochondromas and their cartilaginous components can be assessed and followed. Anterior chest wall irregularities are often due to asymmetric cartilaginous costochondral junctions,[110] readily visible sonographically (**Fig. 32**). Traumatic separation of the costochondral cartilage from rib ends has been reported in child abuse,[111] a finding visible sonographically

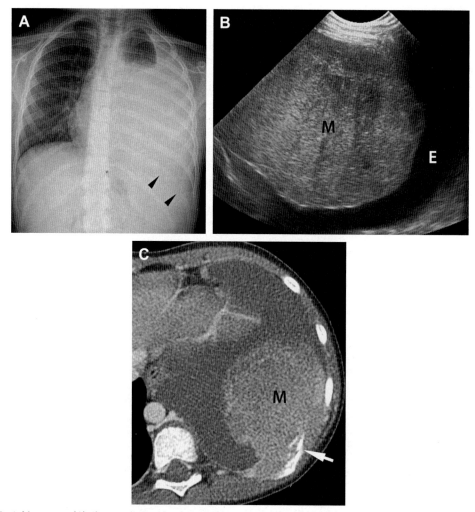

Fig. 34. Askin tumor. (A) Chest radiograph of an 11-year-old girl referred to interventional radiology for drainage of a presumed left parapneumonic effusion. Note the 10th posterior rib erosions (*arrowheads*) not recognized at the referring clinic. (B) Transverse intercostal sonogram shows a large mass (M) protruding form the chest wall into the thorax and an associated effusion (E). Percutaneous biopsy was performed and revealed Askin tumor. (C) Subsequent contrast-enhanced CT confirms the chest wall origin of the mass (M) with associated rib destruction (*arrow*).

but not with plain radiographs. Rib fractures are common after trauma, but radiographic detection may be difficult if there is little fragment displacement.[112] Sonography easily shows the disruption of the rib's cortical surface, and there may be an adjacent hematoma or callous formation depending on the age of the injury (**Fig. 33**).[24,34,113,114] Sternal fractures are also readily detected with US[113] with greater sensitivity and specificity than plain radiographs.[115,116] Costosternal osteocartilaginous injuries can also be seen in children after pectus excavatum surgery.[117]

Malignant chest wall lesions are uncommon in children but include Askin tumor (primitive neuroectodermal tumor of the chest wall) and rhabdomyosarcoma. Echogenicity of these malignant chest wall lesions is variable. The margins of these lesions may be distinct or infiltrative. Color Doppler flow of malignant chest wall lesions is usually increased.[80] Chest wall and rib invasion can be detected as interruption of the normal muscular layers of the chest wall and loss of the normally smooth bony cortical surface (**Fig. 34**).[34] As with most other imaging, US is not histologically specific, and some benign lesions (such as abscesses and hematomas) may have aggressive sonographic appearances (**Fig. 35**).[80] Tissue sampling, often via US-guided biopsy, is usually needed for a definitive diagnosis.

VESSELS

Advances in contrast MR imaging and CT angiography allow superb depiction of the thoracic vasculature. Deep structures, such as the superior vena cava and thoracic aorta, are difficult to evaluate sonographically in older pediatric patients, but US remains a principle method of investigation of vascular disease particularly within the subclavian and jugular vessels. The most common indication for vascular US is the evaluation of suspected venous thrombosis. Acute thrombosis often occurs in association with an indwelling vascular catheter and/or malignancy[118,119] and appears as hypoechoic material expanding the vessel lumen. Because compression of the subclavian and deeper thoracic veins is not possible, color and pulsed Doppler are important in confirming thrombosis. Depending on patient size and anatomy, it may be difficult to directly interrogate medial portions of the subclavian and brachiocephalic veins, and indirect Doppler findings of venous stenosis or occlusion may have to be relied on. Having no valves, the central thoracic veins show the effects of cardiac and respiratory activity, with marked phasicity and even reversal of flow with atrial systole.[120] With central venous occlusion or stenosis, this phasicity is lost or dampened, and interrogation of more lateral segments of the subclavian vein can thus indicate a more central location of abnormality (**Fig. 36**).[121,122] Investigation of both sides is often helpful in uncovering subtle flow differences that may indicate abnormalities.[120] With chronic occlusion, collaterals may become large and give the appearance of normal native vessels. Doppler flow seldom appears normal, however, and typically is dampened and more monophasic than in normal vessels.[121]

Arterial stenoses and aneurysms may occur from trauma, vascular access complications, or one of the arteritides. Inadvertent arterial puncture

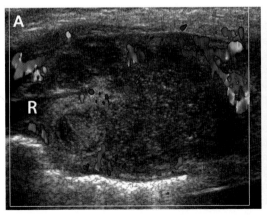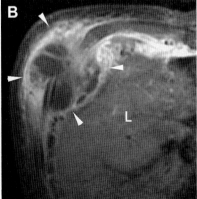

Fig. 35. Rib osteomyelitis. (*A*) Transverse color Doppler sonogram of a teenage boy with right anterolateral chest wall pain and swelling shows destruction of the rib (R) with a large hyperemic mass. (*B*) Axial contrast-enhanced T1-weighted MR imaging with fat saturation shows the rib ending in a complex mass (*arrowheads*) with an enhancing rim and septations the produces mass effect on the liver (L). Subsequent aspiration and biopsy yielded methicillin-resistant *Staphylococcus aureus*.

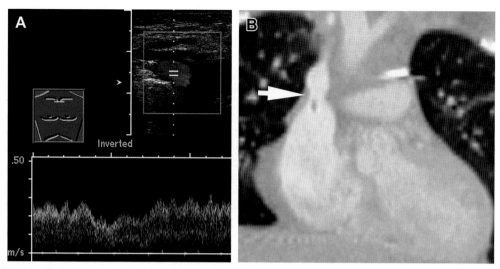

Fig. 36. Superior vena cava stenosis. (A) Duplex Doppler sonogram of the right brachiocephalic vein just cephalad of the superior vena cava in a 1-year-old child with upper extremity swelling after heart transplantation shows a patent vessel but with dampening of transmitted cardiac pulsations. (B) Coronal contrast-enhanced CT image shows stenosis of the superior vena caval anastomosis (arrow).

during line placement can lead to vessel injury or rarely arteriovenous fistula formation. Doppler can detect the abnormal high diastolic arterial flow in arteriovenous fistulas and the elevated and turbulent venous flow. Hyperextension injuries or penetrating trauma can cause intimal disruptions, leading to subclavian arterial occlusion or stenosis. Thoracic arterial stenoses, like those elsewhere in the body, are detectable by elevation of peak systolic flow through the stenosis, delayed systolic upstroke distal to the stenosis, and elevated diastolic flow due to downstream vasodilatation.

Thoracic outlet syndrome produces neurologic or vascular symptoms from compression of neurovascular structures in the upper chest. Anomalous cervical or first thoracic ribs, the anterior scalene muscle, and vascular variants may all contribute and may be seen by US.[123] MR imaging provides exquisite anatomic detail of the thoracic outlet, but duplex US may provide important physiologic information by demonstrating alterations in arterial and/or venous flow, especially during reproduction of the position in which symptoms occur.[124,125] Arterial flow may show acceleration or dampening of flow, depending how proximity to the stenotic segment.[126] Venous flow is more commonly affected, and there may be engorgement of the lateral subclavian and axillary veins and loss of transmitted cardiac waveforms.[120,127] Thrombosis may complicate repetitive venous compression, such as in cases of Paget-Schroetter syndrome, which is readily diagnosable by US.

SUMMARY

Although many pediatric thoracic conditions are adequately evaluated with plain radiographs, further imaging is sometimes required. The beautiful images provided by current CT and MR imaging techniques are aesthetically seductive, but US often provides the clinically necessary information without sedation or radiation exposure. If US cannot provide all the required information in a given case, it may help direct which additional imaging modality that is most definitive or clinically relevant.[29,103,128] Interventional procedures are often best and most safely performed with US guidance, particularly in pediatric patients. As with most US studies, US of the pediatric chest requires more physician involvement than other modalities to yield optimal results. This should not be seen as a negative but as a reason to become better and more facile with US. Understanding proper US techniques and characteristic US imaging appearance of various thoracic diseases in pediatric patients have great potential for early and accurate diagnosis, which in turn, lead to optimal patient care.

REFERENCES

1. Coley BD. Pediatric chest ultrasound. Radiol Clin North Am 2005;43:405–18.
2. Volpicelli G, Silva F, Radeos M. Real-time lung ultrasound for the diagnosis of alveolar consolidation and interstitial syndrome in the emergency department. Eur J Emerg Med 2011;17:63–72.

3. Bouhemad B, Brisson H, Le-Guen M, et al. Bedside ultrasound assessment of positive end-expiratory pressure-induced lung recruitment. Am J Respir Crit Care Med 2011;183(3):341–7.

4. Mallamaci F, Benedetto FA, Tripepi R, et al. Detection of pulmonary congestion by chest ultrasound in dialysis patients. JACC Cardiovasc Imaging 2010;3:586–94.

5. Jambrik Z, Gargani L, Adamicza A, et al. B-lines quantify the lung water content: a lung ultrasound versus lung gravimetry study in acute lung injury. Ultrasound Med Biol 2010;36:2004–10.

6. Lichtenstein DA, Mezière GA, Lagoueyte JF, et al. A-lines and B-lines: lung ultrasound as a bedside tool for predicting pulmonary artery occlusion pressure in the critically ill. Chest 2009;136:1014–20.

7. Chan SS. Comet tail artifacts in emergency chest ultrasound. Am J Emerg Med 2007;25:724–5.

8. Agricola E, Bove T, Oppizzi M, et al. "Ultrasound comet-tail images": a marker of pulmonary edema: a comparative study with wedge pressure and extravascular lung water. Chest 2005;127:1690–5.

9. Cardinale L, Volpicelli G, Binello F, et al. Clinical application of lung ultrasound in patients with acute dyspnea: differential diagnosis between cardiogenic and pulmonary causes. Radiol Med 2009; 114:1053–64.

10. Rosenberg HK. The complementary roles of ultrasound and plain film radiography in differentiating pediatric chest abnormalities. Radiographics 1986;6:427–45.

11. Stein SM, Cox JL, Hernanz-Schulma M, et al. Pediatric chest disease: evaluation by computerized tomography, magnetic resonance imaging, and ultrasonography. South Med J 1992;85:735–42.

12. Zanobetti M, Poggioni C, Pini R. Can chest ultrasonography substitute standard chest radiography for evaluation of acute dyspnea in the emergency department? Chest 2011;139(5):1140–7.

13. Volpicelli G. Usefulness of emergency ultrasound in nontraumatic cardiac arrest. Am J Emerg Med 2011;29(2):216–23.

14. Barillari A, Fioretti M. Lung ultrasound: a new tool for the emergency physician. Intern Emerg Med 2010;5:335–40.

15. Volpicelli G. Sonographic diagnosis of pneumothorax. Intensive Care Med 2011;37(2):224–32.

16. Barillari A, Kiuru S. Detection of spontaneous pneumothorax with chest ultrasound in the emergency department. Intern Emerg Med 2010;5:253–5.

17. Madill JJ. In-flight thoracic ultrasound detection of pneumothorax in combat. J Emerg Med 2010;39: 194–7.

18. Soldati G, Testa A, Sher S, et al. Occult traumatic pneumothorax: diagnostic accuracy of lung ultrasonography in the emergency department. Chest 2008;133:204–11.

19. Ben-Ami TE, O'Donovan JC, Yousefzadeh DK. Sonography of the chest in children. Radiol Clin North Am 1993;31:517–31.

20. Haller JO, Schneider M, Kassner EG, et al. Sonographic evaluation of the chest in infants and children. AJR Am J Roentgenol 1980;134: 1019–27.

21. Kim OH, Kim WS, Min JK, et al. US in the diagnosis of pediatric chest disease. Radiographics 2000;20: 653–71.

22. Koh DM, Burke S, Davies N, et al. Transthoracic US of the chest: clinical uses and applications. Radiographics 2002;22(1):e1.

23. Krejci CS, Trent EJ, Dubinsky T. Thoracic sonography. Respir Care 2001;46:932–9.

24. Mathis G. Thoraxsonography - Part I: chest wall and pleura. Ultrasound Med Biol 1997;23:1131–9.

25. Baron RL, Lee JK, Melson GL. Sonographic evaluation of right juxtadiaphragmatic masses in children using transhepatic approach. J Clin Ultrasound 1980;8:156–9.

26. Cortellaro F, Colombo S, Coen D, et al. Lung ultrasound is an accurate diagnostic tool for the diagnosis of pneumonia in the emergency department. Emerg Med J 2010. [Epub ahead of print].

27. Kocijancic K, Kocijancic I, Vidmar G. Sonography of pleural space in healthy individuals. J Clin Ultrasound 2005;33:386–9.

28. Acunas B, Celik L, Acunas A. Chest sonography: differentiation of pulmonary consolidation from pleural disease. Acta Radiol 1989;30:273–5.

29. Glasier CM, Leithiser RE, Williamson SL, et al. Extracardiac chest ultrasonography in infants and children: radiographic and clinical implications. J Pediatr 1989;114:540–4.

30. Kurian J, Levin TL, Han BK, et al. Comparison of ultrasound and CT in the evaluation of pneumonia complicated by parapneumonic effusion in children. AJR Am J Roentgenol 2009;193:1648–54.

31. Calder A, Owens CM. Imaging of parapneumonic pleural effusions and empyema in children. Pediatr Radiol 2009;39:527–37.

32. Hogan MJ, Coley BD. Interventional radiology treatment of empyema and lung abscesses. Paediatr Respir Rev 2008;9:77–84 [quiz: 84].

33. Coley BD, Hogan MJ. Image-guided interventions in neonates. Eur J Radiol 2006;60:208–20.

34. Sistrom CL, Wallace KK, Gay SB. Thoracic sonography for diagnosis and intervention. Curr Probl Diagn Radiol 1997;26:2–49.

35. Donnelly LF, Taylor CN, Emery KH, et al. Asymptomatic, palpable, anterior chest wall lesions in children: is cross-sectional imaging necessary? Radiology 1997;202:829–31.

36. Yekeler E, Tambag A, Tunaci A, et al. Analysis of the thymus in 151 healthy infants from 0 to 2 years of age. J Ultrasound Med 2004;23:1321–6.

37. Han BK, Yoon HK, Suh YL. Thymic ultrasound: II. Diagnosis of aberrant cervical thymus. Pediatr Radiol 2001;31:480–7.

38. Han BK, Suh YL, Yoon HK. Thymic ultrasound: I. Intrathymic anatomy in infants. Pediatr Radiol 2001;31:474–9.

39. Kocijancic K. Ultrasonographic forms of pleural space in healthy children. Coll Antropol 2007;31:999–1002.

40. Targhetta R, Bourgeois JM, Chavagneux R, et al. Ultrasonographic approach to diagnosing hydropneumothorax. Chest 1992;101:931–4.

41. Stefanidis K, Dimopoulos S, Nanas S. Basic principles and current applications of lung ultrasonography in the intensive care unit. Respirology 2011;16(2):249–56.

42. Kocijancic I, Vidmar K, Ivanovi-Herceg Z. Chest sonography versus lateral decubitus radiography in the diagnosis of small pleural effusions. J Clin Ultrasound 2003;31:69–74.

43. Chiu CY, Wong KS, Huang YC, et al. Echo-guided management of complicated parapneumonic effusion in children. Pediatr Pulmonol 2006;41:1226–32.

44. Yang PC, Luh KT, Chang DB, et al. Value of sonography in determining the nature of pleural effusion: analysis of 320 cases. AJR Am J Roentgenol 1992;159:29–33.

45. Wu RG, Yang PC, Kuo SH, et al. "Fluid color" sign: a useful indicator for discrimination between pleural thickening and pleural effusion. J Ultrasound Med 1995;14:767–9.

46. Yang PC. Applications of colour Doppler ultrasound in the diagnosis of chest diseases. Respirology 1997;2:231–8.

47. Lin FC, Chou CW, Chang SC. Usefulness of the suspended microbubble sign in differentiating empyemic and nonempyemic hydropneumothorax. J Ultrasound Med 2001;20:1341–5.

48. Coley BD. Ultrasound-guided interventional procedures. In: Siegel MJ, editor. Pediatric sonography. Philadelphia: Lippincott Williams & Wilkins; 2002. p. 699–725.

49. Lichtenstein D, Hulot JS, Rabiller A, et al. Feasibility and safety of ultrasound-aided thoracentesis in mechanically ventillated patients. Intensive Care Med 1999;25:955–8.

50. Mitri RK, Brown SD, Zurakowski D, et al. Outcomes of primary image-guided drainage of parapneumonic effusions in children. Pediatrics 2002;110:37–42.

51. Chen KY, Liaw YS, Wang HC, et al. Sonographic septation: a useful prognostic indicator of acute thoracic empyema. J Ultrasound Med 2000;19:837–43.

52. Feola GP, Shaw LC, Coburn L. Management of complicated parapneumonic effusions in children. Tech Vasc Interv Radiol 2003;6:197–204.

53. Wells RG, Havens PL. Intrapleural fibrinolysis for parapneumonic effusion and empyema in children. Radiology 2003;228:370–8.

54. Medford AR, Entwisle JJ. Indications for thoracic ultrasound in chest medicine: an observational study. Postgrad Med J 2010;86:8–11.

55. Chandrasekhar AJ, Reynes CJ, Churchill RJ. Ultrasonically guided percutaneous biopsy of peripheral pulmonary masses. Chest 1976;70:627–30.

56. Sheth S, Hamper UM, Stanley DB, et al. US guidance for thoracic biopsy: a valuable alternative to CT. Radiographics 1999;210:721–6.

57. Fontalvo LF, Amaral JG, Temple M, et al. Percutaneous US-guided biopsies of peripheral pulmonary lesions in children. Pediatr Radiol 2006;36:491–7.

58. Dulchavsky SA, Schwarz KL, Kirkpatrick AW, et al. Prospective evaluation of thoracic ultrasound in the detection of pneumothorax. J Trauma 2001;50:201–5.

59. Lichtenstein D, Meziere G, Biderman P, et al. The "lung point": an ultrasound sign specific to pneumothorax. Intensive Care Med 2000;26:1434–40.

60. McGahan JP, Richards J, Fogata ML. Emergency ultrasound in trauma patients. Radiol Clin North Am 2004;42:417–25.

61. Rowan KR, Kirkpatrick AW, Liu D, et al. Traumatic pneumothorax detection with thoracic US: correlation with chest radiography and CT—initial experience. Radiology 2002;225:210–4.

62. Wilkerson RG, Stone MB. Sensitivity of bedside ultrasound and supine anteroposterior chest radiographs for the identification of pneumothorax after blunt trauma. Acad Emerg Med 2010;17:11–7.

63. Elia F, Ferrari G, Molino P, et al. Lung ultrasound in postprocedural pneumothorax. Acad Emerg Med 2010;17:e81–2.

64. Lim JH, Lee KS, Kim TS, et al. Ring-down artifacts posterior to the right hemidiaphragm on abdominal sonography: sign of pulmonary parenchymal abnormalities. J Ultrasound Med 1999;18:403–10.

65. Zechner PM, Aichinger G, Rigaud M, et al. Prehospital lung ultrasound in the distinction between pulmonary edema and exacerbation of chronic obstructive pulmonary disease. Am J Emerg Med 2010;28:389.e1–2.

66. Reissig A, Kroegel C. Transthoracic sonography of diffuse parenchymal lung disease: the role of comet tail artifacts. J Ultrasound Med 2003;22:173–80.

67. Noble VE, Murray AF, Capp R, et al. Ultrasound assessment for extravascular lung water in patients undergoing hemodialysis. Time course for resolution. Chest 2009;135:1433–9.

68. Copetti R, Cattarossi L. The 'double lung point': an ultrasound sign diagnostic of transient tachypnea of the newborn. Neonatology 2007;91:203–9.

69. Avni EF, Braude P, Pardou A, et al. Hyaline membrane disease in the newborn: diagnosis by US. Pediatr Radiol 1990;20:143–6.

70. Avni EF, Cassart M, de Maertelaer V, et al. Sono-graphic prediction of chronic lung disease in the premature undergoing mechanical ventilation. Pe-diatr Radiol 1996;26:463–9.

71. Bober K, Swietliński J. Diagnostic utility of ultraso-nography for respiratory distress syndrome in neonates. Med Sci Monit 2006;12:CR440–6.

72. Pieper CH, Smith J, Brand EJ. The value of ultra-sound examination of the lungs in predicting bron-chopulmonary dysplasia. Pediatr Radiol 2004;34:227–31.

73. Cattarossi L, Copetti R, Poskurica B, et al. Surfactant administration for neonatal respiratory distress does not improve lung interstitial fluid clearance: echo-graphic and experimental evidence. J Perinat Med 2010;38:557–63.

74. Iuri D, De Candia A, Bazzocchi M. Evaluation of the lung in children with suspected pneumonia: useful-ness of ultrasonography. Radiol Med 2009;114:321–30.

75. Weinberg B, Diakoumakis EE, Kass EG, et al. The air bronchogram: sonographic demonstration. AJR Am J Roentgenol 1986;147:593–5.

76. Mathis G. Thoraxsonography—part II: peripheral pulmonary consolidation. Ultrasound Med Biol 1997;23:1141–53.

77. Lichtenstein D, Mezière G, Seitz J. The dynamic air bronchogram. A lung ultrasound sign of alveolar consolidation ruling out atelectasis. Chest 2009;135:1421–5.

78. Chiu CY, Wong KS, Lai SH, et al. Peripheral hypoe-choic spaces in consolidated lung: a specific diagnostic sonographic finding for necrotizing pneu-monia in children. Turk J Pediatr 2008;50:58–62.

79. Yang PC, Luh KT, Lee YC. Lung abscesses: ultra-sonography and ultrasound-guided transthoracic aspiration. Radiology 1991;180:171–5.

80. Siegel MJ. Chest. In: Siegel MJ, editor. Pediatric sonography. Philadelphia: Lippincott Williams & Wilkins; 2002. p. 167–211.

81. Langston C. New concepts in the pathology of congenital lung malformations. Semin Pediatr Surg 2003;12:17–37.

82. Dhingsa R, Coakley FV, Albanese CT, et al. Prenatal sonography and MR imaging of pulmonary sequestration. AJR Am J Roentgenol 2003;180:433–7.

83. Khosa JK, Leong SL, Borzi PA. Congenital cystic adenomatoid malformation of the lung: indications and timing of surgery. Pediatr Surg Int 2004;20:505–8.

84. Laberge JM, Bratu I, Flageole H. The management of asymptomatic congenital lung malformations. Paediatr Respir Rev 2004;5(Suppl A):S305–12.

85. Hang JD, Guo QY, Chen CX, et al. Imaging approach to the diagnosis of pulmonary sequestra-tion. Acta Radiol 1996;37(6):883–8.

86. Schlesinger AE, DiPietro MA, Statter MB, et al. Utility of sonography in the diagnosis of broncho-pulmonary sequestration. J Pediatr Surg 1994;29:52–5.

87. Fumino S, Iwai N, Kimura O, et al. Preoperative eval-uation of the aberrant artery in intralobar pulmonary sequestration using multidetector computed tomog-raphy angiography. J Pediatr Surg 2007;42:1776–9.

88. Cromi A, Ghezzi F, Raffaelli R, et al. Ultrasono-graphic measurement of thymus size in IUGR fetuses: a marker of the fetal immunoendocrine response to malnutrition. Ultrasound Obstet Gyne-col 2009;33:421–6.

89. Rothstein DH, Voss SD, Isakoff M, et al. Thymoma in a child: case report and review of the literature. Pediatr Surg Int 2005;21:548–51.

90. Jaggers J, Balsara K. Mediastinal masses in chil-dren. Semin Thorac Cardiovasc Surg 2004;16:201–8.

91. Sakai F, Sone S, Kawai T, et al. Ultrasonography of thymoma with pathologic correlation. Acta Radiol 1994;35:25–9.

92. Tomiyama N, Honda O, Tsubamoto M, et al. Ante-rior mediastinal tumors: diagnostic accuracy of CT and MRI. Eur J Radiol 2009;69:280–8.

93. Yağci B, Varan A, Uner A, et al. Thymic Langerhans cell histiocytosis mimicking lymphoma. Pediatr Blood Cancer 2008;51:833–5.

94. Sturm-O'Brien AK, Salazar JD, Byrd RH, et al. Cervical thymic anomalies–the Texas Children's Hospital experience. Laryngoscope 2009;119:1988–93.

95. Kontny HU, Sleasman JW, Kingma DW, et al. Multi-locular thymic cysts in children with human immuno-deficiency virus infection: clinical and pathologic aspects. J Pediatr 1997;131:264–70.

96. Leonidas JC, Berdon WE, Valderrama E, et al. Human immunodeficiency virus infection and multi-locular thymic cysts. Radiology 1996;198:377–9.

97. McKenney JK, Heerema-McKenney A, Rouse RV. Extragonadal germ cell tumors: a review with emphasis on pathologic features, clinical prog-nostic variables, and differential diagnostic consid-erations. Adv Anat Pathol 2007;14:69–92.

98. Wu TT, Wang HC, Chang YC, et al. Mature medias-tinal teratoma: sonographic imaging patterns and pathologic correlation. J Ultrasound Med 2002;21:759–65.

99. Zhang KR, Jia HM, Pan EY, et al. Diagnosis and treatment of mediastinal enterogenous cysts in children. Chin Med Sci J 2006;21:201–3.

100. Bosch-Marcet J, Serres-Créixams X, Borrás-Pérez V, et al. Value of sonography for follow-up of mediastinal lymphadenopathy in children with tuberculosis. J Clin Ultrasound 2007;35:118–24.

101. Akinci D, Akhan O, Ozmen M, et al. Diaphragmatic mesothelial cysts in children: radiologic findings

and percutaneous ethanol sclerotherapy. AJR Am J Roentgenol 2005;185:873–7.

102. Gerscovich EO, Cronan M, McGahan JP, et al. Ultrasonographic evaluation of diaphragmatic motion. J Ultrasound Med 2001;20:597–604.

103. Riccabona M. Thoraxsonographie im neugeborenen- und kindesalter. Radiologe 2003;43:1075–89.

104. Sanchez de Toledo J, Munoz R, Landsittel D, et al. Diagnosis of abnormal diaphragm motion after cardiothoracic surgery: ultrasound performed by a cardiac intensivist vs. fluoroscopy. Congenit Heart Dis 2010;5:565–72.

105. Yazici M, Karaca I, Arikan A, et al. Congenital even- tration of the diaphragm in children: 25 years' experience in three pediatric surgery centers. Eur J Pediatr Surg 2003;13:298–301.

106. Riccabona M. Ultrasound of the chest in children (mediastinum excluded). Eur Radiol 2008;18:390–9.

107. Dubois J, Patriquin HB, Garel L, et al. Soft-tissue hemangiomas in infants and children: diagnosis using color Doppler sonography. AJR Am J Roent- genol 1998;171:247–52.

108. Dubois J, Garel L, David M, et al. Vascular soft- tissue tumors in infancy: distinguishing features on Doppler sonography. AJR Am J Roentgenol 2002;178:1541–5.

109. Shiels WE, Kang DR, Murakami JW, et al. Percuta- neous treatment of lymphatic malformations. Oto- laryngol Head Neck Surg 2009;141:219–24.

110. Donnelly LF, Frush DP. Abnormalities of the chest wall in pediatric patients. AJR Am J Roentgenol 1999;173:1595–601.

111. Smeets AJ, Robben SG, Meradji M. Sonographi- cally detected costo-chondral dislocation in an abused child: a new sonographic sign to the radio- logical spectrum of child abuse. Pediatr Radiol 1990;20:566–7.

112. Kelloff J, Hulett R, Spivey M. Acute rib fracture diagnosis in an infant by US: a matter of child protection. Pediatr Radiol 2009;39:70–2.

113. Bitschnau R, Gehmacher O, Kopf A, et al. Ultra- sound in the diagnosis of rib and sternal fracture. Ultraschall Med 1997;18:158–61.

114. Hurley ME, Keye GD, Hamilton S. Is ultrasound really helpful in the detection of rib fractures? Injury 2004;35:562–6.

115. You JS, Chung YE, Kim D, et al. Role of sonography in the emergency room to diagnose sternal frac- tures. J Clin Ultrasound 2010;38:135–7.

116. Jin W, Yang DM, Kim HC, et al. Diagnostic values of sonography for assessment of sternal fractures compared with conventional radiography and bone scans. J Ultrasound Med 2006;25:1263–8 [quiz: 1269–70].

117. Zeng Q, Lai JY, Wang XM, et al. Costochondral changes in the chest wall after the Nuss procedure: ultrasonographic findings. J Pediatr Surg 2008;43: 2147–50.

118. Ong B, Gibbs H, Catchpole I, et al. Peripherally inserted central catheters and upper extremity deep vein thrombosis. Australas Radiol 2006;50: 451–4.

119. Pinon M, Bezzio S, Tovo PA, et al. A prospective 7- year survey on central venous catheter-related complications at a single pediatric hospital. Eur J Pediatr 2009;168:1505–12.

120. Beidle TR, Letourneau JG. Arm swelling. In: Bluth EI, Arger PH, Benson CB, et al, editors. Ultra- sound: a practical approach to clinical problems. New York: Thieme; 2000. p. 566–82.

121. Nazarian GK, Foshager MC. Color Doppler sonog- raphy of the thoracic inlet veins. Radiographics 1995;15:1357–71.

122. Patel MC, Berman LH, Moss HA, et al. Subclavian and internal jugular veins at Doppler US: abnormal cardiac pulsatility and respiratory phasicity as a predictor of complete occlusion. Radiology 1999;211:579–83.

123. Mangrulkar VH, Cohen HL, Dougherty D. Sonog- raphy for diagnosis of cervical ribs in children. J Ultrasound Med 2008;27:1083–6.

124. Demondion X, Herbinet P, Van Sint Jan S, et al. Imaging assessment of thoracic outlet syndrome. Radiographics 2006;26:1735–50.

125. Demondion X, Vidal C, Herbinet P, et al. Ultrasono- graphic assessment of arterial cross-sectional area in the thoracic outlet on postural maneuvers measured with power Doppler ultrasonography in both asymptomatic and symptomatic populations. J Ultrasound Med 2006;25:217–24.

126. Rose SC. Noninvasive vascular laboratory for eval- uation of peripheral arterial occlusive disease. Part III - clinical applications: nonatherosclerotic lower extremity arterial conditions and upper extremity arterial disesae. J Vasc Interv Radiol 1991;12:11–8.

127. Longley DG, Yedlicka JW, Molina EJ, et al. Thoracic outlet syndrome: evaluation of the subclavian vessels by color duplex sonography. AJR Am J Roentgenol 1992;158:623–30.

128. Durand C, Garel C, Nugues F, et al. L'echographie dans la pathologie thoracique de l'enfant. J Radiol 2001;82:729–37.

Contemporary Perspectives on Pediatric Diffuse Lung Disease

R. Paul Guillerman, MD[a],*, Alan S. Brody, MD[b]

KEYWORDS

- Interstitial lung disease • Diffuse lung disease
- Computed tomography • Surfactant
- Alveolar growth disorder
- Neuroendocrine cell hyperplasia of infancy
- Pulmonary interstitial glycogenosis

Pediatric diffuse lung disease encompasses a heterogeneous group of rare disorders characterized by widespread pulmonary parenchymal pathology and impaired gas exchange. The term interstitial lung disease (ILD) is entrenched in the medical literature as a descriptor of these disorders. However, these disorders may involve not only the pulmonary interstitium but also the airspaces and airways, so that the term diffuse lung disease is more apt. In addition to the anatomic heterogeneity, the injury and repair processes that occur in immature lung differ from those observed in the mature adult lung, and the stage of lung growth and development must be taken into consideration in the diagnostic approach to these disorders.[1]

The American Thoracic Society (ATS)/European Respiratory Society (ERS) International Multidisciplinary Consensus Classification of the Idiopathic Interstitial Pneumonias developed for the adult population[2] is not broadly applicable to children. Fibrosis is more prominent in diffuse lung diseases of adults than in those of children. Usual interstitial pneumonia (UIP), the pathologic correlate of idiopathic pulmonary fibrosis (IPF) and the dominant form of diffuse lung disease in the adult ATS/ERS

scheme, rarely, if ever, occurs in children. The erroneous labeling of poorly defined interstitial disease in children as "UIP" likely accounts for the better outcomes reported in children given this diagnosis. Many pediatric cases of desquamative interstitial pneumonia (DIP) diagnosed before the advent of specific genetic testing were likely attributable to unrecognized mutations in surfactant-related genes.[3] Several forms of pediatric diffuse lung disease exhibit distinct clinical, pathologic, and radiologic patterns not observed in adults, reflecting the influence of the stage of lung growth and development on disease manifestations.[1]

In light of advances in imaging technology, infant pulmonary function testing, molecular genetics, immunopathology, and electron microscopy, a new approach to the recognition and classification of childhood diffuse lung disease has been developed by the collaborative efforts of clinicians, pathologists, and radiologists in the Children's Interstitial Lung Disease (ChILD) Research Cooperative.[4] The overarching goal of this article is to review clinical presentation, classification, imaging technique, and spectrum of characteristic imaging findings of diffuse lung disease in pediatric patients.

Financial disclosure/Conflicts of interest: The authors have nothing to disclose.
[a] Department of Pediatric Radiology, Texas Children's Hospital, Baylor College of Medicine, 6701 Fannin Street, Suite 470, Houston, TX 77030, USA
[b] Department of Radiology, Cincinnati Children's Hospital Medical Center, 3333 Burnet Avenue, MLC 5031, Cincinnati, OH 45229-3039, USA
* Corresponding author.
E-mail address: rpguille@texaschildrens.org

Radiol Clin N Am 49 (2011) 847–868
doi:10.1016/j.rcl.2011.06.004

CLINICAL PRESENTATION AND CLASSIFICATION

Diffuse lung diseases are less common in children than in adults, and are more frequently observed in infants and young children than in older children. The true prevalence of pediatric diffuse lung disease is likely understated in the literature, due to the lack of familiarity with recently characterized disorders and appropriate classification schemes and the more reticent use of diagnostic lung biopsy in children compared with adults. Pediatric diffuse lung disease generally presents either in the neonatal period with dramatic respiratory failure or later in infancy or childhood with an insidious course of respiratory difficulty, failure to thrive, or exercise intolerance. In the latter setting, it may be misattributed for months or even years to another condition, such as asthma, bronchopulmonary dysplasia, congenital heart disease, or recurrent aspiration, but be atypically severe or refractory to treatment. A constellation of symptoms and signs termed "ChILD syndrome" has been proposed to assist clinicians in identifying children that warrant further investigation for possible diffuse lung disease. The ChILD syndrome working definition consists of the following criteria: (1) respiratory symptoms (cough, dyspnea, or exercise intolerance), (2) signs (resting tachypnea, adventitious sounds, retractions, digital clubbing, failure to thrive, or respiratory failure), (3) hypoxemia, and (4) diffuse pulmonary parenchymal abnormality on chest radiograph (CXR) or computed tomography (CT). More than 90% of children diagnosed with diffuse lung disease will satisfy at least 3 of these criteria. The criteria are best applied after more common entities such as asthma, cystic fibrosis, immunodeficiency, congenital heart disease, bronchopulmonary dysplasia, pulmonary infection, and recurrent aspiration have been excluded as the primary etiology.[5]

The specific forms of diffuse lung disease affecting infants and young children with ChILD syndrome are organized by the ChILD Research Cooperative into a novel classification scheme (Table 1).[4] Unlike the adult ATS/ERS scheme that is based primarily on clinicopathologic findings, the scheme for children is largely categorized based on the presumed etiology, and there is overlap of distinct pathologies and clinical disorders among different etiologic categories. For example, pulmonary alveolar proteinosis (PAP), DIP, nonspecific

Table 1
Child research cooperative classification scheme for pediatric diffuse lung disease

Category	Entities
Diffuse developmental disorders	Acinar dysplasia Congenital alveolar dysplasia Alveolar capillary dysplasia with misalignment of the pulmonary veins
Alveolar growth abnormalities	Pulmonary hypoplasia Chronic neonatal lung disease (BPD) Related to genetic disorders or congenital heart disease
Specific disorders of unknown etiology	Neuroendocrine cell hyperplasia of infancy Pulmonary interstitial glycogenosis
Genetic disorders of surfactant metabolism	Mutations of the genes for SP-B, SP-C, ABCA3, TTF-1, SLC747, others
Disorders of the normal host	Postinfectious processes Related to environmental agents Aspiration Eosinophilic lung diseases
Disorders related to systemic disease processes	Immune-mediated disorders (pulmonary capillaritis, collagen-vascular diseases) Storage diseases Langerhans cell histiocytosis
Disorders of the immunocompromised host	Opportunistic infections Related to therapeutic intervention Related to transplantation and rejection syndromes
Disorders masquerading as interstitial lung disease	Arterial, venous, lymphatic disorders Congestive changes related to cardiac dysfunction

interstitial pneumonia (NSIP), and chronic pneumonitis of infancy are distinct lung pathologies that can be attributable to genetic surfactant disorders, and the pathology of NSIP can be observed in disorders of the normal host, disorders related to systemic disease, and genetic surfactant disorders.

Reviews of the correlative findings and diagnostic efficacy of imaging for specific forms of pediatric diffuse lung disease are emerging.[6] In some disorders the imaging findings can be diagnostic, whereas in other disorders the imaging findings are nonspecific and lung biopsy may be needed for diagnosis. The diagnostic efficacy of imaging is a function of the quality of the images obtained and the proficiency of the interpreter. Existing studies on the imaging of diffuse lung disease in children have largely been conducted at academic centers by pediatric subspecialists with a particular interest or expertise in these disorders. Generalization of these observations to the broader community setting is dependent on increased awareness of appropriate pediatric chest-imaging technique and recognition of the salient imaging features of specific forms of pediatric diffuse lung disease.

IMAGING TECHNIQUE

Chest radiographs are usually the first imaging study performed in children with diffuse lung disease. These radiographs are rarely normal, but are neither sensitive nor specific enough to eliminate the need for a CT scan, the current standard noninvasive method of assessing lung structure.[7] The goal of performing CT for diffuse lung disease in children is to provide the necessary image quality to make the diagnosis, or refine the differential diagnosis and guide further diagnostic testing with the least risk to the child. The primary disadvantages of pediatric chest CT are the risks of sedation, anesthesia, and carcinogenesis from exposure to ionizing radiation.

The majority of cases of pediatric diffuse lung disease present in the first year of life, a time when obtaining high-quality CT images of the lungs is particularly difficult because of the rapid respiratory rate, the small size of the anatomic structures, the proclivity for atelectasis, and the inability of the patient to comply with instructions to breath-hold and refrain from motion. If general anesthesia is used to control patient motion and ventilation, it is important to image the patient as soon as possible after induction, and to implement alveolar recruitment maneuvers and adequate positive airway pressure to minimize atelectasis. Reduction of motion artifact and atelectasis can be obtained without general anesthesia or

intubation using a controlled-ventilation technique. By hyperventilating a sedated child with positive pressure applied via face mask, the resultant hypocarbia and stimulation of the Hering-Breuer reflex induce a respiratory pause. During this pause, imaging with and without positive airway pressure provides simulated inspiratory and expiratory images.[8] However, this technique requires coordination with a specialist trained in the required respiratory maneuvers, and is not available at most imaging centers. The use of scanning during quiet breathing and lateral decubitus or prone positioning to reexpand atelectasis and to serve as a surrogate for inspiratory/expiratory series often allows sufficient image quality for diagnostic purposes.[9,10]

Due to the relatively low cross-sectional attenuation of the pediatric chest, the inherent high contrast between air and the lung parenchyma, and the widespread nature of the disease process, a very low radiation dose high-resolution CT (HRCT) technique can be used to evaluate children with suspected diffuse lung disease.[11] Unfortunately, the term HRCT has become confusing, particularly in recent years. HRCT originated more than 2 decades ago as a limited sampling technique entailing the acquisition and display of noncontiguous thin (1–1.5 mm) axial sections of the lungs reconstructed with a high spatial frequency reconstruction algorithm to minimize the scan time and maximize the image detail.[12] The multidetector CT scanners now prevalent permit contiguous high-resolution images of the entire lungs to be rapidly acquired, reducing motion artifact and allowing spirometric gated or dynamic cine imaging through the respiratory cycle.[13] Conventional noncontiguous axial HRCT technique can still be performed on current multidetector scanners to exploit the radiation dose reduction advantage of irradiating only a small portion of the lungs.[14,15] Because each additional breath-hold during a noncontiguous axial HRCT scan becomes more challenging and the lung apices are more resistant to respiratory motion artifact than the lung bases, images should be acquired caudal to cranial.[16] Compared with volumetric multidetector CT, axial noncontiguous HRCT is more technically demanding, has more motion artifact, risks missing abnormalities in skipped areas, makes distinction of small nodules and vessels more difficult, does not allow multiplanar reconstructions, offers limited reproducibility for follow-up, and is more limited for evaluating the mediastinum and central airways.[17,18] Ideally, the radiologist should directly supervise the CT scan and decide whether noncontiguous HRCT is sufficient to minimize radiation dose or whether volumetric CT or additional image series (eg, prone, decubitus, expiratory) are needed.[12]

To optimize visualization of fine lung details at acceptable radiation dose levels, the smallest field of view encompassing the lungs, a high but not necessarily the highest spatial frequency reconstruction algorithm, and thin but not necessarily the thinnest slices should be reconstructed. On some CT scanners, the bone reconstruction algorithm may be preferable to the lung reconstruction algorithm. Image degradation from excessive noise becomes problematic with thinner slices and sharper reconstruction algorithms, particularly with very low radiation dose technique. With slice thicknesses of less than 1 mm on most current CT scanners, the decrease in signal-to-noise ratio mitigates any appreciable improvement in the spatial resolution.[19]

The preferred number of images or image slice spacing for noncontiguous axial HRCT in children involves a trade-off between radiation dose and estimation of disease extent. A commonly selected, albeit arbitrary, interval for inspiratory HRCT is 10 mm for children, with smaller (5–7 mm) intervals reserved for infants. Expiratory HRCT images are obtained primarily to evaluate for air trapping and airway malacia. Expiratory HRCT images are usually acquired at double the inspiratory interval,[7,14] although the precision of estimates of the degree of air trapping has been noted to decrease at sampling densities of less than 10%.[20]

If the clinical setting warrants complete lung or mediastinal coverage so that volumetric technique is indicated, the radiation dose from z-axis overranging can be reduced by using a narrower macrodetector array and lower helical pitch values, but at the expense of slower scan speed and increased motion artifact. Alternatively, a broad macrodetector array and higher pitch should be selected if scan duration and motion artifacts are principal concerns, such as in a tachypneic child incapable of breath-holding.[21] Recently introduced high-pitch helical and very broad macrodetector array volumetric axial CT scanning techniques are capable of subsecond coverage of the entire chest in small children, ameliorating cardiac and respiratory motion artifact and obviating the need for sedation, even in awake agitated patients.[22–24]

The fastest CT gantry rotation setting should generally be used, because the minimization of motion artifact usually more than compensates for the slight degradation of in-plane spatial resolution that occurs with the reduced number of views sampled per gantry rotation.[25] New gemstone-based scintillators improve the in-plane spatial resolution by allowing the sampling of many more views per gantry rotation, thus increasing the conspicuity of the margins of small airways, vessels, and ground-glass opacities.[26]

For CT without iodinated contrast, lowering the tube voltage increases streak and beam-hardening artifact and does not significantly improve soft tissue contrast-to-noise ratio for a given radiation dose.[27,28] Lowering the mAs and using automatic tube modulation tailored to patient size and clinical indication are preferred methods for reducing radiation dose in pediatric HRCT. A universal protocol for imaging pediatric diffuse lung disease is not desirable because the geometry, beam filtration, and detector efficiency varies among different CT scanners. Appropriate patient positioning in the center of the gantry with the arms raised out of the scan field of view is especially important in children to maximize the effectiveness of automatic tube current modulation and avoid undesirable beam attenuation, image noise, and artifacts.[29] Imaging the lungs at a more fully inflated state is an underappreciated method of reducing the radiation dose needed to resolve small lung structures. New iterative reconstruction techniques reduce image noise, permitting the use of lower radiation dose and sharper reconstruction algorithms for better depiction of ground-glass opacities, tiny nodules, and other fine lung details compared with conventional filtered back-projection image reconstruction.[19,30]

With currently available techniques, diagnostic quality volumetric pediatric chest CT scans can be performed with effective doses of less than 1.5 mSv per examination, and several-fold lower doses can be achieved with use of the noncontiguous axial HRCT technique. For certain findings and disorders, a confident diagnosis can be made with CT performed with radiation doses in the range of a few chest radiographs.[31,32] While it is desirable to eliminate unnecessary radiation exposure, it is very important to recognize that the carcinogenic risks of radiation at the doses administered during pediatric chest CT are theoretical, and even on a theoretical basis the risks are usually far smaller than those of erroneous diagnosis and misguided treatment.

SPECTRUM OF IMAGING FINDINGS

The correct interpretation of technically satisfactory images requires understanding of the normal appearance of the immature lung, identification of abnormal findings, and recognition of disease patterns.[14] CT often reveals findings in children that may incorrectly be interpreted as pathologic by the inexperienced observer. The lung parenchyma of infants and toddlers is relatively high in attenuation, simulating the appearance of diffuse ground-glass opacification. This appearance is attributable to the images often being acquired during tidal breathing rather than at deep inspiration, and to the smaller mean alveolar diameter in this age range that results in more alveolar walls relative to air per unit volume and image voxel.[33] The alveoli begin to progressively enlarge around the age of 3 years, accounting for the decrease in normal lung attenuation after early childhood. Normal interlobular septa are occasionally thick enough to be resolved by CT, especially in the lung periphery.[25] The bronchoarterial size ratio normally does not exceed 0.75 in children. Reliance on the adult criterion of a ratio greater than 1 to define airway dilation risks underestimation of the presence and extent of airway disease.[34] Physiologic elevation of the ratio can occur in the setting of high-altitude reflex bronchoconstriction,[33] and a radiologic impression of bronchiectasis should be regarded with caution in children because airway dilation may be transient rather than irreversible.[35]

Although findings on pediatric CT are adequately described by the glossary of terms for thoracic imaging advocated by the Fleischner Society,[36] the diagnostic considerations for diffuse lung disease are very different in children to those in adults. Radiologists involved in the interpretation of pediatric chest imaging examinations should become familiar with the disorders covered under the classification scheme for pediatric diffuse lung disease recently proposed by the ChILD Research Cooperative.[4] Awareness of the distinguishing pathologic, clinical, and radiologic features of disorders allows refinement of the differential diagnosis, guidance of further testing and, in some cases, confident diagnosis and aversion of unnecessary biopsy.

Diffuse Developmental Disorders

The diffuse developmental disorders of the lung are associated with profound impairment of alveolar gas exchange. Acinar dysplasia is characterized by arrest in the pseudoglandular or early canalicular phase of lung development, whereas congenital alveolar dysplasia is characterized by arrest in the late canalicular/early saccular phase of lung development. Alveolar capillary dysplasia with misalignment of the pulmonary veins (ACD/MPV) is characterized by malpositioning of the pulmonary vein branches adjacent to the pulmonary artery branches rather than within the interlobular septae, medial hypertrophy of pulmonary arterioles, reduced alveolar capillary density, and pulmonary lobular maldevelopment.[37]

The typical presentation of the diffuse developmental disorders of the lung is a term neonate of appropriate size for gestational age that develops respiratory failure and severe pulmonary hypertension within a couple days of birth unrelated to usual factors such as meconium aspiration, congenital heart disease, perinatal asphyxia, or sepsis. Death usually ensues within the first month of life, although longer survival is possible if the lung involvement is patchy rather than diffuse or if extracorporeal membrane oxygenation (ECMO) bridging to lung transplantation is available.[38,39] More than 80% of cases of ACD/MPV are associated with extrapulmonary malformations, most commonly hypoplastic left heart syndrome, aortic coarctation, midgut malrotation, alimentary tract atresias, and urinary tract malformations. FOXF1 gene mutations or 16q24.1 microdeletions are a cause of some ACD/MPV cases.[40]

As a consequence of the lung disease severity, imaging of these patients is usually limited to portable chest radiographs. The initial chest radiographs may be unimpressive, but follow-up radiographs usually show progressive hazy pulmonary opacification, evocative of surfactant deficiency of prematurity or genetic surfactant disorders (**Fig. 1**). Air leak in the form of pneumothorax or pneumomediastinum is common and is likely due to barotrauma.[39,41–43]

Alveolar Growth Abnormalities

Alveolar growth abnormalities are the most common cause of diffuse lung disease in infancy. The histopathology of alveolar growth abnormalities is characterized by impaired alveolarization, manifesting as lobular simplification with fewer and larger alveoli with deficient septation and vascularization that can be misinterpreted as

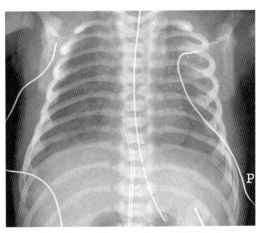

Fig. 1. Alveolar capillary dysplasia with misalignment of the pulmonary veins. Chest radiograph of a term newborn with respiratory distress shows hazy pulmonary opacification.

emphysema. Pulmonary interstitial glycogenosis is often an accompanying finding. The growth abnormality can be prenatal or postnatal in onset, and acquired or genetic.[4,37] The most commonly encountered postnatal form is bronchopulmonary dysplasia (BPD) or chronic neonatal lung disease of prematurity. Advances in perinatal medicine, including antenatal corticosteroid administration, surfactant replacement, and mechanical ventilation refinements, have decreased lung injury from barotrauma and oxygen toxicity and lowered the threshold of viability of premature neonates, so that there has been a transition to "new" BPD distinguished by impaired alveolarization but less fibrosis and airway obstruction than in classic BPD.[44] The best known prenatal form is pulmonary hypoplasia arising from in utero intrathoracic space constraints (eg, congenital diaphragmatic hernia, oligohydramnios, mass lesion, skeletal dysplasia). Alveolar growth abnormalities may also be observed in the setting of congenital heart disease, certain genetic disorders, and as a primary idiopathic disorder in near-term and term infants.[4,37]

Affected children usually present with respiratory difficulties in the neonatal period, and may improve slowly or worsen over time depending on the degree of alveolar abnormality and the ability of the child to develop new alveoli. Most alveolarization occurs from 32 weeks' gestational age to 2 years' postnatal age, and the number of alveoli slowly increases in later childhood, reaching adult levels at around 8 years of age, so that there is only a limited period during which catch-up growth may compensate for prenatal or neonatal disturbances.[45]

Chest radiographs and CT scans of infants with "new" BPD and other alveolar growth abnormalities demonstrate findings ranging from near normal to markedly disordered pulmonary lobules of variable shape and attenuation, thick perilobular reticular opacities, linear subpleural opacities, ground-glass opacities, and hyperlucent areas, some of which are cyst-like (**Fig. 2**). The hyperlucent areas may correspond to enlarged alveoli with reduced septation and vascularization rather than obstructive emphysema.[46] Children with trisomy 21 have been noted to have a diminished number of alveoli and alveolar enlargement, especially in the subpleural region that produces the appearance of subpleural cysts on CT in about one-third of these children (**Fig. 3**).[47] Evaluation for abnormal alveolar growth should be considered in children with trisomy 21 and respiratory difficulties not attributable to congenital heart disease. Abnormal alveolar growth has been also noted in patients with mutations in the filamin A (FLNA) X-linked gene that encodes an actin-binding cytoskeletal protein involved in neuronal migration, cardiovascular development, and connective tissue integrity. Patients with FLNA mutations can have periventricular nodular gray matter heterotopia, vascular aneurysms, skeletal dysplasia, and joint hyperextensibility. The alveolar growth abnormality is especially severe, and causes pulmonary hypertension and progressive respiratory decline in infancy that may require lung transplantation for continued survival. Chest imaging shows central pulmonary artery enlargement, atelectasis, and progressive severe pulmonary hyperinflation coupled with hyperlucency and peripheral pulmonary vascular attenuation simulating emphysema (**Fig. 4**).[6,48]

Specific Disorders of Unknown Etiology

Pulmonary interstitial glycogenosis (PIG), previously known as infantile cellular interstitial pneumonitis,

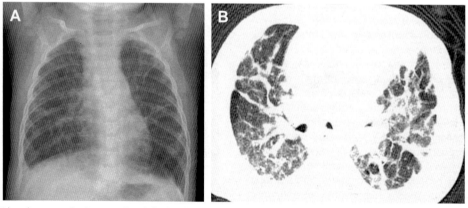

Fig. 2. Alveolar growth abnormality. (*A*) Chest radiograph of a 3-month-old term infant with respiratory insufficiency shows coarse reticular pulmonary opacities. (*B*) CT image of the same patient obtained at 4 months of age demonstrates disordered pulmonary lobules of variable shape and attenuation, thick perilobular reticular opacities, and ground-glass opacities.

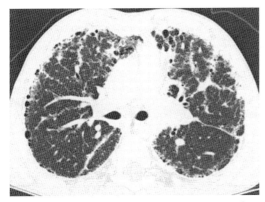

Fig. 3. Alveolar growth abnormality. CT image from a 4-year-old with trisomy 21 reveals numerous subpleural cysts.

is a disorder of unknown etiology characterized histopathologically by infiltration of the interstitium with immature mesenchymal cells that contain abundant cytoplasmic glycogen and stain positive for vimentin. The pneumocytes and endothelial cells are largely unaffected, and inflammation and fibrosis are not prominent features.[49] PIG has not been seen in lung biopsies from children older than 10 months, suggesting a relationship of PIG to lung growth and development.[5,50] Patchy PIG is commonly observed in association with alveolar growth abnormalities.[4]

Most patients with PIG present in the early neonatal period with tachypnea and a requirement for supplemental oxygen. Clinical outcome is usually favorable and depends primarily on the severity of any associated alveolar growth abnormality, although the resolution of histopathologic findings of PIG in conjunction with clinical improvement suggests that PIG has an impact on the patient's respiratory status.[50] PIG can respond favorably to corticosteroid treatment,

possibly due to acceleration of lung maturation rather than inflammatory suppression.[5,50–52]

Findings reported on chest radiographs include hyperinflation and interstitial opacities.[49,51–53] Findings reported on CT include pulmonary architectural distortion, interstitial thickening, hyperlucent areas, and ground-glass opacities.[49,52–54] The common association with alveolar growth abnormalities confounds assessment of the imaging appearance of "pure" PIG, and published reports of the imaging findings of PIG describe changes that could largely be attributable to alveolar growth abnormalities, limiting the value of these reports (**Fig. 5**).

Neuroendocrine cell hyperplasia of infancy (NEHI), originally termed persistent tachypnea of infancy, is a disorder of unknown etiology characterized histopathologically by increased numbers of pulmonary neuroendocrine cells (PNECs) and innervated clusters of PNECs called neuroepithelial bodies in the epithelium of the peripheral airways.[55] Detection of PNECs is facilitated by special staining for bombesin. PNECs play a role in oxygen sensing and fetal lung development, and usually rapidly decline in number after the neonatal period. Increased numbers of PNECs can be also observed in patients with sudden infant death syndrome, bronchopulmonary dysplasia, pulmonary hypertension, and cystic fibrosis, although the histopathologic findings of these disorders are unlikely to be confused for NEHI. Minor patchy inflammation or fibrosis is seen in a small proportion of airways in NEHI.[56] The existence of familial cases of NEHI suggests the possibility of a genetic etiology.[55]

NEHI usually presents in infancy with persistent tachypnea, hypoxemia, and often failure to thrive. Auscultation may reveal crackles, but wheezing is unusual. Symptoms can be precipitated or

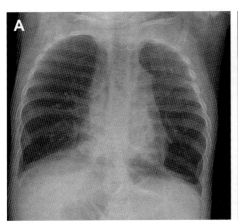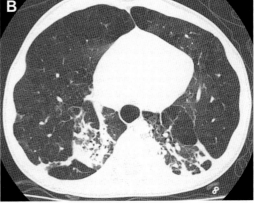

Fig. 4. Alveolar growth abnormality. (*A*) Chest radiograph of a 10-month-old with filamin A mutation shows pulmonary hyperinflation. (*B*) CT image of the same patient obtained at 11 months of age reveals marked multilobar hyperlucency with vascular attenuation resembling emphysema, as well as posterior atelectasis.

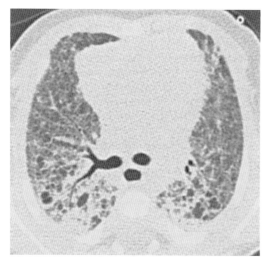

Fig. 5. Pulmonary interstitial glycogenosis and alveolar growth abnormality. CT image from a near-term 4-week-old with respiratory insufficiency demonstrates ground-glass opacification, interstitial thickening, and cyst-like hyperlucent disordered pulmonary lobules.

exacerbated by viral respiratory infections or residence at high altitude.[55] Lung function testing shows profound air trapping with reduced forced expiratory flow and markedly elevated functional residual capacity and residual volume. The severity of small airway obstruction correlates with prominence of PNECs.[56] Treatment is largely supportive, and focused on oxygen supplementation and nutritional support. Bronchodilators and corticosteroids have not been shown to be beneficial except for treatment of superimposed viral infections. Although NEHI is not a life-threatening condition, most patients require supplemental oxygen for many years, and air trapping and exercise intolerance may persist into adolescence.[5,55]

On chest radiographs, NEHI presents with hyperinflation resembling bronchiolitis or reactive airways disease. CT findings of diffuse air trapping, mosaic attenuation, and geographic ground-glass opacities of the right middle lobe, lingula, and paramediastinal lung regions are highly characteristic, approaching 100% specificity when interpreted by pediatric radiologists familiar with the disorder (**Fig. 6**). Septal thickening, cysts, bronchiectasis, and peribronchial thickening are not typically seen. With a sensitivity of 80%, CT is unable to exclude NEHI, and misdiagnoses can occur when other pulmonary abnormalities are present and the distribution of ground-glass opacities differs from the classic pattern.[31] Due to intersubject and intrasubject variability in PNEC number, pathologic confirmation of the diagnosis is not always reliable, especially if airway sampling is limited.[56] A confident

diagnosis of NEHI can be made if the clinical presentation and CT findings are typical, averting the need for lung biopsy.[5,56]

Genetic Disorders of Surfactant

Genetic disorders affecting surfactant metabolism are the most common cause of unexplained fatal respiratory distress syndrome (RDS) of term newborns, and are increasingly identified as a cause of chronic diffuse lung disease later in childhood. The most frequent disease-causing mutations involve the adenosine triphosphate binding cassette A3 (ABCA3) gene. Other disease-causing mutations involve the genes encoding surfactant protein C (SP-C), surfactant protein B (SP-B), granulocyte-macrophage colony stimulating factor receptor alpha subunit (GM-CSF-Rα), thyroid transcription factor 1 (TTF-1), and solute carrier 747 (SLC747).[57]

In early infancy, PAP is typical, and the presence of diffuse alveolar epithelial hyperplasia and foamy macrophages without hyaline membrane formation are distinguishing features from adult PAP and neonatal RDS, respectively. In older infants, children, and adolescents, there is chronic lobular remodeling with variable interstitial fibrosis, interstitial inflammation, and lesser amounts of alveolar proteinosis material, corresponding to the pattern of chronic pneumonitis of infancy, DIP, or NSIP. Endogenous lipoid pneumonia can also be observed. Electron microscopy is useful for identifying abnormal lamellar bodies characteristic of ABCA3 mutations.[37]

The clinical presentation and imaging findings vary with age. Term neonates with inability to produce SP-B due to their autosomal recessive mutations develop severe respiratory distress within hours of birth. Chest radiographs show diffuse hazy granular pulmonary opacification resembling RDS of prematurity. Unlike RDS of prematurity, most affected infants develop progressive respiratory failure unresponsive to exogenous surfactant administration or ECMO, and die within a few months of birth unless lung transplantation is performed. The diagnosis can be established by the identification of disease-causing mutations on both alleles. In rare cases of mutations that allow some SP-B production the clinical course may be milder, with survival for months to years.[57,58]

Autosomal recessive ABCA3 mutations and inherited or spontaneous autosomal dominant SP-C mutations are associated with very variable phenotypes that range from acute severe RDS in term newborns to chronic diffuse lung disease in children or even adults.[59–61] The most common

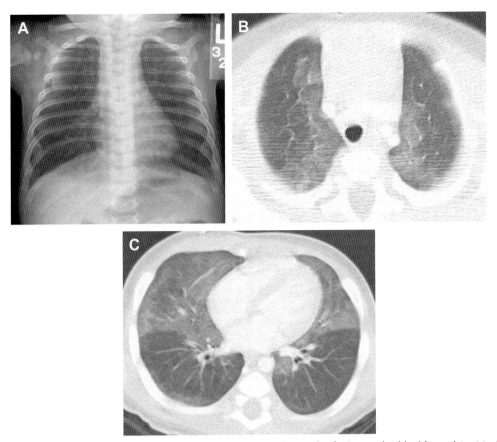

Fig. 6. Neuroendocrine cell hyperplasia of infancy. (*A*) Chest radiograph of a 3-month-old with persistent tachypnea shows pulmonary hyperinflation. (*B, C*) CT images display geographic ground-glass opacities of the right middle lobe, lingula, and paramediastinal lung regions.

childhood clinical presentation of respiratory disease related to ABCA3 or SP-C mutations is cough, tachypnea, hypoxemia, and failure to thrive, beginning in infancy. Some patients treated with corticosteroids or hydroxychloroquine show improvement and a few even become asymptomatic, but it is unclear whether this is attributable to the therapy or the natural history of the disease.[5,57,61] Chest radiographs in young infants with disease-causing ABCA3 or SP-C mutations show diffuse or patchy hazy granular pulmonary opacities, while CT scans reveal diffuse ground-glass or consolidating opacity, septal thickening, and crazy paving (**Fig. 7**).[59,62–65] In older infants and children, findings evolve to include ground-glass opacities that decrease in extent with age, and thin-walled parenchymal cysts that increase in number and size with age. Septal thickening and consolidation may also be observed.[59,66] Pectus excavatum frequently develops in those surviving infancy, possibly related to the effect of chronic restrictive lung disease on the growing chest wall (**Fig. 8**).[59] Changes in CT findings do not correlate with lung function or

outcome, suggesting that routine imaging studies are not warranted after the diagnosis is established. Recognition of these clinical and radiographic patterns is important, since genetic testing of blood or buccal swab-derived samples for surfactant gene mutations has become available at selected clinical and research laboratories and can avert the need for lung biopsy. Lung biopsy may still be warranted if the genetic testing is nondiagnostic, or if awaiting genetic testing results would delay diagnosis in patients with rapidly progressive disease but possibly eligible for lung transplantation.[59,66]

Knowledge of the spectrum of genetic defects causing surfactant dysfunction and pediatric diffuse lung disease continues to expand. GM-CSF-Rα mutations or deletions that severely reduce GM-CSF receptor signaling result in impaired alveolar macrophage function and PAP. Affected children present with tachypnea, failure to thrive, diffuse pulmonary opacities on chest radiographs, and crazy paving on chest CT (**Fig. 9**).[67,68] Thyroid transcription factor-1 (TTF-1),

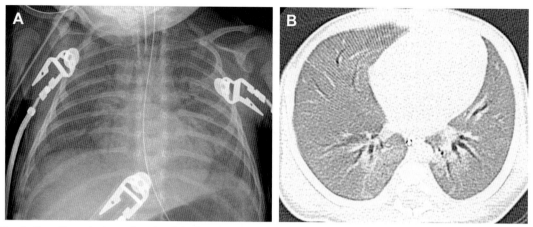

Fig. 7. Genetic surfactant disorder. (A) Chest radiograph of a 5-week-old with SP-C mutation, grunting, and failure to thrive shows diffuse hazy granular pulmonary opacification. (B) CT image demonstrates diffuse ground-glass pulmonary opacification.

also known as NK2 homeobox 1 (NKX2-1), is expressed in the forebrain, thyroid, and lung, and is a critical regulator of SP-B and SP-C gene transcription. TTF-1 mutations lead to maldevelopment of the basal ganglia and thyroid and decreased production of SP-B and SP-C, resulting in "brain-lung-thyroid syndrome" (congenital hypothyroidism, hypotonia, chorea, and diffuse lung disease). Clinical manifestations range from mild asthma to severe neonatal respiratory distress. Chest CT in cases with neonatal presentation shows diffuse ground-glass opacities from PAP. The thyroid abnormalities are not appreciable by ultrasonography.[69] Lysinuric protein intolerance (LPI) is an autosomal recessive disease attributable to SLC747 mutations. Although it affects many organ systems, the only life-threatening complication in children is acute progressive respiratory insufficiency attributable to PAP and pulmonary hemorrhage.[70] In LPI patients with respiratory

insufficiency, chest radiographs and CT show widespread pulmonary airspace opacities. Prior to the onset of respiratory symptoms or abnormal pulmonary function tests, CT can reveal subtle abnormalities such as septal thickening, nodules, and subpleural cysts, and serve as a sensitive method for early diagnosis of lung involvement.[71]

PAP in children is not always attributable to genetic disorders. The catabolism of surfactant by alveolar macrophages can be impaired by several processes, including autoimmune disorders, leukemia, and toxic exposures.[37] Autoimmune PAP, characterized by autoantibodies to GM-CSF that interfere with alveolar macrophage signaling, is the most common cause of sporadic PAP in adults and occasionally manifests in adolescents. The CT findings of ground-glass opacities, septal thickening, and crazy paving are the same as those of other causes of PAP. Autoimmune PAP is amenable to treatment with whole

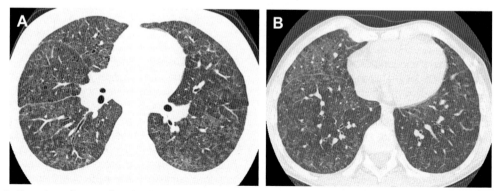

Fig. 8. Genetic surfactant disorder. (A, B) CT images from a 9-year-old with chronic diffuse lung disease related to ABCA3 mutations show patchy ground-glass pulmonary opacities, tiny parenchymal cysts, and pectus excavatum.

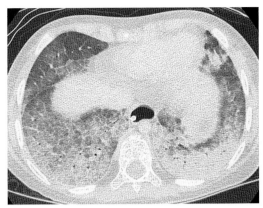

Fig. 9. Genetic surfactant disorder. CT image from a 3-year-old with GM-CSF-Rα defect displays pulmonary consolidation, ground-glass opacification, septal thickening, and crazy paving.

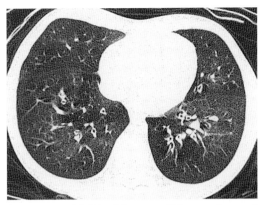

Fig. 10. Bronchiolitis obliterans. CT images from a 4-year-old with a history of adenovirus respiratory tract infection shows predominantly hyperlucent mosaic lung attenuation, bronchiectasis, and bronchial wall thickening.

lung lavage and aerosolized GM-CSF, and CT can be used to monitor the response to therapy.[72]

Disorders of the Normal Host

These processes affect previously healthy children and include postinflammatory responses, reactions to environmental agents, eosinophilic pneumonia, and aspiration. Constrictive or obliterative bronchiolitis is the histopathologic correlate for the clinical syndrome of bronchiolitis obliterans (BO) and is characterized by a fibroblastic reparative response to injury to the small airways, leading to luminal occlusion. The injurious event is typically a respiratory viral infection (especially adenovirus or influenza) with extensive airway mucosal necrosis. Other preceding conditions include graft-versus-host disease, chronic airway rejection in lung transplant patients, and Stevens-Johnson syndrome.[37] The interval between the infection and the onset of obstructive lung disease symptoms is variable, and may be as short as a few months. Chest radiographs may show hyperinflation, but are nonspecific and insensitive.[73] CT findings of pediatric BO include bronchiectasis, bronchial wall thickening, mosaic attenuation, parenchymal hyperlucency, pulmonary vascular attenuation, and expiratory air trapping (Fig. 10).[73,74] The combination of hyperlucency and pulmonary vascular attenuation is highly specific for moderate or severe nontransplant BO.[75] A confident diagnosis of BO can be made in children with a suggestive clinical history, fixed obstructive pattern on pulmonary function testing, and characteristic CT findings, allowing lung biopsy to be avoided in most patients. The heterogeneous distribution of airway involvement can lead to false negative biopsies from sampling error.[76] The sensitivity of CT for moderate or severe nontransplant BO is only modest, so that it is not an effective screening test for excluding BO.[75] CT may be useful as a prognostic tool, because severe abnormalities on CT in children younger than 3 years with postinfectious BO predict poor lung function several years later.[77]

The characteristic histopathologic features of hypersensitivity pneumonitis are lymphocytic infiltration of the bronchioles and adjacent interstitium, and giant cells and poorly formed granulomas distributed around the bronchioles. NSIP, interstitial fibrosis, and cystic remodeling of the lung may be observed in the chronic setting.[37] In childhood, the mean age at diagnosis is 10 years, and the most common precipitating agents are avian antigens and molds. Highly reactive low molecular weight compounds found in spray paints, glues, epoxy resins, and insecticides, as well as drugs such as methotrexate, can also cause hypersensitivity pneumonitis.[78] A detailed environmental exposure history is the most important step in the clinical evaluation. Serum-precipitating antibodies against the inciting antigen are not sensitive enough for their absence to exclude the diagnosis.[58,78] Chest radiographs are also limited in sensitivity. On CT, the acute phase is exemplified by consolidation or ground-glass opacities that can simulate infection or edema. Ill-defined centrilobular nodules, ground-glass opacities, and low-attenuation foci of air trapping typify the subacute phase. The chronic phase is characterized by irregular linear or reticular opacities, architectural distortion, and honeycombing related to fibrosis (Fig. 11). The findings of more than one phase may be observed if there is ongoing exposure to the inciting antigen. Following cessation

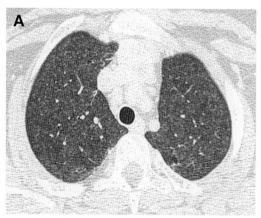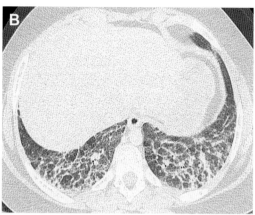

Fig. 11. Hypersensitivity pneumonitis. (A) CT image of a 10-year-old with cough, fatigue, and repetitive bird exposure demonstrates numerous ill-defined ground-glass centrilobular pulmonary opacities involving the upper lobes. (B) CT image of the lung bases shows reticular interstitial thickening.

of exposure, imaging findings associated with the acute and subacute phases regress, but the chronic changes of fibrosis persist.[79,80]

The eosinophilic lung diseases are a diverse group of disorders that are usually, but not always, associated with peripheral eosinophilia. These diseases can be acute or chronic, idiopathic or secondary to parasitic infections or drug reactions, or associated with vasculitis. The CT findings of ground-glass opacities, septal thickening, and pleural effusions in acute eosinophilic pneumonia can mimic pulmonary edema or acute RDS. Allergic bronchopulmonary aspergillosis manifests with bilateral central bronchiectasis with or without mucoid impaction, while chronic eosinophilic pneumonia and drug reactions classically exhibit peripheral consolidations (**Fig. 12**). Simple pulmonary eosinophilia and idiopathic hypereosinophilic syndrome are characterized on CT by nodules with ground-glass halos. The CT findings in Churg-Strauss syndrome include subpleural consolidation, centrilobular nodules, bronchial wall thickening, and septal thickening. Bronchocentric granulomatosis typically shows focal masses or consolidation.[81] CT is helpful in assessing response to therapy.[82]

Although aspiration is a common condition, it is often unsuspected clinically and may present as unexplained diffuse lung disease in children. Silent aspiration can occur in even developmentally normal children and present with nonspecific symptoms such as cough, tachypnea, or fever. The finding of increased lipid-laden macrophages on bronchoalveolar lavage or biopsy is not specific for aspiration and can be seen in association with several other pulmonary conditions, including resolving hemorrhage, pneumonia, and surfactant disorders. The diagnosis of aspiration is often difficult, and CT may play a key role in suggesting the diagnosis. The presence of bronchiectasis and tree-in-bud centrilobular opacities, more marked posteriorly and on the right, should raise the suspicion of aspiration. Exogenous lipoid pneumonia is most frequently seen in children given mineral oil for chronic constipation, and characteristically presents on CT as consolidations, sometimes with fatty (−30 to −150 HU) attenuation, ground-glass opacities, and crazy paving (**Fig. 13**). However, fatty attenuation may not be evident because of volume averaging with surrounding inflammatory exudates, and volume averaging of inflammatory exudates and air can simulate fatty attenuation on CT.[83,84]

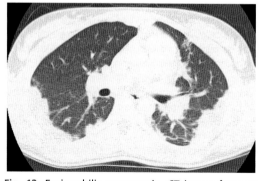

Fig. 12. Eosinophilic pneumonia. CT image from an 18-year-old with an adverse reaction to minocycline prescribed for acne shows bilateral peripheral pulmonary consolidation.

Disorders Related to Systemic Disease Processes

A large and diffuse group of systemic diseases processes may be associated with diffuse lung disease in children. The clinical presentations

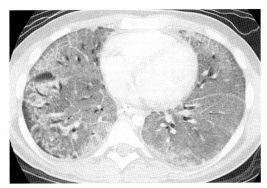

Fig. 13. Exogenous lipoid pneumonia. CT image of a 17-year-old with repetitive aspiration of mineral oil administered for chronic constipation shows diffuse ground-glass opacification, septal thickening, and crazy paving.

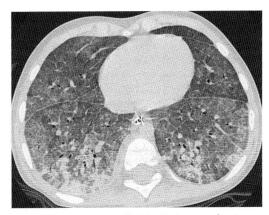

Fig. 14. Pulmonary capillaritis. CT image of a 4-year-old with anemia and elevated ANCA levels demonstrates patchy consolidation, ground-glass opacities, and septal thickening related to repetitive pulmonary hemorrhage.

and imaging appearances of these diseases are varied but may suggest a specific etiology in certain settings. Pulmonary capillaritis is an under-recognized cause of pulmonary hemorrhage and is often misdiagnosed as the rarer entity of idiopathic pulmonary hemosiderosis.[78] Pulmonary capillaritis is characterized histopathologically by inflammatory disruption of the alveolar interstitial capillary network. Pulmonary capillaritis can be a primary disorder or associated with another vasculitis, such as Wegener granulomatosis, microscopic polyangiitis, Goodpasture disease, or systemic lupus erythematosus (SLE). If vasculitis is not identified, other causes of chronic pulmonary hemorrhage should be considered, such as pulmonary venous hypertension, idiopathic pulmonary hemosiderosis, Heiner syndrome, and coagulation disorders.[37,85] Most pediatric patients with pulmonary capillaritis have anemia on presentation, but only a minority has hemoptysis.[86] Antineutrophilic cytoplasmic antibodies (ANCA) and nephropathy are often present.[78] Children with diffuse pulmonary hemorrhage disorders typically have nonspecific bilateral airspace or interstitial opacities on chest radiographs.[85] Acute hemorrhage into the airspaces results in patchy ground-glass opacities and consolidation on CT. With repetitive hemorrhage, aggregates of hemosiderin-laden macrophages cause septal thickening and produce crazy paving when coupled with ground-glass opacities (Fig. 14). Tiny parenchymal or juxtapleural cysts may be observed in the chronic setting.[6,86,87] While the presence of fluffy centrilobular opacities suggest angiocentric inflammation and hemorrhage from pulmonary capillaritis,[88] it is difficult to differentiate capillaritis from idiopathic pulmonary hemosiderosis and other causes of diffuse pulmonary hemorrhage by imaging or

clinical features, and lung biopsy is often required for differentiation. Definitive diagnosis is crucial because successful treatment of pulmonary capillaritis often requires aggressive therapy with immunosuppressants. Response to therapy is corroborated by improvement in the CT findings.[78]

The collagen-vascular diseases have a high prevalence of diffuse lung disease that can involve multiple compartments, including the interstitium, vasculature, airways, and pleura. NSIP is the most commonly associated histopathologic pattern, with pulmonary lymphoid hyperplasia, organizing pneumonia, vasculopathy, and pleuritis also occurring.[37] The histopathologic and imaging patterns observed in the lungs usually do not permit reliable discrimination between the different collagen-vascular diseases. For example, NSIP can be seen in various collagen-vascular diseases, including juvenile-onset systemic sclerosis (JSS), juvenile-onset dermatomyositis (JDMS), and mixed connective tissue disease (MCTD). Recognition of extrapulmonary findings, such as a dilated esophagus in JSS, can assist diagnosis. Respiratory symptoms or signs may be minimal or absent, underscoring the important role of imaging in detecting disease.

At initial assessment, about half of children with JSS have CT evidence of pulmonary involvement, which may be a negative prognostic factor because it occurs more frequently and earlier in JSS patients who die from the disease.[89] The most common findings in JSS relate to NSIP and include ground-glass opacities and fine intralobular reticular opacities, predominantly at the lung periphery. Tiny nodules and clusters of cysts resembling honeycombing can also be seen

(Fig. 15).[90] The finding of pulmonary arterial enlargement out of proportion to the severity of the lung disease suggests the presence of serious arterial vasculopathy.[25,37] The severity of CT abnormalities correlates inversely with values FEV_1 (forced expiratory volume in 1 second), forced vital capacity (FVC), and lung diffusion capacity for carbon monoxide (D_LCO), but there is no correlation between the duration of illness and the severity of the diffuse lung disease in JSS, and pulmonary fibrosis may progress to an advanced state in the absence of symptoms.[89,90] With the advent of new and more effective treatment regimens, low radiation dose surveillance CT examinations may be useful for early detection of clinically silent lung disease in JSS and prevention of irreversible fibrosis or vasculopathy.[89,90] Pulmonary involvement, most commonly NSIP or pulmonary lymphoid hyperplasia, occurs in 10% to 20% of JDMS cases. JDMS also has a greater proclivity for organizing pneumonia than other collagen-vascular diseases. Although pulmonary involvement most often occurs after the diagnosis of JDMS, it can be a presenting sign or precede the diagnosis.[78] Evidence of pulmonary involvement is found on CT in 25% of patients with MCTD. The findings are indistinguishable from those that can be seen in JSS and JDMS, but typically mild.[91]

Manifestations of SLE range from acute pneumonitis, pulmonary vasculitis, and pleuritis to chronic NSIP and pleural fibrosis.[37] In distinction to adult SLE, diffuse lung disease is unusual in childhood SLE, with fewer than 10% of patients having abnormal findings on CT, suggesting that CT is not needed in asymptomatic children.[92] The most severe manifestation is acute lupus pneumonitis, which exhibits diffuse alveolar damage on pathology and has a mortality rate of 70% to 90%. The diagnosis is often unsuspected because it has an incidence of less than 5%, half of the cases are the initial presenting manifestation of SLE, and chest imaging shows widespread airspace opacification mimicking infectious pneumonia. The progression to respiratory failure and death is rapid without prompt corticosteroid therapy.[78]

The most common thoracic manifestation of sarcoidosis in children is bilateral hilar lymphadenopathy. Pulmonary parenchymal disease occurs in approximately two-thirds of cases, usually in association with lymphadenopathy. Isolated pulmonary parenchymal involvement is found in only 11%.[93] A typical CT finding of pulmonary sarcoidosis in children is nodular beading of the bronchovascular bundles, interlobular septae, and fissures.[94]

Langerhans cell histiocytosis (LCH) is characterized by the proliferation of CD1a+ histiocytes (Langerhans cells) in various organs. These histiocytes form granulomas and may later be replaced by fibrosis and cysts. Pulmonary LCH in children is usually seen only in the context of multisystem LCH, and childhood pulmonary LCH is a different disease from adult pulmonary LCH, the former being clonal and not associated with smoking. Because only half of patients with lung involvement at presentation have respiratory symptoms, chest imaging is recommended in all newly diagnosed LCH patients, even in the absence of respiratory symptoms. Although the lungs are designated as a risk organ in the Histiocyte Society protocols, the severity of lung involvement does not predict outcome. The most common appearance on chest radiographs is diffuse nodular interstitial opacities. CT better demonstrates the nodules, which may cavitate to form cysts of unusual shape (Fig. 16).[95] Spontaneous pneumothorax can ensue from cyst rupture.[96] A

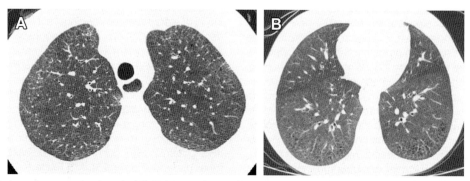

Fig. 15. Juvenile systemic sclerosis. (A) CT image obtained in a 12-year-old patient without respiratory symptoms shows fine reticular and ground-glass opacities at the periphery of the lungs, along with esophageal dilation. (B) CT image of the same patient at 18 years of age shows clusters of cysts at the lung periphery, resembling honeycombing.

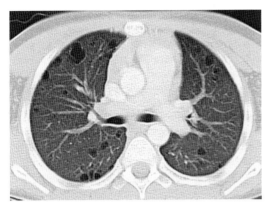

Fig. 16. Langerhans cell histiocytosis. CT image from an 8-year-old displays numerous cysts of variable size and shape.

specific appearance of LCH on CT is thymic enlargement with intrathymic calcification or cavitation.[97] Recognition of these findings is important, because the diagnosis may be able to be confirmed and lung biopsy avoided by biopsy of an accompanying rash or by detection of elevated numbers of CD1a[+] cells in bronchoalveolar lavage fluid.[58] Despite successful treatment, the effects of cytokines may result in pulmonary fibrosis, and 6% of patients have asymptomatic lung involvement a mean of 15 years after treatment.[95]

Gaucher disease is the most common lysosomal storage disorder, and is caused by a hereditary deficiency of glucocerebrosidase resulting in glucocerebroside accumulation in various organs. Lung pathology is caused directly by infiltration of Gaucher cells and indirectly by hepatopulmonary syndrome, chronic aspiration, and recurrent infection. Symptomatic lung involvement is rare at presentation, but occurs later in the disease course in some patients, particularly those with neuronopathic type III Gaucher disease, in which respiratory failure is second only to hepatic failure as a cause of death. Chest radiographs can show reticulonodular opacities, and CT demonstrates a range of abnormalities including ground-glass opacities, consolidation, interstitial thickening, bronchial wall thickening, thymic enlargement, and lymphadenopathy. Chest radiographs are currently recommended as part of a radiographic survey every 24 months to periodically evaluate the lungs.[98] The pulmonary abnormalities gradually improve with enzyme replacement therapy, although complete normalization is usually not achieved.[99]

Niemann-Pick disease is a lysosomal storage disorder in which lipid-laden "foamy" macrophages accumulate in various organs. The type

B form of the disease is most often associated with lung involvement and is characterized histopathologically by lipid-laden macrophages infiltrating the alveolar walls, peribronchovascular lymphatics, and subpleural and interlobular connective tissues. This appearance accounts for the pattern of diffuse interstitial thickening on chest radiographs and chest CT (**Fig. 17**). The imaging findings are not predictive of outcome, and the lung disease usually slowly progresses.[100] The type 2C form of Niemann-Pick disease typically presents in infancy with hepatosplenomegaly, failure to thrive, and respiratory distress. Impaired cholesterol transport in this disorder leads to the accumulation of cholesterol-laden dysfunctional surfactant in the air spaces, and PAP.[101] CT performed on affected infants often shows crazy paving.[6]

Disorders of the Immunocompromised Host

Infections are the most common disorders in this group. As community-acquired bacterial pneumonias do not usually present as suspected diffuse lung disease, the infections in this group are usually atypical and opportunistic. The immunocompromised state is most frequently attributable to therapeutic intervention, either immunosuppressant therapy for bone marrow or organ transplantation or autoimmune disorders, or chemotherapy for malignancies. In addition to infection, some of the primary and acquired pediatric immunodeficiency disorders are associated with pulmonary lymphoid hyperplasia and unique forms of chronic diffuse lung disease.

Follicular bronchitis/bronchiolitis and lymphocytic interstitial pneumonitis (LIP) are overlapping

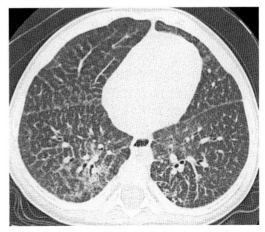

Fig. 17. Niemann-Pick type B. CT image of a 22-month-old shows diffuse thickening of the pulmonary interstitium.

disorders in the spectrum of pulmonary lymphoid hyperplasia. The histopathology of follicular bronchitis/bronchiolitis is characterized by prominent peribronchial/peribronchiolar lymphoid follicles, whereas LIP is characterized by interstitial lymphocytic infiltrate.[102] Pulmonary lymphoid hyperplasia is associated with viruses (especially Epstein-Barr virus, human immunodeficiency virus [HIV], and human herpesvirus [HHV]-6), autoimmune diseases (especially Sjögren syndrome), and immunodeficiency.[37] Childhood follicular bronchitis/bronchiolitis usually presents by 6 to 8 weeks of age, with respiratory distress and fever. Chest radiographs show pulmonary hyperinflation and peribronchial thickening resembling lower airway infection or reactive airways disease. This pattern may transition over several months to peribronchial nodules and pulmonary interstitial thickening.[103] LIP occurs in up to 30% to 40% of HIV-infected children, classically presenting in those older than 2 years with chronic or recurrent cough and mild hypoxemia.[104] Chest radiographs in pediatric LIP show a diffuse nodular or reticulonodular pattern.[105] CT reveals nodules in a subpleural, septal, centrilobular, or peribronchial distribution, and ground-glass opacities without or with lymphadenopathy that can simulate tuberculosis (Fig. 18).[106] Bronchiectasis and cystic dilated air spaces have also been described in LIP.[105,107] Spontaneous clinical and radiographic resolution of LIP in children in the absence of antiretroviral or corticosteroid therapy does not necessarily herald immunologic deterioration and HIV progression.[104]

Chronic granulomatous disease (CGD) is a heterogeneous group of disorders in which phagocytic cells are unable to generate the respiratory burst that produces reactive oxygen species to destroy engulfed microbes. The X-linked form tends to present earlier and have more severe disease than the less common autosomal recessive forms. Most patients with X-linked CGD develop failure to thrive, severe bacterial adenitis, osteomyelitis, or soft tissue abscesses within the first year of life, although the mean age at diagnosis is 3 years. CGD patients are particularly at risk of recurrent infection from catalase-producing *Staphylococcus*, *Burkholderia*, *Serratia*, *Aspergillus*, *Nocardia*, *Mycobacterium*, and *Candida*. Intracellular persistence of microbes leads to a chronic inflammatory response and granuloma formation. The myriad of pulmonary CT findings include consolidation, ground-glass opacities, tree-in-bud opacities, centrilobular or random nodules, bronchiectasis, septal thickening, air trapping, cysts, fibrosis, and honeycombing. Suppurative or nonsuppurative hilar and mediastinal lymphadenopathy, pleural thickening, empyema, vertebral or rib osteomyelitis, and chest wall invasion are also common (Fig. 19).[108,109] CGD is treated with lipophilic antibiotics, antifungals, interferon-γ, abscess drainage, surgical resection, and stem cell transplantation. CT is less reliable than [18F]fluorodeoxyglucose positron emission tomography for discriminating active from quiescent disease sites.[110]

Common variable immunodeficiency (CVID) is characterized by failure of terminal differentiation of B cells, resulting in low plasma cell and immunoglobulin levels. Patients with CVID are subject not only to recurrent infection but also to a unique diffuse lung disease termed granulomatous-lymphocytic interstitial lung disease (GLILD), consisting of both granulomatous and lymphoproliferative

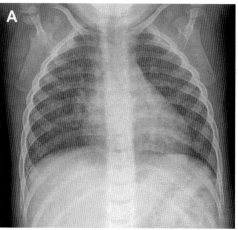
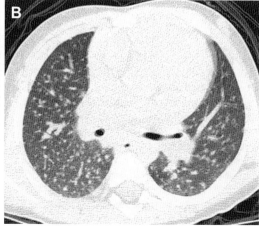

Fig. 18. Lymphocytic interstitial pneumonitis. (A) Chest radiograph of a 19-month-old shows multiple pulmonary nodules. (B) CT image obtained from the same patient at 21 months of age demonstrates multiple small pulmonary nodules located in both lungs.

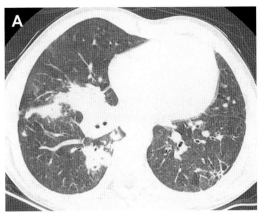 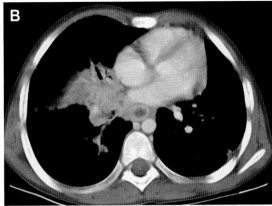

Fig. 19. Chronic granulomatous disease. (A) CT image of a 9-year-old demonstrates patchy consolidation, ill-defined ground-glass opacities, nodules, bronchiectasis, and linear fibrosis. (B) CT image displayed at soft tissue windows reveals consolidation of the right lung, suppurative mediastinal lymphadenopathy, and left pleural thickening.

histopathology. HHV-8 infection, splenomegaly, dyspnea, a restrictive pattern on pulmonary function testing, and a decreased survival rate are associated with GLILD. Findings on chest imaging are similar to those in pulmonary lymphoid hyperplasia, with nodules, consolidation, and reticular and ground-glass opacities (Fig. 20). GLILD may respond to immunosuppressants.[111] Chest CT is recommended at initial diagnosis and for follow-up, but there is no consensus on optimal surveillance intervals.[112]

Ataxia-telangiectasia (AT) is attributable to mutations in the Ataxia Telangiectasia Mutated (ATM) gene leading to impaired DNA double-strand break repair. Patients with AT demonstrate a markedly elevated cancer rate (especially leukemia and lymphoma), cerebellar ataxia, telangiectasias, noninfectious granulomatous inflammation, recurrent pulmonary infections, bronchiectasis, and a unique chronic ILD. AT-associated interstitial lung disease (AT-ILD) is characterized histopathologically by fibrosis, acute and chronic lymphocytic

infiltration, and bizarre atypical cells in the lung epithelium and interstitium. AT-ILD presents with chronic nonproductive cough, dyspnea, fever, and a restrictive pattern on pulmonary function testing. Radiographic findings include interstitial thickening, bronchiectasis, pleural thickening/effusion, and pneumothorax (Fig. 21). Progressive clinical deterioration and death within 2 years after the appearance of AT-ILD is typical, although AT-ILD may show clinical and radiographic improvement in response to corticosteroids given within a year of onset, underscoring the importance of early

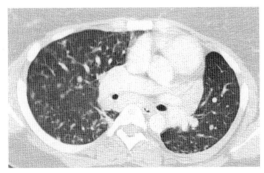

Fig. 20. Granulomatous-lymphocytic interstitial lung disease. CT image from a 20-year-old with common variable immunodeficiency reveals multiple small pulmonary nodules.

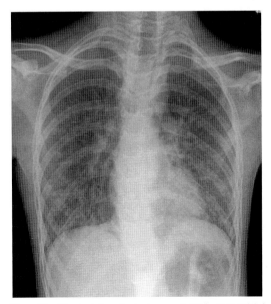

Fig. 21. Ataxia-telangiectasia-associated interstitial lung disease. Chest radiograph of a 15-year-old demonstrates bronchiectasis and interstitial opacities.

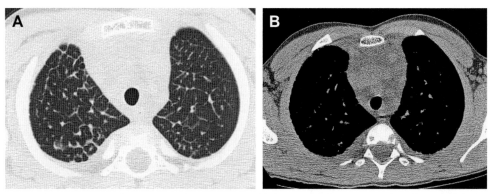

Fig. 22. Lymphangiomatosis. (*A*) CT image from a 6-year-old shows interlobular septal thickening. (*B*) CT image displayed at soft tissue window reveals mediastinal edema.

diagnosis. It has been recommended that chest radiographs should be obtained in any AT patient with pulmonary symptoms that do not resolve after vigorous antibiotic and bronchodilator therapy.[113] Unfortunately, apprehension over the risk of radiation-induced malignancy may lead to unwarranted diagnostic delay.[113]

Disorders Masquerading as Diffuse Lung Disease

In the ChILD Research Cooperative diffuse lung disease classification,[4] vascular or lymphatic disorders with clinical and imaging features that can prompt lung biopsy for suspected diffuse lung disease are categorized as masquerading disorders. Some are congenital left-sided obstructive cardiovascular disorders that secondarily affect the lung parenchyma via congestive vasculopathy, whereas others such as primary pulmonary lymphangiectasia and lymphangiomatosis can be construed as true ILDs.[58] These "masqueraders" should be kept in mind when diffuse lung disease is suspected.

Pulmonary lymphangiectasia is characterized by dilation of the lymphatics draining the pulmonary interstitial and subpleural spaces. The primary form can be restricted to the lungs or involve extrapulmonary structures. The secondary form is due to pulmonary lymphatic or venous congestion such as from total anomalous pulmonary venous return, pulmonary vein stenosis, pulmonary vein atresia, cor triatriatum, hypoplastic left heart syndrome, or heart failure. Pulmonary lymphangiectasia classically presents as severe respiratory distress in a term neonate with diffuse hazy opacification of the lungs on chest radiographs, resembling the findings of surfactant deficiency of prematurity or genetic surfactant

disorders. CT shows smooth thickening of the septae and bronchovascular bundles, patchy ground-glass opacities, and pleural effusions, often chylous.[114] In surviving neonates or those presenting later in infancy, the pulmonary opacities are less diffuse, the septal thickening is less marked, and hyperinflation becomes a consistent finding.[115] In lymphangiomatosis, there is proliferation of complex anastomosing lymphatic channels with secondary lymphatic dilation. Pulmonary lymphangiomatosis can be difficult to differentiate from pulmonary lymphangiectasia, because the histopathologic and radiographic findings in the lungs are very similar and chylous pleural effusions are common in both (**Fig. 22**).[116] In distinction to lymphangiectasia, lymphangiomatosis tends to present later in childhood and frequently involves extrapulmonary tissues, with mediastinal soft tissue edema and lytic bone lesions commonly observed.[114,117,118]

SUMMARY

The diffuse lung diseases are a rare but important cause of childhood morbidity and mortality. Recent insights have improved the ability to identify and properly treat these disorders, but much remains to be learned about their underlying etiology, clinical phenotypes, and natural history in the context of the growing and developing lung. For the radiologist, acquiring diagnostic quality images of the lungs in children is only a prerequisite. Developing a clear understanding of the novel classification of pediatric diffuse lung disease and characteristic imaging findings is paramount, in order to promote recognition of specific disorders, facilitate communication between clinicians, and provide a foundation for future research.

REFERENCES

1. Clement A, Eber E. Interstitial lung diseases in infants and children. Eur Respir J 2008;31:658–66.
2. American Thoracic Society, European Respiratory Society. American Thoracic Society/European Respiratory Society International Multidisciplinary Consensus Classification of the Idiopathic Interstitial Pneumonias. Am J Respir Crit Care Med 2002;165:277–304.
3. Fan LL, Deterding RR, Langston C. Pediatric interstitial lung disease revisited. Pediatr Pulmonol 2004;38:369–78.
4. Deutsch GH, Young LR, Deterding RR, et al. Diffuse lung disease in young children: application of a novel classification scheme. Am J Respir Crit Care Med 2007;176:1120–8.
5. Deterding RR. Infants and young children with children's interstitial lung disease. Pediatr Allergy Immunol Pulmonol 2010;23:25–31.
6. Guillerman RP. Imaging of childhood interstitial lung disease. Pediatr Allergy Immunol Pulmonol 2010;23:43–68.
7. Clement A, ERS Task Force. Task force on chronic interstitial lung disease in immunocompetent children. Eur Respir J 2004;24:686–97.
8. Long FR, Castile RG. Technique and clinical applications of full-inflation and end-exhalation controlled-ventilation chest CT in infants and young children. Pediatr Radiol 2001;31:413–22.
9. Lucaya J, Piqueras J, Garcia-Pena P, et al. Low-dose high-resolution CT of the chest in children and young adults: dose, cooperation, artifact incidence, and image quality. AJR Am J Roentgenol 2000;175:985–92.
10. Choi SJ, Choi BK, Kim HJ, et al. Lateral decubitus HRCT: a simple technique to replace expiratory CT in children with air trapping. Pediatr Radiol 2002;32:179–82.
11. Valentin J, International Commission on Radiological Protection. ICRP Publication 102: managing patient dose in multi-detector computed tomography (MDCT). Ann ICRP 2007;37:1–79, iii.
12. Garcia-Pena P, Lucaya J. HRCT in children: technique and indications. Eur Radiol 2004;14:L13–30.
13. Goo HW, Kim HJ. Detection of air trapping on inspiratory and expiratory phase images obtained by 0.3-second cine CT in the lungs of free-breathing young children. AJR Am J Roentgenol 2006;187:1019–23.
14. Brody AS. Imaging considerations: interstitial lung disease in children. Radiol Clin North Am 2005;43:391–403.
15. Funama Y, Awai K, Taguchi K, et al. Cone-beam technique for 64-MDCT of lung: image quality comparison with stepwise (step-and-shoot) technique. AJR Am J Roentgenol 2009;192:273–8.
16. Bastos M, Lee EY, Strauss KJ, et al. Motion artifact on high-resolution CT images of pediatric patients: comparison of volumetric and axial CT methods. AJR Am J Roentgenol 2009;193:1414–8.
17. Studler U, Gluecker T, Bongartz G, et al. Image quality from high-resolution CT of the lung: comparison of axial scans and of sections reconstructed from volumetric data acquired using MDCT. AJR Am J Roentgenol 2005;185:602–7.
18. Vikgren J, Johnsson AA, Flinck A, et al. High-resolution computed tomography with 16-row MDCT: a comparison regarding visibility and motion artifacts of dose-modulated thin slices and "step and shoot" images. Acta Radiol 2008;49:755–60.
19. Prakash P, Kalra MK, Ackman JB, et al. Diffuse lung disease: CT of the chest with adaptive statistical iterative reconstruction technique. Radiology 2010;256:261–9.
20. Goris ML, Robinson TE. Sampling density for the quantitative evaluation of air trapping. Pediatr Radiol 2009;39:221–5.
21. Tzedakis A, Damilakis J, Perisinakis K, et al. Influence of z overscanning on normalized effective doses calculated for pediatric patients undergoing multidetector CT examinations. Med Phys 2007;34:1163–75.
22. Kroft LJ, Roelofs JJ, Geleijns J. Scan time and patient dose for thoracic imaging in neonates and small children using axial volumetric 320-detector row CT compared to helical 64-, 32-, and 16-detector row CT acquisitions. Pediatr Radiol 2010;40:294–300.
23. Lell MM, May M, Deak P, et al. High pitch spiral computed tomography: effect on image quality and radiation dose in pediatric chest computed tomography. Invest Radiol 2011;46:116–23.
24. Baumueller S, Alkadhi H, Stolzmann P, et al. Computed tomography of the lung in the high-pitch mode. Is breath holding still required? Invest Radiol 2011;46:240–5.
25. Zompatori M, Sverzellati N, Poletti V, et al. High-resolution CT in diagnosis of diffuse infiltrative lung disease. Semin Ultrasound CT MR 2005;26:332–47.
26. Yanagawa M, Tomiyama N, Honda O, et al. Multidetector CT of the lung: image quality with garnet-based detectors. Radiology 2010;255:944–54.
27. Kalender WA, Buchenau S, Deak P, et al. Technical approaches to the optimisation of CT. Phys Med 2008;24:71–9.
28. Vollmar SV, Kalender WA. Reduction of dose to the female breast as a result of spectral optimisation for high-contrast thoracic CT imaging: a phantom study. Br J Radiol 2009;82:920–9.
29. Li J, Udayasankar UK, Toth TL, et al. Automatic patient centering for MDCT: effect on radiation dose. AJR Am J Roentgenol 2007;188:547–52.

30. Pontana F, Pagniez J, Flohr T, et al. Chest computed tomography using iterative reconstruction vs. filtered back projection (Pt 1): evaluation of image noise reduction in 32 patients. Eur Radiol 2011;21:627–35.

31. Brody AS, Guillerman RP, Hay TC, et al. Neuroendocrine cell hyperplasia of infancy: diagnosis with high-resolution CT. AJR Am J Roentgenol 2010; 194:1–7.

32. O'Connor OJ, Vandeleur M, McGarrigle AM, et al. Development of low-dose protocols for thin-section CT assessment of cystic fibrosis in pediatric patients. Radiology 2010;257:820–9.

33. Hansell DM. Thin-section CT of the lungs: the hinterland of normal. Radiology 2010;256:695–711.

34. Kapur N, Masel JP, Watson D, et al. Bronchoarterial ratio on high resolution CT scan of the chest in children without pulmonary pathology – need to redefine bronchial dilation. Chest 2011;139(6):1445–50.

35. Gaillard EA, Carty H, Heaf D, et al. Reversible bronchial dilation in children: comparison of serial high-resolution computed tomography scans of the lungs. Eur J Radiol 2003;47:215–20.

36. Hansell DM, Bankier AA, MacMahon H, et al. Fleischner society: glossary of terms for thoracic imaging. Radiology 2008;246:697–722.

37. Dishop MK. Diagnostic pathology of diffuse lung disease in children. Pediatr Allergy Immunol Pulmonol 2010;23:69–85.

38. Sen P, Thakur N, Stockton DW, et al. Expanding the phenotype of alveolar capillary dysplasia. J Pediatr 2004;145:646–51.

39. Michalsky MP, Arca MJ, Groenman F, et al. Alveolar capillary dysplasia: a logical approach to a fatal disease. J Pediatr Surg 2005;40:1100–5.

40. Stankiewicz P, Sen P, Bhatt SS, et al. Genomic and genic deletions of the FOX gene cluster on 16q24.1 and inactivating mutations of FOXF1 cause alveolar capillary dysplasia and other malformations. Am J Hum Genet 2009;84:780–91.

41. Hugosson CO, Salama HM, Al-Dayel F, et al. Primary alveolar capillary dysplasia (acinar dysplasia) and surfactant protein B deficiency: a clinical, radiological and pathological study. Pediatr Radiol 2005;35:311–6.

42. Gillespie LM, Fenton AC, Wright C. Acinar dysplasia: a rare cause of neonatal respiratory failure. Acta Paediatr 2004;93:712–3.

43. Newman B, Yunis E. Primary alveolar capillary dysplasia. Pediatr Radiol 1990;21:20–2.

44. Bhandari A, Bhandari V. Pitfalls, problems, and progress in bronchopulmonary dysplasia. Pediatrics 2009;123:1562–73.

45. Owens C. Radiology of diffuse interstitial pulmonary disease in children. Eur Radiol 2004;14:L2–12.

46. Mahut B, De Blic J, Emond S, et al. Chest computed tomography findings in bronchopulmonary dysplasia and correlation with lung function. Arch Dis Child Fetal Neonatal Ed 2007;92:F459–64.

47. Biko DM, Schwartz M, Anupindi SA, et al. Subpleural lung cysts in Down syndrome: prevalence and association with coexisting diagnoses. Pediatr Radiol 2008;38:280–4.

48. Taylor PA, Dishop MK, Lotze TE, et al. Congenital multilobar emphysema: a characteristic lung growth disorder attributable to Filamin A gene mutations. Pediatr Radiol 2009;39(Suppl 3):S516.

49. Smets K, Dhaene K, Schelstraete P, et al. Neonatal pulmonary interstitial glycogen accumulation disorder. Eur J Pediatr 2004;163:408–9.

50. Deutsch GH, Young LR. Pulmonary interstitial glycogenosis: words of caution. Pediatr Radiol 2010; 40:1471–5.

51. Canakis AM, Kutz E, Manson D, et al. Pulmonary interstitial glycogenosis: a new variant of interstitial neonatal lung disease. Am J Respir Crit Care Med 2002;165:1557–75.

52. Onland W, Molenaar JJ, Leguit RJ, et al. Pulmonary interstitial glycogenosis in identical twins. Pediatr Pulmonol 2005;40:362–6.

53. Lanfranchi M, Allbery SM, Wheelock L. Pulmonary interstitial glycogenosis. Pediatr Radiol 2010;40: 361–5.

54. Castillo M, Vade A, Lim-Dunham JE, et al. Pulmonary interstitial glycogenosis in the setting of lung growth abnormality: radiographic and pathologic correlation. Pediatr Radiol 2010;40:1562–5.

55. Popler J, Gower WA, Mogayzel PJ Jr, et al. Familial neuroendocrine cell hyperplasia of infancy. Pediatr Pulmonol 2010;45:749–55.

56. Young LR, Brody AS, Inge TH, et al. Neuroendocrine cell distribution and frequency distinguish neuroendocrine cell hyperplasia of infancy from other pulmonary disorders. Chest 2011;139(5): 1060–71.

57. Nogee LM. Genetic basis of children's interstitial lung disease (ChILD). Pediatr Allergy Immunol Pulmonol 2010;23:15–24.

58. Clement A, Nathan N, Epaud R, et al. Interstitial lung diseases in children. Orphanet J Rare Dis 2010;5:22.

59. Doan ML, Guillerman RP, Dishop MK, et al. Clinical, radiological and pathological features of ABCA3 mutations in children. Thorax 2008;63:366–73.

60. Guillot L, Epaud R, Thouvenin G, et al. New surfactant protein CT gene mutations associated with diffuse lung disease. J Med Genet 2009;46:490–4.

61. Thouvenin G, Taam RA, Flamein F, et al. Characteristics of disorders associated with genetic mutations of surfactant protein C. Arch Dis Child 2010; 95:449–54.

62. Olsen ØE, Sebire NJ, Jaffe A, et al. Chronic pneumonitis of infancy: high-resolution CT findings. Pediatr Radiol 2004;34:86–8.

63. Stevens PA, Pettenazzo A, Brasch F, et al. Nonspecific interstitial pneumonia, alveolar proteinosis, and abnormal proprotein trafficking resulting from a spontaneous mutation in the surfactant protein C gene. Pediatr Res 2005;57:89–98.

64. Prestridge A, Wooldridge J, Deutsch G, et al. Persistent tachypnea and hypoxia in a 3-month-old term infant. J Pediatr 2006;149:702–6.

65. Soraisham AS, Tierney AJ, Amin HJ. Neonatal respiratory failure associated with mutation in the surfactant protein C gene. J Perinatol 2006;26: 67–70.

66. Mechri M, Epaud R, Emond S, et al. Surfactant protein C gene (SFTPC) mutation-associated lung disease: high-resolution computed tomography (HRCT) findings and its relation to histological analysis. Pediatr Pulmonol 2010;45:1021–9.

67. Suzuki T, Sakagami T, Rubin BK, et al. Familial pulmonary alveolar proteinosis caused by mutations in CSF2RA. J Exp Med 2008;205:2703–10.

68. Martinez-Moczygemba M, Doan ML, Elidemir O, et al. Pulmonary alveolar proteinosis caused by deletion of the GM-CSFRα gene in the X chromosome pseudoautosomal region 1. J Exp Med 2008;205:2711–6.

69. Guillot L, Carre A, Szinnai G, et al. NKX2-1 mutations leading to surfactant protein promoter dysregulation cause interstitial lung disease in "brain-lung-thyroid" syndrome. Hum Mutat 2010; 31:E1146–62.

70. Parto K, Svedström E, Majurin ML, et al. Pulmonary manifestations in lysinuric protein intolerance. Chest 1993;104:1176–82.

71. Santamaria F, Parenti G, Guidi G, et al. Early detection of lung involvement in lysinuric protein intolerance: role of high-resolution computed tomography and radioisotopic methods. Am J Respir Crit Care Med 1996;153:731–5.

72. Robinson TE, Trapnell BC, Goris ML, et al. Quantitative analysis of longitudinal response to aerosolized granulocyte-macrophage colony-stimulating factor in two adolescents with autoimmune pulmonary alveolar proteinosis. Chest 2009;135:842–8.

73. Yalcin E, Dog D, Halilog M, et al. Postinfectious bronchiolitis obliterans in children: clinical and radiological profile and prognostic factors. Respiration 2003;70:371–5.

74. Zhang L, Irion K, da Silva Porto N, et al. High-resolution computed tomography in pediatric patients with postinfectious bronchiolitis obliterans. J Thorac Imaging 1999;14:85–9.

75. Smith KJ, Dishop MK, Fan LL, et al. Diagnosis of bronchiolitis obliterans with computed tomography in children. Pediatr Allergy Immunol Pulmonol 2011;23:253–9.

76. Moonnumakal SP, Fan LL. Bronchiolitis obliterans in children. Curr Opin Pediatr 2008;20:272–8.

77. Mattiello R, Sarria EE, Mallol J, et al. Post-infectious bronchiolitis obliterans: can CT scan findings at early age anticipate lung function? Pediatr Pulmonol 2010;45(4):315–9.

78. Vece TJ, Fan LL. Interstitial lung disease in children older than 2 years. Pediatr Allergy Immunol Pulmonol 2010;23:33–41.

79. Hartman TE. The HRCT features of extrinsic allergic alveolitis. Semin Respir Crit Care Med 2003;24: 419–26.

80. MacDonald S, Müller NL. Insights from HRCT: how they affect the management of diffuse parenchymal lung disease. Semin Respir Crit Care Med 2003;24:357–64.

81. Jeong YJ, Kim KI, Seo IJ, et al. Eosinophilic lung diseases: a clinical, radiologic, and pathologic overview. Radiographics 2007;27:617–37.

82. Oermann CM, Panesar KS, Langston C, et al. Pulmonary infiltrates with eosinophilia syndromes in children. J Pediatr 2000;136:351–8.

83. Zanetti G, Marchiori E, Gasparetto TD, et al. Lipoid pneumonia in children following aspiration of mineral oil used in the treatment of constipation: high-resolution CT findings in 17 patients. Pediatr Radiol 2007;37:1135–9.

84. Marchiori E, Zanetti G, Mano CM, et al. Lipoid pneumonia in 53 patients after aspiration of mineral oil: comparison of high-resolution computed tomography findings in adults and children. J Comput Assist Tomogr 2010;34:9–12.

85. Susarla S, Fan LL. Diffuse alveolar hemorrhage syndromes in children. Curr Opin Pediatr 2007;19: 314–20.

86. Fullmer JJ, Langston C, Dishop MK, et al. Pulmonary capillaritis in children: a review of eight cases with comparison to other alveolar hemorrhage syndromes. J Pediatr 2005;146:376–81.

87. Ravenel JG, McAdams HP. Pulmonary vasculitis: CT features. Semin Respir Crit Care Med 2003;24:427–36.

88. Connolly B, Manson D, Eberhard A, et al. CT appearance of pulmonary vasculitis in children. AJR Am J Roentgenol 1996;167:901–4.

89. Panigada S, Ravelli A, Silvestri M, et al. HRCT and pulmonary function tests in monitoring of lung involvement in juvenile systemic sclerosis. Pediatr Pulmonol 2009;44:1226–34.

90. Seely JM, Jones LT, Wallace C, et al. Systemic sclerosis: using high-resolution CT to detect lung disease in children. AJR Am J Roentgenol 1998; 170:691–7.

91. Aaløkken TM, Lilleby V, Søyseth V, et al. Chest abnormalities in juvenile-onset mixed connective tissue disease: assessment with high-resolution computed tomography and pulmonary function tests. Acta Radiol 2009;50:430–6.

92. Lilleby C, Aaløkken TM, Johansen B, et al. Pulmonary involvement in patients with childhood-onset

systemic lupus erythematosus. Clin Exp Rheumatol 2006;24:203–8.

93. Keesling CA, Frush DP, O'Hara SM, et al. Clinical and imaging manifestations of pediatric sarcoidosis. Acad Radiol 1998;5:122–32.

94. Milman N, Hoffmann AL, Byg KE. Sarcoidosis in children. Epidemiology in Danes, clinical features, diagnosis, treatment and prognosis. Acta Paediatr 1998;87:871–8.

95. Odame I, Li P, Lau L, et al. Pulmonary Langerhans cell histiocytosis: a variable disease in childhood. Pediatr Blood Cancer 2006;47:889–93.

96. Ha SY, Helms P, Fletcher M, et al. Lung involvement in Langerhans' cell histiocytosis: prevalence, clinical features, and outcome. Pediatrics 1992;89:466–9.

97. Crawley AJ, Guillerman RP. Langerhans cell histiocytosis with intrathymic calcifications and cavitation. Pediatr Radiol 2010;40(Suppl 1):S162.

98. McHugh K, Olsen ØE, Vellodi A. Gaucher disease in children: radiology of non-central nervous system manifestations. Clin Radiol 2004;59:117–23.

99. Goitein O, Elstein D, Abrahamov A, et al. Lung involvement and enzyme replacement therapy in Gaucher's disease. QJM 2001;94:407–15.

100. Guillemot N, Troadec C, de Villemeur TB, et al. Lung disease in Niemann-Pick disease. Pediatr Pulmonol 2007;42:1207–14.

101. Griese M, Brasch F, Aldana VR, et al. Respiratory disease in Niemann-Pick type C2 is caused by pulmonary alveolar proteinosis. Clin Genet 2010;77:119–30.

102. Nicholson AG. Lymphocytic interstitial pneumonia and other lymphoproliferative disorders in the lung. Semin Respir Crit Care Med 2001;22:409–22.

103. Bramson RT, Cleveland R, Blickman JG, et al. Radiographic appearance of follicular bronchitis in children. AJR Am J Roentgenol 1996;166:1447–50.

104. Theron S, Andronikou S, George R, et al. Non-infective pulmonary disease in HIV-positive children. Pediatr Radiol 2009;39:555–64.

105. Pitcher RD, Beningfield SJ, Zar HJ. Chest radiographic features of lymphocytic interstitial pneumonitis in HIV-infected children. Clin Radiol 2010;65:150–4.

106. Becciolini V, Gudinchet F, Cheseaux J-J, et al. Lymphocytic interstitial pneumonia in children with AIDS: high-resolution CT findings. Eur Radiol 2001;11:1015–20.

107. Marks MJ, Haney PJ, McDermott MP, et al. Thoracic disease in children with AIDS. Radiographics 1996;16:1349–62.

108. Towbin AJ, Chaves I. Chronic granulomatous disease. Pediatr Radiol 2010;40:657–68.

109. Khanna G, Kao SC, Kirby P, et al. Imaging of chronic granulomatous disease in children. Radiographics 2005;25:1183–95.

110. Gungor T, Engel-Bicik I, Eich G, et al. Diagnostic and therapeutic impact of whole body positron emission tomography using fluorine-18-fluoro-2-deoxy-D-glucose in children with chronic granulomatous disease. Arch Dis Child 2001;85:341–5.

111. Park JH, Levinson AI. Granulomatous-lymphocytic interstitial lung disease (GLILD) in common variable immunodeficiency (CVID). Clin Immunol 2010;134:97–103.

112. Touw CM, van de Ven AA, de Jong PA, et al. Detection of pulmonary complications in common variable immunodeficiency. Pediatr Allergy Immunol 2010;21:793–805.

113. Schroeder SA, Swift M, Sandoval C, et al. Interstitial lung disease in patients with ataxia-telangiectasia. Pediatr Pulmonol 2005;39:537–43.

114. Esther CR Jr, Barker PM. Pulmonary lymphangiectasia: diagnosis and clinical course. Pediatr Pulmonol 2004;38:308–13.

115. Barker PM, Esther CR Jr, Fordham LA, et al. Primary pulmonary lymphangiectasia in infancy and childhood. Eur Respir J 2004;24:413–9.

116. Copley SJ, Coren M, Nicholson AG, et al. Diagnostic accuracy of thin-section CT and chest radiography of pediatric interstitial lung disease. AJR Am J Roentgenol 2000;174:549–54.

117. Faul JL, Berry GJ, Colby TV, et al. Thoracic lymphangiomas, lymphangiectasis, lymphangiomatosis, and lymphatic dysplasia syndrome. Am J Respir Crit Care Med 2000;161:1037–46.

118. Swenson SJ, Hartman TE, Mayor JR, et al. Diffuse pulmonary lymphangiomatosis: CT findings. J Comput Assist Tomogr 1995;19:348–52.

Multidetector Computed Tomography of Pediatric Large Airway Diseases: State-of-the-Art

Edward Y. Lee, MD, MPH[a,b,]*, S. Bruce Greenberg, MD[c],
Phillip M. Boiselle, MD[d]

KEYWORDS
- Multidetector computed tomography
- Large airway diseases • Pediatric patients

Recent advances in multidetector computed tomography (MDCT) technology have revolutionized the noninvasive imaging evaluation of the large airways in pediatric patients. Compared with single-detector CT scanners, MDCT provides faster acquisition times, increased anatomic coverage, and decreased need for sedation, which are particularly beneficial for imaging the large airways in children. In addition, superb-quality multiplanar (MPR) two-dimensional (2D) and three-dimensional (3D) reconstructions have enabled MDCT to become an essential noninvasive imaging tool for assessing the full spectrum of congenital and acquired large airway diseases in pediatric patients. Furthermore, paired inspiratory-expiratory MDCT imaging, cine MDCT imaging, and newer four-dimensional (4D) MDCT imaging have substantially enhanced the evaluation of dynamic large airway disease such as tracheobronchomalacia (TBM). This article reviews imaging techniques and clinical applications of MDCT for assessing large airway diseases in children.

ADVANCES IN PEDIATRIC LARGE AIRWAY IMAGING WITH MDCT: IMAGING EVOLUTION AND REVOLUTION

Continued rapid advances in CT technology have revolutionized the noninvasive imaging of the large airways in pediatric patients, particularly over the past 2 decades.[1–5] The development of MDCT with multiple arrays of detectors, which can simultaneously obtain multiple channels of information with each gantry rotation, substantially increased the speed of data collection compared with single-detector CT. When this innovative multidetector CT technology was combined with the advent of decreased gantry rotation times and

[a] Division of Thoracic Imaging, Department of Radiology, Children's Hospital Boston and Harvard Medical School, 330 Longwood Avenue, Boston, MA 02115, USA
[b] Pulmonary Division, Department of Medicine, Children's Hospital Boston and Harvard Medical School, 330 Longwood Avenue, Boston, MA 02115, USA
[c] Departments of Radiology and Pediatrics, University of Arkansas for Medical Sciences, Arkansas Children's Hospital, 1 Children's Way, Slot #105, Little Rock, AR 72202, USA
[d] Department of Radiology, Beth Israel Deaconess Medical Center and Harvard Medical School, 330 Brookline Avenue, Boston, MA 02215, USA
* Corresponding author. Division of Thoracic Imaging, Department of Radiology, Children's Hospital Boston and Harvard Medical School, 330 Longwood Avenue, Boston, MA 02115.
E-mail address: Edward.Lee@childrens.harvard.edu

Radiol Clin N Am 49 (2011) 869–893
doi:10.1016/j.rcl.2011.06.006

increased craniocaudal volume coverage, modern MDCT scanners with the capacity to produce high spatial resolution thin-section images of the entire large airways in seconds were subsequently developed (**Fig. 1**). The latest wide-detector MDCT scanners, which are currently offered with 256 to 320 detectors, have made real-time, dynamic imaging of the large airways a reality, even for non-sedated infants and young children. Recent advances in radiation dose-reduction strategies have further solidified the pivotal role of MDCT as an attractive noninvasive imaging technique for assessing large airway disease in pediatric patients.

MDCT TECHNIQUE: IMAGE OPTIMIZATION

Infants and young children pose several unique challenges for large airway imaging with MDCT, including patient motion, inability to follow breathing instructions, and greater sensitivity to radiation.[1] Such problems can be minimized by appropriate use of sedation, intubation, breathing techniques, and by closely following the ALARA principle of "as low as reasonably achievable" tailored to each individual pediatric patient as detailed in the following sections.

Patient Preparation

Sedation
Although the frequency with which sedation is required for infants and young children in

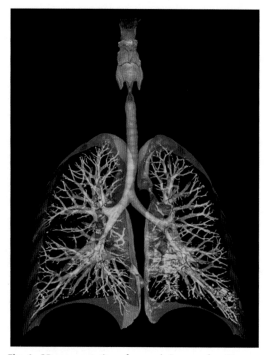

Fig. 1. 3D segmentation of normal airways of an 11-year-old boy obtained using a 320-detector MDCT scanner.

evaluating central airways has decreased with MDCT because of its fast CT scanning times, sedation is still generally necessary for uncooperative infants and young children (≤5 years old) unless using state-of-the-art, 320-detector MDCT scanners.[1,3,6,7] Light sedation, which allows patients to continuously maintain a patent airway independently and respond appropriately to physical stimulation and /or verbal commands with a minimal depressed level of consciousness, is nearly always recommended for MDCT studies in infants and young children.[1,3,6,7] Oral chloral hydrate and intravenous pentobarbital sodium are the most commonly used drugs of choice for light sedation.[1,7]

Breathing instruction, coughing technique, and breath-hold technique
Older children (>5 years old) are usually able to follow instructions for various respiratory maneuvers (end-inspiration, end-expiration, forced expiration, and coughing) after a practice session before the CT scan. Careful attention to patient breathing or coughing instructions and practice is essential because inadvertent imaging during submaximal inspiration, expiration, or coughing can result in underdiagnosis or misdiagnosis. To ensure a high-quality CT study, either the radiologists or CT technologists should review and practice breathing or coughing instructions with the patient before the CT study. In infants and young children (≤5 years old), a controlled ventilation technique (ie, breath-hold) is required to obtain end-inspiratory and end-expiratory phases of an MDCT airway study after sedation and intubation.[7] By alternatively applying and withholding positive pressure (15–20 cm H_2O) ventilation during inspiration and expiration, respectively, end-inspiratory and end-expiratory phases of a CT study can be successfully obtained.[7] For dynamic 4D MDCT imaging, CT scanning can be obtained during real-time breathing in infants and children without sedation or intubation. In sedated and intubated patients, respiratory rate should be set at 40 breaths per minute, and tidal volumes should be as large as practical.

Intravenous contrast material
Intravenous contrast material is not necessary for the routine assessment of the large airways. However, it is recommended when simultaneously evaluating suspected mediastinal vascular anomalies (eg, innominate artery compression, vascular rings, and pulmonary artery sling), extrinsic mediastinal masses (eg, foregut duplication cysts, lymphadenopathy), or central airway neoplasms (eg, hemangioma) that can result in central airway

abnormalities.[1,3,5,7,8] Nonionic low-osmolar contrast material (2 mL/kg, not to exceed 4 mL/kg or 125 mL) can be administered either by hand injection or mechanical injection depending on the size of the intravenous catheter and the stability of intravenous catheter placement.[1,7] Although contrast material may be administered manually in infants and young children with a small-caliber catheter (<22 gauge) or a central access line, mechanical injection of contrast material is the preferred method, because it generally provides more homogeneous vascular contrast enhancement.[1,7] Mechanical administration of intravenous contrast material can be performed at 1.5 to 2.5 mL/s for a 22-gauge catheter or 2.0 to 4.0 mL/s for a 20-gauge catheter.[1,7]

MDCT PARAMETERS: BALANCING IMAGE QUALITY AND RADIATION DOSE
Types of MDCT Techniques

There are currently 5 main types of MDCT techniques that can be used for evaluating the large airways in pediatric patients including: (1) single acquisition, end-inspiratory study; (2) paired end-inspiratory/end-expiratory study; (3) paired end-inspiratory/dynamic expiratory study; (4) cine study; and (5) dynamic 4D study.

Whereas anatomic imaging of the large airways is performed at end-inspiration, an additional expiratory imaging sequence should be performed when there is known or suspected TBM. There are 2 options for expiratory imaging.[7,9] In end-expiratory imaging, CT images are obtained at the end of exhalation; however, in dynamic expiratory imaging, CT images are acquired during a forced exhalation.[7,9] In the latter method, patients are instructed to take a deep breath in and to blow it out during the CT acquisition, which is coordinated to start at the initiation of the patient's forced expiratory effort. MDCT imaging during dynamic expiration (ie, forced expiration) results in a greater degree of central airway collapse compared with imaging during a static end-expiratory maneuver, because of the higher intrathoracic pressures that can be generated during dynamic expiration.[7,10]

Therefore, the dynamic expiratory MDCT technique is currently recommended for pediatric patients who can follow breathing instructions.[10]

With 64-detector MDCT, which can provide anatomic coverage up to 4 cm in the z-axis, a cine MDCT technique can be helpful for imaging pediatric patients with focal TBM.[7] By using a coughing maneuver, which is known to elicit an even higher level of intrathoracic-extratracheal pressure than forced exhalation, the sensitivity of detecting TBM can be increased with cine

MDCT.[7,11] Dynamic large airway imaging has recently been further advanced by the advent of state-of-the-art 320 MDCT scanners. Such scanners can image the large airways (up to 16 cm craniocaudal coverage) in real time and provide 4D information of large airway dynamics without the need for sedation or intubation in infants and young children (see **Fig. 1**).[12,13]

MDCT parameters

To acquire an optimal MDCT data set, one should carefully select proper MDCT parameters, including tube current (milliampere-seconds [mAs]), kilovoltage peak (kVp), table speed, detector collimation, and reconstruction thickness (for 2D and 3D reconstructions), maintaining the lowest radiation dose as possible.

Parameters for end-inspiratory and expiratory helical MDCT acquisitions Guidelines for determining mAs and kVp based on patient weight are listed in **Table 1**, which can be used for most available MDCT scanners with more than 4 rows. Because of the inherent natural contrast between the air-filled large airways and adjacent mediastinal soft tissues, low radiation dose technique is possible for imaging the large airways in children.[7,14] For example, a recent study showed that the radiation dose of paired inspiratory-expiratory MDCT study can be reduced by 23% with decreasing mAs by 50% during expiratory

Table 1
Tube current and kilovoltage by patient weight for static central airway MDCT, paired inspiratory-expiratory MDCT, and paired inspiratory-dynamic expiratory MDCT

Weight (kg)	Tube Current (mAs) Inspiratory/ Expiratory	Kilovoltage
<10	40/20	80
10–14	50/25	80
15–24	60/30	80
25–34	70/35	80
35–44	80/40	80
45–54	90/40	90
55–70	100–120/40	100–120

For tube current and kilovoltage by patient weight for end-expiratory MDCT examination, mAs should be reduced by 50% to a maximum of 40 mAs, maintaining the same level of kilovoltage for end-inspiratory MDCT examination.
Data from Lee EY and Boiselle PM. Tracheobronchomalacia in infants and children: multidetector CT evaluation. Radiology 2009;252:7–22.

MDCT imaging while maintaining similar diagnostic confidence for assessment of the tracheal lumen compared with standard-dose technique in pediatric patients.[14]

A rapid CT acquisition based on a gantry rotation time of 1 second or less and a pitch of 1.0 to 1.5 is recommended. In general, recommended detector collimation values are: 1.0 to 1.5 mm for 4-row MDCT; 0.625 to 1.0 mm for 8-row to 16-row MDCT; and 0.5 to 0.6 mm for 64-row MDCT.[1,7] To optimize the appearance of 2D and 3D reconstructions, a reconstruction interval (RI) that provides approximately 50% overlap (eg, a 3-mm section thickness at a 2-mm RI or a 2-mm section thickness at a 1-mm RI) should be selected when collimation thickness is greater than 1.0 mm.[1,7] However, because the use of very thin collimation (eg, 0.5–1.0 mm) produces an isotropic data set with spatial resolution that is the same when CT images are reviewed in transverse and various MPR axes, it is not necessary to provide overlapping RIs in this setting.[15]

Parameters for cine MDCT Optimal MDCT parameters for cine MDCT are based on: (1) weight-based mAs and kVp (see **Table 1**); (2) gantry rotation of 0.5 second or less; (3) detector collimation of 0.5 to 0.625 mm; and (4) image reconstruction at 8-mm collimation in a standard algorithm, creating 4 contiguous cine data sets from a single acquisition.[7]

Parameters for dynamic 4D MDCT The recommended MDCT parameters for a dynamic 4D MDCT study include: (1) mA determined by the formula ([(kg $\times$ 2.5) + 5] $\div$ 0.35 = mA); (2) 80 kVp; (3) continuous scanning for 1.4 seconds (4 cycles at 350 ms/rotation); and (4) image reconstructions of 8 phases of obtained CT data set for image review in cine mode.

Postprocessing Techniques: Beyond Axial CT Imaging

MPR 2D imaging

2D MPR images are single-voxel-thick CT images that can be created and displayed along any selected planes such as the coronal, sagittal, or oblique plane.[1,7] Such 2D images can be created easily at the CT console or at a remote postprocessing station. For evaluation of the large airways that are not linear structures, curved reformation along the long axis of the large airways is a valuable 2D postprocessing technique.[7] By following a reference line though the center of the airway on sagittal MPR CT images, a curved coronal MPR can be reconstructed (**Fig. 2**). Such images provide a more accurate measurement of the large airway, because they provide a straightened view that allows for a more precise measurement of the distance between 2 points. Accurate measurements are particularly important for preoperative evaluation before a surgical or interventional procedure.

When multiple adjacent thin slices are added together, a thick slab or MPR volume reformation image (which can be adjusted to any thickness dimension) is generated. For large airway imaging, such slabs typically vary from 3 to 10 mm thickness and are the mainstay of postprocessing techniques because they combine the high spatial resolution of MPR images with the anatomic display of thicker sections.[6,7,16] In addition, minimum intensity projection (MinIP) volume-rendering images, which are reconstructed by selecting the lowest attenuation voxels, can enhance the visibility of the large airways within the mediastinum and the lung parenchyma (see **Fig. 2**).[17,18] Such images are also helpful for detecting subtle small airway disease, often manifested by air-trapping.[19]

3D Imaging

Volume rendering, which is reconstructed based on an edge detection image processing system using entire information from all voxels in the available data set, is the most widely used 3D reconstruction technique for evaluation of the large airways.[1,7] Major advantages of this technique are its ability to maintain the original spatial relationships of the volumetric data and reconstruct lifelike 3D images by adding depth information, enhancing detail, and clarifying complex 3D relationships. This technique provides both external (ie, virtual bronchography) and internal (ie, virtual bronchoscopy) renderings of the large airways using the initial axial CT data (**Fig. 3**).[1,7]

Whereas external 3D rendering of the large airways displays the outer surface of the airways and its relationship with adjacent structures, internal 3D rendering of the large airways provides endoluminal views of the large airways similar to that of conventional bronchoscopy. Virtual bronchoscopy is particularly useful for: (1) visualizing airways distal to an area of high-grade stenosis beyond which a flexible bronchoscopy cannot be passed; (2) facilitating guidance of bronchoscopic interventions; and (3) providing a noninvasive method for postprocedural surveillance.[20,21] The evaluation of large airway anomalies and abnormalities with 3D MDCT reconstruction images is particularly useful in infants and young children in whom conventional bronchoscopy is often avoided because of its invasiveness and need for general anesthesia.[22–24]

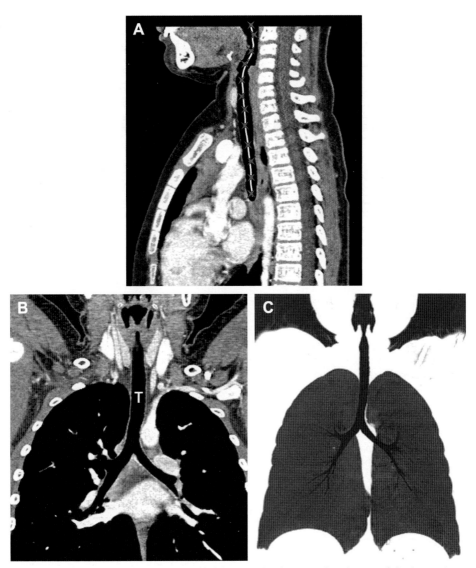

Fig. 2. Normal large airways of an 8-year-old girl. (*A*) Sagittal reformatted CT image of the large airways shows a reference line through the center of the airway for reconstruction of a curved coronal reformatted image. (*B*) Curved coronal reformatted CT image shows a straightened view of the entire trachea (T). (*C*) MinIP image shows normal trachea and bronchi.

4D imaging

With recent advancements in MDCT technology, newer methods of evaluating the large airways in children in real time are being developed.[12,13] 4D MDCT of the large airways represents a real-time moving 3D representation of the large airways. With state-of-the-art 320 MDCT scanners, true isometric, isophasic, and isovolumetric 4D imaging in a real-time respiratory cycle up to 16-cm-long craniocaudal extent of the large airways can be generated.[2,13] The craniocaudal coverage of 16 cm with 320 MDCT scanners can capture the entire airways in infants and the large airways in most older children.[7,12,13] By combining real-time

motion information with anatomic details from 3D volume-rendering CT images, dynamic 4D MDCT can provide physiologic information that complements anatomic information from 3D imaging. This innovative technique is particularly helpful for evaluating dynamic large airway disease processes such as TBM in nonsedated infants and young children.[12,13]

IMAGE INTERPRETATION
Axial CT Images

Interpretation of the large airways should begin with a review of the axial CT images, which provide

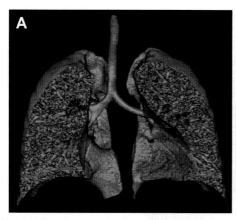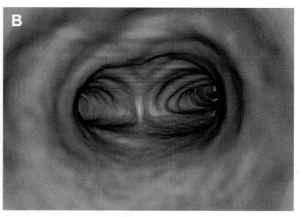

Fig. 3. 3D volume rendering of the large airways in a 6-year-old girl. (*A*) 3D external volume-rendered image shows patent trachea and bilateral bronchi. (*B*) 3D internal volume-rendered image obtained at the level of carina. Bilateral main stem bronchi are patent.

a comprehensive review of the entire thoracic structures. Thin-section axial (ie, transverse) CT images acquired by MDCT can provide essential information about the large airways regarding: (1) the size and shape of the airway lumen; (2) the presence and distribution of airway wall thickening; (3) the relationship of the large airways to adjacent mediastinal, hilar, or pulmonary parenchymal structures; and (4) the presence of artifacts that may simulate disease on 2D or 3D reconstruction MDCT images.[1,7] The initial evaluation of the large airways with the axial CT images allows the recognition of major abnormalities and also provides guidance for subsequently selecting the optimal type of postprocessing techniques for better displaying the abnormality to enhance the diagnosis.

MPR (2D) and 3D Images: Added Diagnostic Value

Axial CT images alone are no longer the reference standard for assessing large airway anatomy and disease. Such images are inadequate for assessment of: (1) subtle stenosis; (2) craniocaudal extent of airway disease; (3) airways obliquely located to the axial plane; and (4) complex airway anatomy.[25–29] 2D and 3D MDCT reconstruction images, which are now easily and interactively generated in real time at the CT console or workstation, can overcome these limitations by providing a display that is more visually accessible and often more anatomically meaningful (see **Figs. 2 and 3**). Such images can increase the accuracy of detecting large airway stenosis, enhance the assessment of the craniocaudad extent of airway disorders, and clarify complex congenital airway abnormalities. For example, external 3D reconstruction images, when compared with axial CT images alone, provided important additional information regarding airway stenoses in 16 (34%) of 47 patients in a study by Remy-Jardin and colleagues.[25] In recent years, virtual bronchoscopy has emerged as a particularly useful postprocessing imaging technique for evaluating tracheobronchial stenosis. When compared with flexible bronchoscopy, MDCT with 2D and 3D reconstruction images has been shown to be highly sensitive for detecting large airway stenoses, with reported sensitivities ranging from 87% to 92% in children.[24,30] Furthermore, diagnostic confidence of interpretation and communication among radiologists, clinicians, and patients can be also improved when 2D and 3D reconstruction MDCT images are used to complement the axial CT images for evaluating the large airways.[1,7,20] 2D and 3D reconstructions should be integrated into study interpretation along with the axial CT images, but are not a replacement for axial CT images. All axial CT images in addition to 2D and 3D reconstruction MDCT images should be thoroughly reviewed for a complete evaluation.

Dynamic Large Airway Images: TBM

Although static anatomic imaging of the large airways is obtained at end-inspiration, an additional expiratory imaging sequence is required for evaluating dynamic large airway disease such as TBM, which can be missed on routine end-inspiratory CT images.[7,9,31] The standard CT criterion of at least 50% expiratory reduction in the cross-sectional luminal area of the trachea or bronchi for the diagnosis of TBM has been found to correlate well with the results of bronchoscopy in pediatric patients with TBM.[31,32] In addition, cine MDCT and dynamic 4D MDCT studies, which can display the caliber change of the large airways in real time, can enhance the diagnosis and extent of TBM.[11]

CLINICAL APPLICATIONS: MDCT FOR PEDIATRIC LARGE AIRWAY EVALUATION

MDCT with 2D and 3D reconstruction images is increasingly being considered as an essential, one-stop imaging evaluation for pediatric patients with clinically suspected large airway anomalies and abnormalities. The common clinical indications for the use of MDCT in assessing the large airways in the pediatric population include: (1) evaluation of congenital tracheobronchial anomalies; (2) diagnosis of acquired large airway abnormalities; and (3) detection or confirmation of suspected TBM.[1,7]

Congenital Malformations

Nonvascular lesions
Congenital anomalies of tracheobronchial branching Ectopic and supernumerary bronchi are the 2 most common congenital anomalies of tracheobronchial branching.[1] An ectopic bronchus is more common than a supernumerary bronchus.[1] Tracheal bronchus, also known as bronchial suis, is the most common type of ectopic bronchus (**Fig. 4**). In this condition, an anomalous upper lobe bronchus arises directly from the lateral

wall of the trachea (typically <2 cm above the carina) instead of from the main bronchus.[33–36] Tracheal bronchus may supply the entire upper lobe or its apical segment. Patients with this anomaly are usually asymptomatic but the diagnosis of tracheal bronchus should be considered in cases of persistent or recurrent upper lobe air-trapping, atelectasis, or pneumonia.[1,33] One of the most common supernumerary bronchi is the cardiac bronchus, which arises from the medial wall of the bronchus intermedius (**Fig. 5**). Cardiac bronchus can be blind-ending or connected with a hypoplastic lobe.[1,37,38] Supernumerary bronchus can also arise directly from the main bronchus. Although ectopic and supernumerary bronchi are often detected incidentally in asymptomatic children, surgical resection may be required in cases associated with recurrent infection or hemoptysis.[33,38,39] Whereas axial CT images are usually sufficient for evaluating atelectasis or consolidation often associated with ectopic or supernumerary bronchi, 2D and 3D reconstruction MDCT images are helpful for precisely localizing the origin and assessing the size of the ectopic or supernumerary bronchi for preoperative evaluation (see **Figs. 4 and 5**).[38,40]

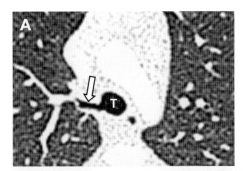

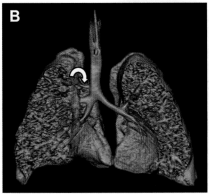
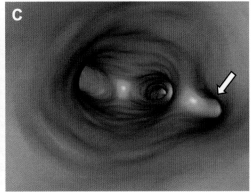

Fig. 4. Tracheal bronchus in a 6-month-old girl who presented with a history of recurrent right upper lobe infection. Subsequently obtained bronchoscopy confirmed abnormal bronchus arising from the right lateral wall of the trachea. (*A*) Axial CT image shows an anomalous right upper lobe bronchus (*arrow*), tracheal bronchus, arises directly from the lateral wall of the trachea (T). (*B*) 3D external volume-rendered image of the large airways and lungs confirms the origin and course of the tracheal bronchus (*curved arrow*). (*C*) 3D internal volume-rendered image shows an opening (*arrow*) of the tracheal bronchus located above the carina.

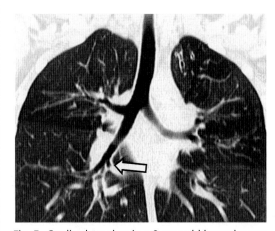

Fig. 5. Cardiac bronchus in a 9-year-old boy who presented with recurrent shortness of breath. Coronal CT image shows an anomalous, cardiac bronchus (*arrow*), which arises from the medial wall of the bronchus intermedius. Subsequently obtained bronchoscopy confirmed the presence of cardiac bronchus.

Bronchial agenesis, aplasia, and hypoplasia Bronchial agenesis, aplasia, and hypoplasia represent the spectrum of congenital underdevelopment of the bronchus.[1,33] The cause and embryonic pathophysiology of congenital underdevelopment of the bronchi are currently unknown. In bronchial agenesis, there is a complete absence of the bronchus, lung, and vascular supply (**Fig. 6**). Bronchial agenesis can be either unilateral or bilateral. Bronchial aplasia represents a bronchial malformation characterized by a rudimentary bronchus and incomplete development of lung. In bronchial hypoplasia, which is the most commonly encountered anomaly of underdeveloped lung parenchyma, the bronchus is rudimentary and the affected portion of the lung is hypoplastic.[1,33] The development of vascular supply in bronchial aplasia and hypoplasia can be absent or hypoplastic. MDCT with 2D and 3D reconstruction images can show detailed anatomic information of the large airways, vessels, and lungs in pediatric patients with bronchial agenesis, aplasia, or hypoplasia (see **Fig. 6**).[6,41]

Congenital tracheal stenosis Congenital tracheal stenosis is a rare anomaly in which a tracheal cartilage ring is associated with absent or deficient tracheal membranes.[1,3,42] This malformation results in a fixed narrowing, and affected patients usually present with biphasic stridor, wheezing, and recurrent pneumonia during the first year of life.[1,3,42] Congenital tracheal stenoses are focal in 50%, diffuse in 30%, and funnel-shaped in 20% of cases (**Figs. 7** and **8**).[43] Accurate determination of the location and extent of congenital tracheal

stenosis is essential for proper patient management.[40] Although chest radiographs and fluoroscopy may show narrowing of the trachea in patients with tracheal stenosis, CT is able to more accurately characterize the tracheal stenosis and precisely evaluate its extent. In addition, MDCT can also correctly diagnose other congenital cardiovascular anomalies often associated with congenital tracheal stenosis. The management of tracheal stenosis in symptomatic patients is surgical resection and end-to-end anastomosis for short stenosis (≤5 cm) and a patch or tracheal autograft repair in longer stenosis (>5 cm).[44]

Vascular lesions
Congenital mediastinal vascular anomalies such as vascular rings and sling are common causes of respiratory distress in pediatric patients that result from extrinsic compression on the large airways.[45] Such airway narrowing because of mediastinal vascular anomalies can be now successfully evaluated with submillisievert low-dose MDCT imaging strategies in pediatric patients.

Double aortic arch Double aortic arch is the most primitive form of aortic arch anomaly and is also the most frequently symptomatic.[40,45] In this condition, the ascending aortic arch bifurcates into 2 aortic arches (ie, right and left aortic arches), which join together to form a descending aorta. Both aortic arches encircle the trachea and esophagus, which results in extrinsic tracheal and esophageal compression. Affected patients typically present with inspiratory stridor, wheezing, and dysphagia in the neonatal period or infancy.[40,45] The size and location of aortic arches is usually asymmetric. The right aortic arch is usually larger and higher in location than the left aortic arch. Either aortic arch can be atretic. Whereas the descending aorta is positioned on the same side as the location of the larger aortic arch, the ductus arteriosus is located on the opposite side. Other congenital heart diseases associated with double aortic arch include tetralogy of Fallot, ventricular septal defect, and transposition of the great arteries. Although chest radiographs and esophagrams have been traditionally used for evaluating vascular rings such as double aortic arch in infants and young children in the past, MDCT has assumed a role of diagnostic imaging modality of choice for evaluating double aortic arch in symptomatic pediatric patients in recent years.[1,3,8,40,46,47] Unlike other currently available imaging modalities, MDCT can provide comprehensive anatomic information of vascular, airway, and lung anomalies in pediatric patients with double aortic arch (**Fig. 9**).[1,3,8,40] MDCT with 2D

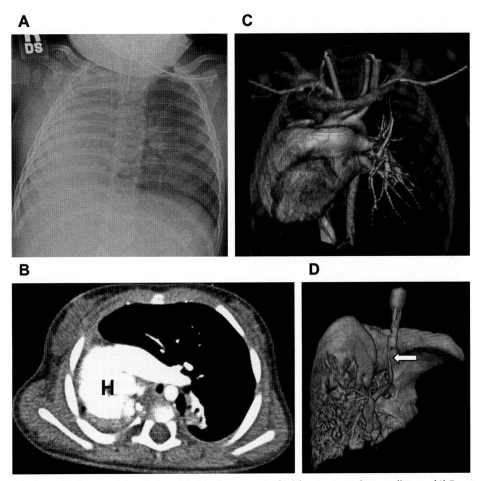

Fig. 6. Right bronchial agenesis in a 2-day-old girl who presented with severe respiratory distress. (*A*) Frontal chest radiograph shows an opacity of the entire right hemithorax associated with mediastinal structures shifted to the right hemithorax. Endotracheal tube and nasogastric tube are also seen. (*B*) Axial CT image shows an absence of the right lung and compensatory hyperinflation of the left lung. The mediastinal structures including heart (H) are located in the right hemithorax. (*C*) 3D external volume-rendered image shows the absence of the right lung and mediastinal structure located within the right hemithorax. (*D*) 3D external volume-rendered image of the large airways and lungs shows the absent right bronchus, severe tracheal stenosis (*arrow*), and hyperinflated left lung.

and 3D reconstruction images are often necessary for a complete evaluation of such structures because the entire anatomic structures are rarely visualized in a single axial view. The correct identification of the smaller arch is important because current management of double aortic arch involves surgical division of the smaller of the 2 aortic arches.[48,49] Using a paired inspiratory-expiratory MDCT technique, concomitant tracheomalacia often associated with double aortic arch can be reliably diagnosed in infants and children (see **Fig. 9**).[31,32,50] The presence of severe tracheomalacia in patients with double aortic arch may require a direct surgical repair of the trachea in addition to surgical division of double aortic arch. Thus, it has been recommended that paired inspiratory-expiratory MDCT be performed routinely

in the preoperative assessment of patients with double aortic arch.[32,50]

Right aortic arch with aberrant left subclavian artery In this condition, an aberrant origin of the left subclavian artery originates as the last branch of the right-sided aortic arch.[1,45] A vascular ring is formed by a left-sided ductus (or its remnant ligamentum arteriosum) when it connects the aberrant left subclavian artery to the proximal left pulmonary artery. Affected patients typically present with respiratory distress and dysphagia, particularly when the ligamentum arteriosum is tight or they have a large diverticulum of Kommerell, which is a dilated origin of the aberrant left subclavian artery.[1,45] MDCT with 2D and 3D reconstruction images can accurately show the origin and course

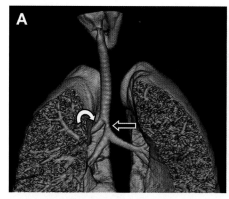
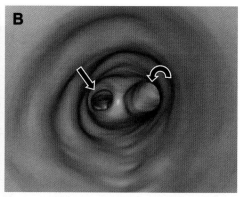

Fig. 7. Focal congenital tracheal stenosis in a 5-year-old boy who presented with worsening biphasic stridor and cough. (A) 3D external volume-rendered image shows a short-segment tracheal stenosis (*straight arrow*) located just above the carina. Also noted is a right tracheal bronchus (*curved arrow*). (B) 3D internal volume-rendered image shows a tracheal stenosis (*arrow*) and an opening of the right tracheal bronchus (*curved arrow*).

of an anomalous left subclavian artery and associated tracheal narrowing before surgical division of this type of vascular ring in children (**Fig. 10**).[1,3]

Pulmonary artery sling Pulmonary artery sling is a rare congenital mediastinal vascular anomaly that is caused by involution of the proximal left sixth arch.[1,6,41,45] In this condition, an anomalous left pulmonary artery arises from the posterior aspect of the right main pulmonary artery, courses dorsal to the right main stem bronchus, and passes between the trachea and esophagus to reach the left lung (**Fig. 11**). Such a course of an anomalous left pulmonary artery often results in extrinsic compression on the trachea or right main bronchus and causes respiratory distress.[1,6,41,45] In addition to extrinsic compression, intrinsic large airway anomalies such as congenital tracheal stenosis or

tracheomalacia can further potentiate the large airway obstruction.[1,6,41,45] The early and correct diagnosis of vascular and large airway anomalies in pediatric patients with pulmonary artery sling is best performed with MDCT with 2D and 3D reconstruction images using a paired inspiratory-expiratory MDCT technique (see **Fig. 11**). A comprehensive preoperative assessment with MDCT can provide detailed anatomic information that is required to successfully perform surgical re-implantation of the left pulmonary artery and tracheal reconstruction in pediatric patients with pulmonary artery sling.[51,52]

Innominate artery compression syndrome Innominate artery compression syndrome, which was first described by Gross and Neuhauser in 1948, occurs when an aberrant innominate artery originates anomalously on the left side of the aortic

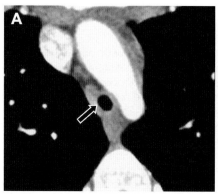
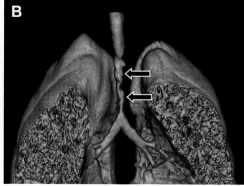

Fig. 8. Diffuse congenital tracheal stenosis in an 11-year-old girl who presented with severe stridor and wheezing. (A) Axial CT shows a narrowed trachea (*arrow*). (B) 3D external volume-rendered image shows a long segment tracheal stenosis (*arrows*). The location, degree, and extent of the long segment tracheal stenosis are better shown with the 3D volume-rendered image than the axial CT (see Fig. 8A) image.

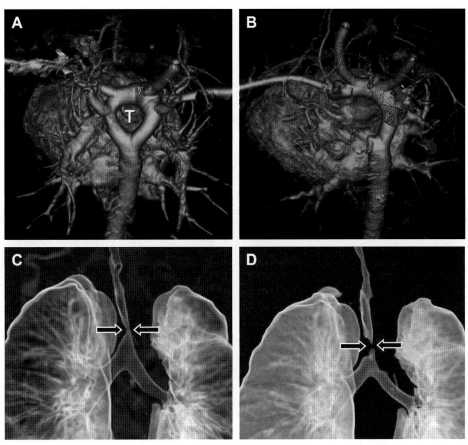

Fig. 9. Double aortic arch with tracheomalacia in a 2-month-old female infant who presented with stridor and repeated apnea. The patient underwent MDCT study for preoperative evaluation. Because of the persistent stridor and apnea after surgery, the patient subsequently underwent a second MDCT study using paired inspiratory-expiratory imaging technique. (A) Preoperative 3D external volume-rendered image shows vascular ring formed by double aortic arch that encircles the trachea (T). (B) Postoperative 3D external volume-rendered image shows discontinuation and splaying of vascular ring after surgery. (C) Postoperative 3D external volume-rendered image obtained at end-inspiration shows a narrowing (arrows) of the trachea at the level of the double aortic arch. (D) Postoperative 3D external volume-rendered image obtained at end-expiration shows a focal collapse (arrows) of the trachea at the level of the double aortic arch consistent with a severe focal tracheomalacia. (Reprinted from Chan MS, Chu WC, Cheung KL, et al. Angiography and dynamic airway evaluation with MDCT in the diagnosis of double aortic arch associated with tracheomalacia. AJR Am J Roentgenol 2005;185:1249, 1250; with permission.)

arch and courses obliquely from left to right hemithorax, resulting in an anterior compression of the trachea.[53] The precise cause of innominate artery compression is unknown. However, some investigators have postulated that innominate artery compression syndrome is more likely to arise in children with a crowded superior mediastinum, such as in those patients with congenital heart disease.[54,55] Although most pediatric patients with mild anterior tracheal compression by an aberrant innominate artery are asymptomatic, severe tracheal compression is often associated with expiratory stridor, cough, recurrent bronchopulmonary infections, and occasionally apnea.[56] The diagnosis of innominate artery compression syndrome

can be facilitated with MDCT.[1,31,32] Although the measurement of tracheal narrowing caused by innominate artery compression is best performed on axial CT images, sagittal 2D images are helpful for assessing the craniocaudal extent and coronal 2D images are useful for visualizing the entire course of the innominate artery crossing the trachea from left to right (Fig. 12). A recent study with paired inspiratory-expiratory MDCT showed that concomitant tracheomalacia associated with an innominate artery compression can be accurately diagnosed in pediatric patients.[32] Such preoperative information has the potential to assist current surgical correction of severe innominate artery compression syndrome, which includes

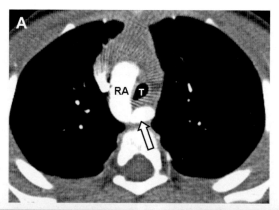

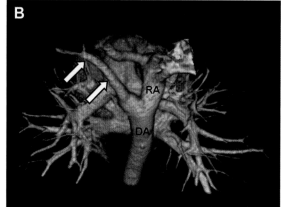

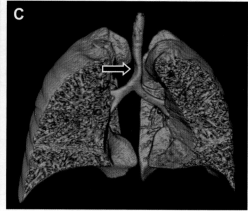

Fig. 10. Right aortic arch with an aberrant left subclavian artery in a 3-year-old boy who presented with respiratory distress and dysphagia. (*A*) Axial CT image shows a right aortic arch (RA) with an aberrant left subclavian artery (*arrow*) resulting in tracheal compression. T, trachea. (*B*) 3D external volume-rendered image of the mediastinal vessels shows a right aortic arch (RA) with an aberrant left subclavian artery (*arrows*). DA, descending aorta. The size and the entire course of an aberrant left subclavian artery are better visualized with the 3D external volume-rendered image than the axial CT image (see Fig. 10A). (*C*) 3D external volume-rendered image of the large airways shows exact location, degree, and extent of the tracheal compression (*arrow*) caused by a right aortic arch and an aberrant left subclavian artery.

arteriopexy or reimplantation of the innominate artery.[57,58]

Acquired Large Airway Lesions

Neoplasm

Tumors of the large airways are rare in children. Because of their rarity and often nonspecific clinical symptoms, missed or delayed diagnoses of large airway tumors is common in pediatric patients. Unlike in adults, most primary large airway neoplasms in pediatric patients are benign. Neoplasms of the large airways can be divided into 2 categories: (1) primary neoplasms directly arising from the airways; and (2) secondary neoplasms located outside but adjacent to the large airways, causing airway narrowing as a result of extrinsic compression or less often by direct invasion. MDCT plays an important role in the detection, staging, and preoperative planning of primary and secondary large airway neoplasms in pediatric patients. Although conventional bronchoscopy is useful for diagnosis because it allows direct visualization of the tumor and makes a histologic diagnosis by biopsy, the true extent of the tumor is often difficult to accurately assess. MDCT can be useful for determining whether a tumor is amenable to complete surgical resection in addition to guiding the approach, type, and extent of surgical resection.

Primary airway neoplasms In general, benign neoplasms of the large airways occur more frequently in the upper trachea, whereas malignant tumors more commonly affect the distal large airways.[1] Benign neoplasms of the large airways typically present as a focal, well-defined intraluminal lesion without tracheal wall or adjacent mediastinal invasion.[59] Hemangioma and papilloma are the 2 most common benign tumors of the large

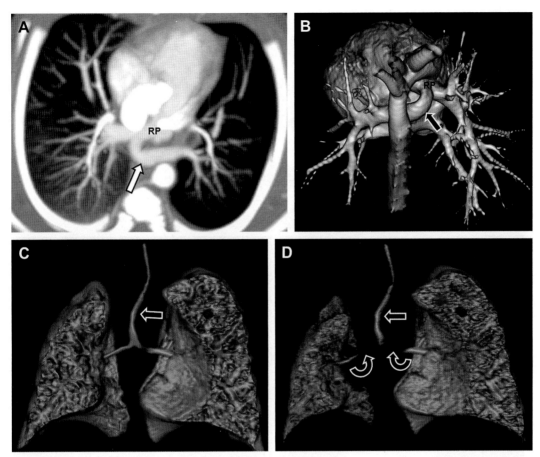

Fig. 11. Pulmonary artery sling in a 3-day-old boy who presented with severe respiratory distress. (A) Axial maximum-intensity projection image shows an anomalous left main pulmonary artery (arrow) arising from the right main pulmonary artery (RP). (B) 3D external volume-rendered image of the mediastinal vessels shows the global anatomic relationship between the left main pulmonary artery (arrow), which arises from the right main pulmonary artery (RP). (C) 3D external volume-rendered image of the large airways obtained at end-inspiration show a T- shaped carina with a tracheal stenosis (arrow). (D) 3D external volume-rendered image of the large airways obtained at end-expiration shows a tracheal stenosis (arrow) with severe bilateral broncho-malacia (curved arrow).

airways in children.[59,60] Hemangioma, typically found either in the subglottic region or in the upper trachea, usually present at birth.[1,59] Affected patients present with symptoms related to airway obstruction or recurrent hemoptysis.[1,7,60] Characteristic CT imaging findings of hemangioma in the large airways are a round and well-circumscribed soft tissue mass with marked contrast enhancement usually arising from the posterolateral aspect of the subglottic trachea (Fig. 13).[1,61] The precise location, size, and extent of hemangioma can be best visualized with MDCT with 2D and 3D reconstruction images before laser treatment (see Fig. 13).[1,3,61] Juvenile or multiple laryngotracheal papillomatosis, which is caused by human papillomavirus (types 6 and 11) infection and acquired during delivery through the birth canal, usually

occurs in the larynx and trachea.[62] Juvenile laryngotracheal papillomatosis usually presents as multiple laryngeal or tracheal lesions typically occurring in children younger than 4 years old.[63] Affected children often present with stridor and changes in voice. CT is not only valuable for detecting papilloma in the large airways but also its spread into the lung parenchyma, which can occur in up to 5% of children affected with this disorder.[62] The current treatments for juvenile laryngotracheal papillomatosis are aimed at: (1) slowing the rate of papilloma growth using antiviral and cytotoxic agents; and (2) excision of endoluminal lesions using electrocautery, cryotherapy, and CO_2 laser.

The 2 most common malignant tumors of the large airways in children include carcinoid tumor

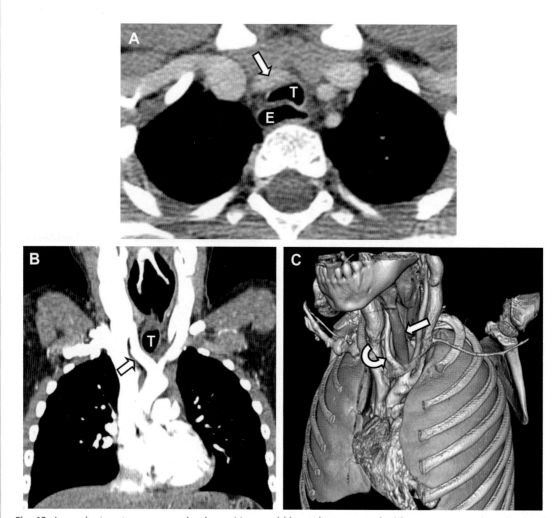

Fig. 12. Innominate artery compression in an 11-year-old boy who presented with recurrent cough and episodic severe respiratory distress. Bronchoscopy showed an anterior tracheal compression by a pulsating mass. (*A*) Axial CT image shows an anterior compression of the trachea (T) by an innominate artery (*arrow*). E, esophagus. (*B*) Coronal CT image shows the entire course of the innominate artery (*arrow*) crossing the trachea (T) from left to right obliquely. (*C*) 3D external volume-rendered image of the large airways and lungs shows the detailed anatomic relationship between the trachea (*straight arrow*) and the innominate artery (*curved arrow*).

and mucoepidermoid carcinoma.[64] Carcinoid tumors, pathologically characterized by neuroendocrine differentiation, account for most malignant large airway neoplasms in the first 2 decades of life.[64–67] As neuroendocrine neoplasms, carcinoid tumors can excrete hormones and neuroamines such as corticotrophin (adrenocorticotropic hormone), serotonin, somatostatin, and bradykinin. These neoplasms typically arise within the main stem or lobar bronchi.[64–67] Affected children typically present with cough, wheeze, chest pain, recurrent pneumonia, and atelectasis caused by airway obstruction.[64–67] Hemoptysis may also occur because of the hypervascularity of these neoplasms. Carcinoid tumor located in the main stem bronchi is often best visualized with curved coronal 2D reformation MDCT images before

surgical resection (**Fig. 14**). Mucoepidermoid carcinoma, which arises from the minor salivary glands of the tracheobronchial tree, is the second most common type of malignant airway neoplasms in pediatric patients.[64,68–70] It typically occurs in a main bronchus or proximal portion of a lobar bronchus.[64,68–70] The tumor is usually polypoid and covered with intact respiratory epithelium. It typically measures 1 to 4 cm in diameter.[70] Mucoepidermoid carcinoma is typically classified into 2 different types based on cellular differentiation and mitotic activity: low-grade and high-grade lesions.[71] In pediatric patients, mucoepidermoid carcinoma is almost always a low-grade lesion, with an excellent prognosis after complete surgical resection. MDCT is not only helpful for diagnosing malignant large

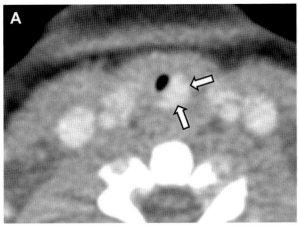
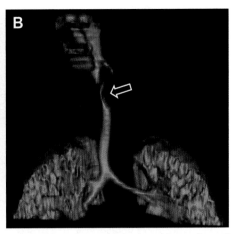

Fig. 13. Subglottic hemangioma in a 3-month-old boy who presented with recurrent biphasic stridor and cough. Bronchoscopy confirmed subglottic hemangioma. (*A*) Axial CT image shows markedly enhancing subglottic mass (*arrows*) arising from the left posterolateral aspect of the subglottic trachea. (*B*) 3D external volume-rendered image better shows the degree, location, and extent of the subglottic airway narrowing (*arrow*).

airway neoplasms but also for detecting local and distal metastasis, thereby enhancing tumor staging. Furthermore, the presence of postobstructive complications from the tumor such as air-trapping, atelectasis, and pneumonia are well evaluated with MDCT.

Secondary airway neoplasms Primary lymphoma and metastatic lymphadenopathy within the mediastinum are the 2 most common secondary airway neoplasms that can affect the large airways either by mass effect or less commonly by direct invasion. Hematogenous metastases to the large

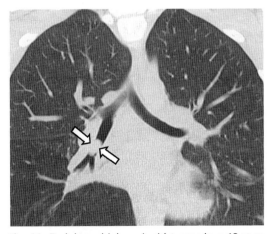

Fig. 14. Endobronchial carcinoid tumor in a 13-year-old boy who presented with respiratory distress and right lower lobe pneumonia. Coronal CT image shows an oval intrabronchial mass (*arrows*) located in the bronchus intermedius. Surgical examination of this mass confirmed the diagnosis of endobronchial carcinoid.

airways from distant neoplasm are extremely rare in pediatric patients. Lymphoma is the most common mediastinal mass in children, which is classified into 2 types: Hodgkin and non-Hodgkin.[72,73] While Hodgkin lymphoma is more common in the first decade of life, non-Hodgkin lymphoma occurs equally in the first and second decades. Large mediastinal lymphoma often extrinsically narrows the large airways, resulting in symptoms such as dyspnea and cough (**Fig. 15**). A recent study showed that CT is valuable imaging modality for assessing the degree of tracheal narrowing in children who present with presumed mediastinal lymphoma.[74] The identification of tracheal narrowing of more than 50% caused by mediastinal lymphoma is reportedly associated with a high risk of developing cardiopulmonary failure under sedation during biopsy for histologic diagnosis. Therefore, in children with a critical large airway compromised (>50%) by a large mediastinal mass, it is encouraged that a diagnosis of lymphoma be obtained by biopsy techniques using local anesthesia or thoracentesis of pleural effusion rather than under general anesthesia.[74] In children, metastatic mediastinal lymphadenopathy can also result in large airway narrowing. Metastatic mediastinal lymphadenopathy can arise from various primary tumors in the abdomen and pelvis such as neuroblastoma, Wilms tumor, testicular neoplasms, and various sarcomas in pediatric patients. On CT, metastatic mediastinal lymphadenopathy usually presents as homogeneous soft tissue masses from a conglomeration of nodes.[1,3] Aggressive metastatic lymphadenopathy has the potential to not only extrinsically compress but also to invade the large airways (**Fig. 16**).

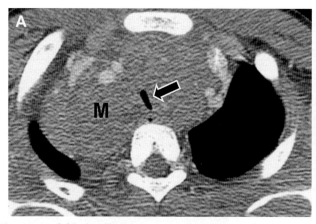
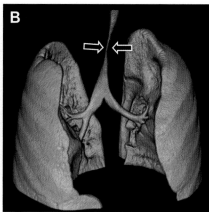

Fig. 15. Hodgkin lymphoma in a 10-year-old boy who presented with supraclavicular lymphadenopathy and chronic fatigue. (A) Axial CT image shows a large heterogeneous mediastinal mass (M) narrowing (*arrow*) the trachea. (B) 3D external volume-rendered image shows a marked tracheal narrowing (*arrows*). The exact location, degree, and extent of airway narrowing are well displayed with the 3D external volume-rendered image.

Infection

Various infections can affect the large airways in pediatric patients. The 2 most common infectious diseases that can substantially narrow the large airways are tuberculosis and fibrosing mediastinitis caused by histoplasmosis infection.[1]

Tuberculosis Tuberculosis (TB), most often caused by *Mycobacterium tuberculosis*, is a common and often deadly infectious disease affecting more than 250,000 children each year worldwide.[75] Large airway involvement by TB can occur by direct infection of the tracheobronchial wall via peribronchial lymphatic pathways or from extrinsic compression by adjacent infected and enlarged mediastinal lymph nodes.[1] The distal trachea and proximal main bronchi are the most common locations.[1] Direct large airway infection by TB in the acute stage of infection is characterized by thickened tracheobronchial walls and airway narrowing caused by lymphocytic infiltration, edema of the airway submucosa, and tubercle formation. As the infection progresses to the late stage of disease without proper treatment, tracheobronchial thickening and narrowing can become irreversible, with fibrotic luminal stenosis caused from destruction of normal mucosa by granulation tissues. Extrinsic compression of the large airway by infected and enlarged lymph nodes in the mediastinum can also obstruct the large airways (**Fig. 17**). However, such obstruction usually resolves, and patency of the large airways can be

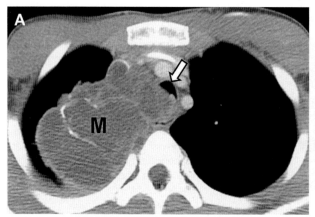
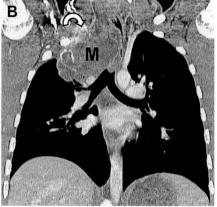

Fig. 16. Metastatic mediastinal lymphadenopathy with tracheal invasion in a 14-year-old boy with a history of embryonal rhabdomyosarcoma of the prostate who presented with dyspnea, right ptosis, myosis, and anhidrosis affecting the right side of the face and upper extremity. (A) Axial CT image shows large heterogeneously enhancing mediastinal mass (M), which invades and narrows the trachea (*arrow*). (B) A coronal CT image better shows the degree and extent of tracheal invasion by mediastinal mass (M) than an axial CT image (see Fig. 16A). Also noted is an invasion (*curved arrow*) of the right lung apex by the metastatic mediastinal mass.

subsequently regained after treatment. CT provides a comprehensive assessment of the large airways, mediastinal lymph nodes, and lung parenchymal abnormalities caused by TB infection.[1,3,76]

Fibrosing mediastinitis Fibrosing mediastinitis, also known as sclerosing mediastinitis or mediastinal fibrosis, is a disorder that is characterized by abnormal proliferation of dense acellular collagen and fibrous tissue in the mediastinum.[77] Although the exact cause for developing fibrosing mediastinitis is unknown, it has been postulated that it may be caused by an immunologic reaction to an infection or other allergens.[77] Among various known causes of fibrosing mediastinitis, *Histoplasma capsulatum* is the most common cause in pediatric patients in the United States.[1,77] Symptoms in patients with fibrosing mediastinitis are usually related to obstruction and compression of

mediastinal structures such as central airways, esophagus, or mediastinal large vessels.[77] Large airway involvement of fibrosing mediastinitis typically occurs at the level of carina and main bronchi.[77,78] On CT, fibrosing mediastinitis can present as 2 different patterns: focal or diffuse. The focal pattern (82%) usually presents as a soft tissue mass, which is often associated with calcification (63%) and may be localized in the right paratracheal, subcarinal, or hilar regions. In contrast, the diffuse pattern (18%) is characterized by a diffusely infiltrating mass without calcification and may affect entire mediastinal compartments (**Fig. 18**).[77,78] Focal pattern of fibrosing mediastinitis is known to be associated with histoplasmosis infection, whereas diffuse pattern is seen in patients with other idiopathic fibrosing disorders such as retroperitoneal fibrosis.[77,78] Current management for fibrosing mediastinitis includes

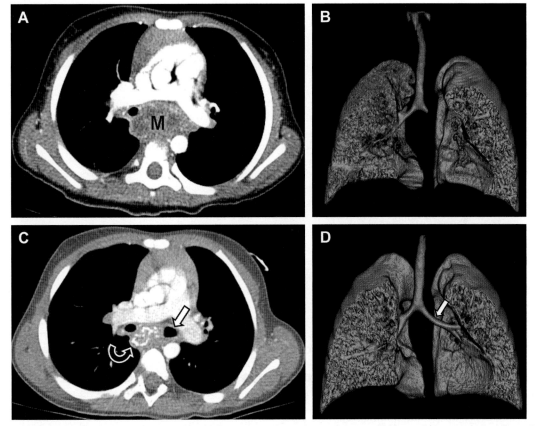

Fig. 17. TB infection with an obstruction of left mainstem bronchus in a 1-year-old boy who presented with respiratory distress, cough, fever, and abnormal chest radiographs. (*A*) Axial CT images show a complete obstruction of the left main stem bronchus by the heterogeneously enhancing subcarinal mass (M). (*B*) 3D external volume-rendered image shows an obstruction of left main stem bronchus. (*C*) Axial CT image obtained 1 year after treatment shows an interval resolution of the previously noted obstruction of the left main stem bronchus (*straight arrow*). Previously noted subcarinal lymphadenopathy (*curved arrow*) has been decreased in size and now partially calcified. (*D*) 3D external volume-rendered image obtained 1 year after treatment shows a patent left main stem bronchus (*arrow*).

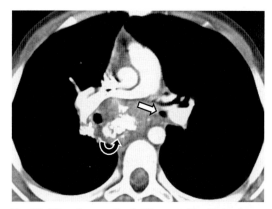

Fig. 18. Fibrosing mediastinitis caused by *Histoplasma capsulatum* infection in a 9-year-old girl who presented with 1-month history of cough and dyspnea. Axial CT image shows narrowing of the left main stem bronchus (*straight arrow*) from heterogeneously enhancing and partially calcified subcarinal soft tissue mass (*curved arrow*).

systemic antifungal or corticosteroid treatment, surgical resection, and local therapy for complications. CT can help correctly show the location and extent of airway narrowing caused by fibrosing mediastinitis before surgical resection.[1,3,77]

Acquired tracheobronchial stenoses

Acquired tracheobronchial stenoses in children are usually caused by previous instrumentation or surgery.[1] Most tracheal stenoses in pediatric patients are caused by previous long-term placement of an endotracheal tube or tracheostomy tube. Such stenoses occur secondary to initial pressure necrosis followed by subsequent development of ischemia and fibrosis of trachea at the level of the endotracheal tube balloon or tracheostomy stoma. On CT, focal proximal tracheal narrowing with eccentric or concentric soft tissue thickening caused by intimal hyperplasia is often seen (**Fig. 19**). The sensitivity and specificity of detecting postintubation stenosis with MDCT are 92% and 100% when compared with bronchoscopy.[79] Bronchial stenosis in children often occurs after lung transplantation at the site of surgical anastomosis.[80,81] MDCT with 2D and 3D reconstruction images can show the precise location and extent of tracheobronchial stenosis before surgical resection and end-to-end anastomosis or stent placement (**Fig. 20**). Obliquely located bronchial stenosis, which may be difficult to be completely evaluated with axial CT images alone, can be clearly visualized with 2D and 3D reconstruction MDCT images. MDCT with 2D and 3D reconstruction images can also provide

a noninvasive method for following up patients after surgery or interventional procedure.

Foreign body aspiration

Aspiration of a foreign body into the tracheobronchial airway remains a common cause of potentially serious respiratory distress in pediatric patients, particularly between 6 months and 3 years.[82,83] Factors that predispose children in this age group to aspirate foreign bodies include: (1) the tendency to insert small objects in their mouths; (2) the increased frequency to cry, run, and play with objects in the mouths; and (3) the lack of molars to adequately chew certain foods before swallowing.[82,83] Aspirated foreign bodies lodge in the bronchus more commonly than in the trachea. When located in the bronchus, the right side is more often affected than the left side. Although affected children may present with the classic clinical history of an acute choking episode followed by coughing, wheezing, and even stridor, children with foreign body aspiration sometimes are asymptomatic at presentation. Therefore, it is imperative to thoroughly evaluate both symptomatic and asymptomatic children with a reliable history of foreign body aspiration.[82,83]

Chest radiographs remain the initial imaging study of choice for evaluating foreign body aspiration in children.[83] Radiopaque foreign bodies, accounting for approximately 10% of all aspirated foreign bodies in the pediatric population, may be obvious on chest radiographs.[84] However, most foreign bodies aspirated by children are radiolucent, which limits the role of chest radiographs in many cases. The sensitivity and specificity of accurately detecting foreign body aspiration with chest radiographs in children are only 68% to 74% and 45% to 67%, respectively.[85,86] CT is the most sensitive diagnostic imaging modality for detecting foreign body aspiration in children. However, to avoid unnecessary ionizing radiation exposure, CT should be reserved for cases in which chest radiograph findings are negative or equivocal.

Several recent studies support the nearly 100% diagnostic accuracy of CT for correctly diagnosing foreign body aspiration in the tracheobronchial airway in children.[23,87,88] On CT, an aspirated foreign body typically presents as an obstructing mass with various attenuation within the tracheobronchial airway (**Fig. 21**). Secondary imaging findings of foreign body aspiration on CT include postobstructive air-trapping, atelectasis, and consolidation. MDCT with low radiation dose technique combined with postprocessing techniques such as 2D and 3D reconstruction images as well as cine imaging technique have been found to be highly accurate (100%) in correctly diagnosing

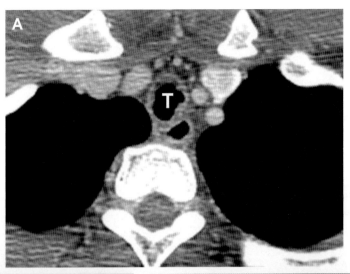

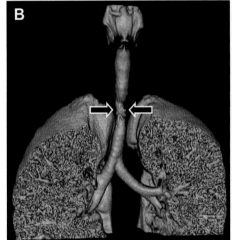
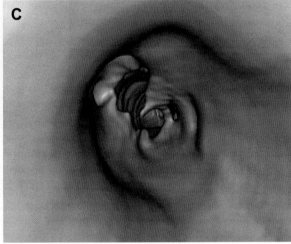

Fig. 19. Acquired tracheal stenosis caused by previous long-term placement of endotracheal tube in a 15-year-old boy. Diagnosis was confirmed by endoscopy. (*A*) Axial CT image shows an irregular thickening and narrowing of the trachea (T). (*B*) 3D external volume-rendered image shows short-segment narrowing (*arrows*) at the thoracic inlet level. (*C*) 3D internal volume-rendered image shows an irregular narrowing of the trachea.

foreign body aspiration in the tracheobronchial airway in pediatric patients.[88,89] Furthermore, a recent study in 9 children by Shin and colleagues[84] with either single-detector CT (55%) or MDCT (45%) reported that CT after bronchoscopy can provide additional diagnostic information regarding the presence and pattern of bronchial obstruction in children with a suspected residual foreign body.

Dynamic Large Airway Abnormality

TBM

TBM is a condition characterized by excessive expiratory collapse of the trachea or bronchi caused by underlying weakening of the airway walls or supporting cartilage.[90] There are 2 different types of TBM: primary (congenital) and secondary (acquired). Whereas the primary type in pediatric patients is usually associated with prematurity, congenital tracheoesophageal fistula or congenital abnormalities of cartilages, the secondary type is associated with previous endotracheal intubation, infection, surgery, and extrinsic compression from mediastinal vascular anomalies.[7,90]

Although TBM has recently been increasingly recognized as an important cause of chronic respiratory symptoms, this condition is still widely underdiagnosed because it escapes the detection with routine end-inspiratory CT imaging.[7] Therefore, it is important to obtain both inspiratory and

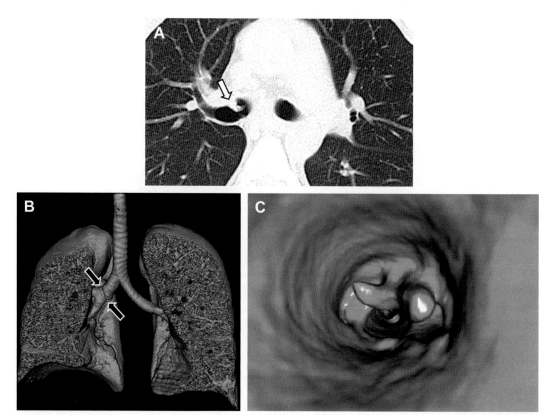

Fig. 20. Acquired bronchial stenosis in a 15-year-old girl with cystic fibrosis who presented with progressively worsening respiratory distress 2 years after lung transplantation. Bronchoscopy confirmed the right bronchial stenosis. (*A*) Axial CT image shows narrowing of the right main stem bronchus because of surgical scar and associated granulation tissue (*arrow*). (*B*) 3D external volume-rendered image shows surgical changes (*arrows*) of the right main stem bronchus. However, surgical scar and associated granulation tissue protruding into the airway lumen seen on axial CT image (see Fig. 20A) are not well shown. (*C*) 3D internal volume-rendered image shows the shape and size of the surgical scar and associated granulation tissue located inside the bronchial lumen.

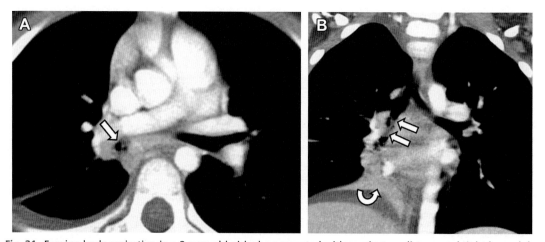

Fig. 21. Foreign body aspiration in a 3-year-old girl who presented with respiratory distress and right lower lobe opacity on chest radiographs. Endoscopy confirmed retained peanut fragments. (*A*) Axial CT image shows endoluminal low-attenuation materials (*arrow*) within the right bronchus intermedius. (*B*) Coronal CT image show endoluminal low-attenuation materials (*straight arrow*) within the right bronchus intermedius and postobstructive atelectasis (*curved arrow*). (*Case courtesy of* Ricardo Restrepo, MD, Miami Children's Hospital.)

expiratory MDCT images in children suspected of having TBM. The current CT diagnosis of TBM in pediatric patients is based on tracheobronchial collapse greater than 50% in the cross-sectional luminal area on expiration, which is the same criterion applied at bronchoscopy (**Fig. 22**).[7,9,31,32]

Although chest radiographs and fluorosocopy have historically been used for evaluating TBM in pediatric patients, these techniques are limited, particularly for precisely assessing the extent of the disease. Objective and quantitative assessment of TBM can now be accurately obtained with MDCT. MDCT can provide a comprehensive

evaluation of TBM by precisely localizing the site of malacia, determining the degree and extent of disease, identifying predisposing conditions, and providing objective preoperative and postoperative assessments (see **Fig. 22**).[7]

Recently, paired inspiratory-expiratory MDCT study has been shown to be a reliable technique for diagnosing TBM in pediatric patients with mediastinal aortic anomalies. In a series of 9 symptomatic pediatric patients with mediastinal aortic anomalies who had bronchoscopically proven malacia, Lee and colleagues[32] showed that paired inspiratory-expiratory MDCT correctly diagnosed

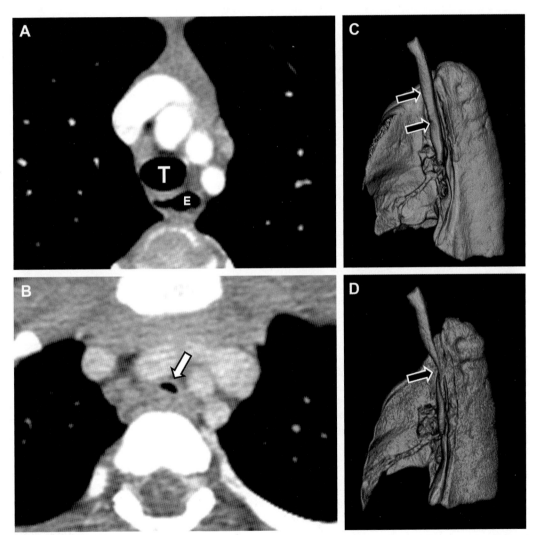

Fig. 22. Tracheomalacia in an 11-year-old boy who presented with recurrent respiratory distress and pneumonia. Endoscopy showed marked tracheomalacia in the mid-to-distal trachea. (*A*) Axial CT image obtained at end-inspiration shows patent trachea (T). E, esophagus. (*B*) Axial CT image obtained at end-expiration shows an almost complete collapse of trachea (*arrow*) consistent with CT diagnosis of tracheomalacia. (*C*) Sagittal view of the 3D external volume-rendered image shows patent trachea (*arrows*). (*D*) Sagittal view of the 3D external volume-rendered image shows a focal collapse of the trachea (*arrow*). Also noted is decreased overall lung volume at end-expiration.

tracheomalacia in all cases. The results of this study showed the need for potential routine use of paired inspiratory-expiratory MDCT in the preoperative evaluation of pediatric patients with mediastinal aortic anomalies.

In addition to evaluating the large airways, CT is also helpful for assessing air-trapping, which has recently been found to be associated with the presence of tracheomalacia in children.[91]

Although paired inspiratory-expiratory MDCT imaging technique is the mainstay of imaging in pediatric patients with suspected TBM, recent advances in MDCT have paved the way for cine imaging with 64 MDCT scanners and dynamic 4D imaging with state-of-the-art 320 MDCT scanners. Such new imaging techniques may play an important role in evaluating dynamic large airway disease such as TBM in pediatric patients. Future studies are needed focusing on optimal radiation dose reduction techniques and the added diagnostic value of these techniques in comparison with traditional inspiration–expiration methods for evaluating TBM in children.

SUMMARY

Recent advances in MDCT technology have given rise to dramatic improvements in the noninvasive and comprehensive assessment of the large airways in pediatric patients. In particular, superb-quality 2D and 3D reconstruction MDCT images have revolutionized the display of large airways and substantially enhanced the ability to diagnose various large airway diseases in children. Furthermore, the recent advent of the 320 MDCT scanner, which can provide combined detailed anatomic and dynamic functional information assessment of the large airways, is highly promising for the accurate assessment of dynamic large airway diseases such as TBM. Understanding the proper MDCT and postprocessing imaging techniques, as well as the characteristic MDCT imaging appearance of various large airway diseases in children, will aid in accurate diagnosis and thus contribute to optimal patient care.

REFERENCES

1. Lee EY. Pediatric airways disorders: large airways. In: Lynch DA, Boiselle PM, editors. CT of the airways. Totowa (NJ): Humana; 2008. p. 351.
2. Lee EY. Advancing CT and MR imaging of the lungs and airways in children: imaging into practice. Pediatr Radiol 2008;38(Suppl 2):S208.
3. Lee EY, Siegel MJ. MDCT of tracheobronchial narrowing in pediatric patients. J Thorac Imaging 2007;22:300.
4. Papaioannou G, Young C, Owens CM. Multidetector row CT for imaging the paediatric tracheobronchial tree. Pediatr Radiol 2007;37:515.
5. Siegel MJ. Multiplanar and three-dimensional multidetector row CT of thoracic vessels and airways in the pediatric population. Radiology 2003;229:641.
6. Lee EY, Boiselle PM, Cleveland RH. Multidetector CT evaluation of congenital lung anomalies. Radiology 2008;247:632.
7. Lee EY, Boiselle PM. Tracheobronchomalacia in infants and children: multidetector CT evaluation. Radiology 2009;252:7.
8. Lee EY, Siegel MJ, Hildebolt CF, et al. MDCT evaluation of thoracic aortic anomalies in pediatric patients and young adults: comparison of axial, multiplanar, and 3D images. AJR Am J Roentgenol 2004;182:777.
9. Lee EY, Litmanovich D, Boiselle PM. Multidetector CT evaluation of tracheobronchomalacia. Radiol Clin North Am 2009;47:261.
10. Baroni RH, Feller-Kopman D, Nishino M, et al. Tracheobronchomalacia: comparison between end-expiratory and dynamic expiratory CT for evaluation of central airway collapse. Radiology 2005;235:635.
11. Boiselle PM, Lee KS, Lin S, et al. Cine CT during coughing for assessment of tracheomalacia: preliminary experience with 64-MDCT. AJR Am J Roentgenol 2006;187:W175.
12. Wagnetz U, Roberts HC, Chung T, et al. Dynamic airway evaluation with volume CT: initial experience. Can Assoc Radiol J 2010;61:90.
13. Kroft LJ, Roelofs JJ, Geleijns J. Scan time and patient dose for thoracic imaging in neonates and small children using axial volumetric 320-detector row CT compared to helical 64-, 32-, and 16-detector row CT acquisitions. Pediatr Radiol 2010; 40:294.
14. Lee EY, Strauss KJ, Tracy DA, et al. Comparison of standard-dose and reduced-dose expiratory MDCT techniques for assessment of tracheomalacia in children. Acad Radiol 2010;17:504.
15. Honda O, Johkoh T, Yamamoto S, et al. Comparison of quality of multiplanar reconstructions and direct coronal multidetector CT scans of the lung. AJR Am J Roentgenol 2002;179:875.
16. Salvolini L, Bichi Secchi E, Costarelli L, et al. Clinical applications of 2D and 3D CT imaging of the airways–a review. Eur J Radiol 2000;34:9.
17. Beigelman-Aubry C, Brillet PY, Grenier PA. MDCT of the airways: technique and normal results. Radiol Clin North Am 2009;47:185.
18. Lee KS, Boiselle PM. Multidetector computed tomography of the central airways. In: Ernst A, editor. Introduction to bronchoscopy. New York: Cambridge University Press; 2009. p. 17.
19. Wittram C, Batt J, Rappaport DC, et al. Inspiratory and expiratory helical CT of normal adults:

comparison of thin section scans and minimum intensity projection images. J Thorac Imaging 2002;17:47.

20. Lee KS, Boiselle PM. Update on multidetector computed tomography imaging of the airways. J Thorac Imaging 2010;25:112.

21. Javidan-Nejad C. MDCT of trachea and main bronchi. Radiol Clin North Am 2010;48:157.

22. Sodhi KS, Aiyappan SK, Saxena AK, et al. Utility of multidetector CT and virtual bronchoscopy in tracheobronchial obstruction in children. Acta Paediatr 2010;99:1011.

23. Adaletli I, Kurugoglu S, Ulus S, et al. Utilization of low-dose multidetector CT and virtual bronchoscopy in children with suspected foreign body aspiration. Pediatr Radiol 2007;37:33.

24. Honnef D, Wildberger JE, Das M, et al. Value of virtual tracheobronchoscopy and bronchography from 16-slice multidetector-row spiral computed tomography for assessment of suspected tracheobronchial stenosis in children. Eur Radiol 2006;16:1684.

25. Remy-Jardin M, Remy J, Artaud D, et al. Volume rendering of the tracheobronchial tree: clinical evaluation of bronchographic images. Radiology 1998; 208:761.

26. Naidich DP, Gruden JF, McGuinness G, et al. Volumetric (helical/spiral) CT (VCT) of the airways. J Thorac Imaging 1997;12:11.

27. Boiselle PM, Ernst A. Recent advances in central airway imaging. Chest 2002;121:1651.

28. Boiselle PM, Reynolds KF, Ernst A. Multiplanar and three-dimensional imaging of the central airways with multidetector CT. AJR Am J Roentgenol 2002; 179:301.

29. Remy-Jardin M, Remy J, Artaud D, et al. Tracheobronchial tree: assessment with volume rendering–technical aspects. Radiology 1998;208:393.

30. Heyer CM, Nuesslein TG, Jung D, et al. Tracheobronchial anomalies and stenoses: detection with low-dose multidetector CT with virtual tracheobronchoscopy–comparison with flexible tracheobronchoscopy. Radiology 2007;242:542.

31. Lee EY, Mason KP, Zurakowski D, et al. MDCT assessment of tracheomalacia in symptomatic infants with mediastinal aortic vascular anomalies: preliminary technical experience. Pediatr Radiol 2008;38:82.

32. Lee EY, Zurakowski D, Waltz DA, et al. MDCT evaluation of the prevalence of tracheomalacia in children with mediastinal aortic vascular anomalies. J Thorac Imaging 2008;23:258.

33. Berrocal T, Madrid C, Novo S, et al. Congenital anomalies of the tracheobronchial tree, lung, and mediastinum: embryology, radiology, and pathology. Radiographics 2004;24:e17.

34. Bennett EC, Holinger LD. Congenital malformations of the trachea and bronchi. In: Bluestone CD,

Stool SE, editors. Pediatric otolaryngology. 4th edition. Philadelphia: Saunders; 2002. p. 1473.

35. Ghaye B, Szapiro D, Fanchamps JM, et al. Congenital bronchial abnormalities revisited. Radiographics 2001;21:105.

36. O'Sullivan BP, Frassica JJ, Rayder SM. Tracheal bronchus: a cause of prolonged atelectasis in intubated children. Chest 1998;113:537.

37. Ghaye B, Kos X, Dondelinger RF. Accessory cardiac bronchus: 3D CT demonstration in nine cases. Eur Radiol 1999;9:45.

38. McGuinness G, Naidich DP, Garay SM, et al. Accessory cardiac bronchus: CT features and clinical significance. Radiology 1993;189:563.

39. Freeman SJ, Harvey JE, Goddard PR. Demonstration of supernumerary tracheal bronchus by computed tomographic scanning and magnetic resonance imaging. Thorax 1995;50:426.

40. Lee EY, Boiselle PM, Shamberger RC. Multidetector computed tomography and 3-dimensional imaging: preoperative evaluation of thoracic vascular and tracheobronchial anomalies and abnormalities in pediatric patients. J Pediatr Surg 2010;45:811.

41. Lee EY. MDCT and 3D evaluation of type 2 hypoplastic pulmonary artery sling associated with right lung agenesis, hypoplastic aortic arch, and long segment tracheal stenosis. J Thorac Imaging 2007; 22:346.

42. Webb WR. The trachea. In: Webb WR, Higgins CB, editors. Thoracic imaging. 1st edition. Philadelphia: Lippincott Williams & Wilkins; 2005. p. 411.

43. Beasley SW, Qi BQ. Understanding tracheomalacia. J Paediatr Child Health 1998;34:209.

44. Laing MR, Albert DM, Quinney RE, et al. Tracheal stenosis in infants and young children. J Laryngol Otol 1990;104:229.

45. Berdon WE. Rings, slings, and other things: vascular compression of the infant trachea updated from the midcentury to the millennium–the legacy of Robert E. Gross, MD, and Edward B. D. Neuhauser, MD. Radiology 2000;216:624.

46. Oguz B, Haliloglu M, Karcaaltincaba M. Paediatric multidetector CT angiography: spectrum of congenital thoracic vascular anomalies. Br J Radiol 2007; 80:376.

47. Predey TA, McDonald V, Demos TC, et al. CT of congenital anomalies of the aortic arch. Semin Roentgenol 1989;24:96.

48. Alsenaidi K, Gurofsky R, Karamlou T, et al. Management and outcomes of double aortic arch in 81 patients. Pediatrics 2006;118:e1336.

49. Backer CL, Mavroudis C, Rigsby CK, et al. Trends in vascular ring surgery. J Thorac Cardiovasc Surg 2005;129:1339.

50. Chan MS, Chu WC, Cheung KL, et al. Angiography and dynamic airway evaluation with MDCT in the diagnosis of double aortic arch associated with

tracheomalacia. AJR Am J Roentgenol 2005;185: 1248.

51. Oshima Y, Yamaguchi M, Yoshimura N, et al. Management of pulmonary artery sling associated with tracheal stenosis. Ann Thorac Surg 2008;86: 1334.

52. Kagadis GC, Panagiotopoulou EC, Priftis KN, et al. Preoperative evaluation of the trachea in a child with pulmonary artery sling using 3-dimensional computed tomographic imaging and virtual bronchoscopy. J Pediatr Surg 2007;42:E9.

53. Gross RE, Neuhauser EB. Compression of the trachea by an anomalous innominate artery; an operation for its relief. Am J Dis Child 1948;75:570.

54. Strife JL, Baumel AS, Dunbar JS. Tracheal compression by the innominate artery in infancy and childhood. Radiology 1981;139:73.

55. Berdon WE, Baker DH, Bordiuk J, et al. Innominate artery compression of the trachea in infants with stridor and apnea. Radiology 1969;92:272.

56. Wiatrak BJ. Congenital anomalies of the larynx and trachea. Otolaryngol Clin North Am 2000;33:91.

57. Hawkins JA, Bailey WW, Clark SM. Innominate artery compression of the trachea. Treatment by reimplantation of the innominate artery. J Thorac Cardiovasc Surg 1992;103:678.

58. Adler SC, Isaacson G, Balsara RK. Innominate artery compression of the trachea: diagnosis and treatment by anterior suspension. A 25-year experience. Ann Otol Rhinol Laryngol 1995;104:924.

59. McCarthy MJ, Rosado-de-Christenson ML. Tumors of the trachea. J Thorac Imaging 1995;10:180.

60. Shikhani AH, Jones MM, Marsh BR, et al. Infantile subglottic hemangiomas. An update. Ann Otol Rhinol Laryngol 1986;95:336.

61. Koplewitz BZ, Springer C, Slasky BS, et al. CT of hemangiomas of the upper airways in children. AJR Am J Roentgenol 2005;184:663.

62. Pransky SM, Kang DR. Tumors of the larynx, trachea, and bronchi. In: Bluestone CD, Stool SE, Alper CM, et al, editors. Pediatric otolaryngology. 4th edition. Philadelphia: Saunders; 2002. p. 1558.

63. Benjamin B, Parsons DS. Recurrent respiratory papillomatosis: a 10 year study. J Laryngol Otol 1988; 102:1022.

64. Bellah RD, Mahboubi S, Berdon WE. Malignant endobronchial lesions of adolescence. Pediatr Radiol 1992;22:563.

65. Chong S, Lee KS, Chung MJ, et al. Neuroendocrine tumors of the lung: clinical, pathologic, and imaging findings. Radiographics 2006;26:41.

66. Connor GF, Fishman EK. Endobronchial carcinoid in a child: depiction with three-dimensional volume rendering. Pediatr Radiol 2004;34:1008.

67. Yikilmaz A, Lee EY. CT imaging of mass-like nonvascular pulmonary lesions in children. Pediatr Radiol 2007;37:1253.

68. Granata C, Battistini E, Toma P, et al. Mucoepidermoid carcinoma of the bronchus: a case report and review of the literature. Pediatr Pulmonol 1997; 23:226.

69. Lee EY, Vargas SO, Sawicki GS, et al. Mucoepidermoid carcinoma of bronchus in a pediatric patient: (18)F-FDG PET findings. Pediatr Radiol 2007;37: 1278.

70. Kim TS, Lee KS, Han J, et al. Mucoepidermoid carcinoma of the tracheobronchial tree: radiographic and CT findings in 12 patients. Radiology 1999;212:643.

71. Colby TV, Koss MN, Travis WD. Carcinoid and other neuroendocrine tumors. In: Colby TV, Koss MN, Travis WD, editors, Atlas of tumor pathology: tumors of the lower respiratory tract, vol. 13. Washington, DC: Armed Forces Institute of Pathology; 1995. p. 287.

72. Merten DF. Diagnostic imaging of mediastinal masses in children. AJR Am J Roentgenol 1992; 158:825.

73. Blickman JG, Parker BR, Barnes PD: In Pediatric radiology: the requisites. Philadelphia: Mosby Elsevier; 2009. p. 45.

74. Perger L, Lee EY, Shamberger RC. Management of children and adolescents with a critical airway due to compression by an anterior mediastinal mass. J Pediatr Surg 2008;43:1990.

75. WHO. Communicable diseases, tuberculosis, factsheets. Available at: http://www.searo.who.int/en/ Section10/Section2097/Section2106_10681.htm. Accessed March 1, 2011. WHO Regional Office for South-East Asia 2010, 2006, vol. 2011; 2011.

76. du Plessis J, Goussard P, Andronikou S, et al. Comparing three-dimensional volume-rendered CT images with fibreoptic tracheobronchoscopy in the evaluation of airway compression caused by tuberculous lymphadenopathy in children. Pediatr Radiol 2009;39:694.

77. Rossi SE, McAdams HP, Rosado-de-Christenson ML, et al. Fibrosing mediastinitis. Radiographics 2001; 21:737.

78. Sherrick AD, Brown LR, Harms GF, et al. The radiographic findings of fibrosing mediastinitis. Chest 1994;106:484.

79. Sun M, Ernst A, Boiselle PM. MDCT of the central airways: comparison with bronchoscopy in the evaluation of complications of endotracheal and tracheostomy tubes. J Thorac Imaging 2007;22:136.

80. McAdams HP, Palmer SM, Erasmus JJ, et al. Bronchial anastomotic complications in lung transplant recipients: virtual bronchoscopy for noninvasive assessment. Radiology 1998;209:689.

81. Medina LS, Siegel MJ, Glazer HS, et al. Diagnosis of pulmonary complications associated with lung transplantation in children: value of CT vs histopathologic studies. AJR Am J Roentgenol 1994;162:969.

82. Reilly JS, Cook SP, Stool D, et al. Prevention and management of aerodigestive foreign body injuries in childhood. Pediatr Clin North Am 1996;43:1403.

83. Rovin JD, Rodgers BM. Pediatric foreign body aspiration. Pediatr Rev 2000;21:86.

84. Shin SM, Kim WS, Cheon JE, et al. CT in children with suspected residual foreign body in airway after bronchoscopy. AJR Am J Roentgenol 2009;192:1744.

85. Silva AB, Muntz HR, Clary R. Utility of conventional radiography in the diagnosis and management of pediatric airway foreign bodies. Ann Otol Rhinol Laryngol 1998;107:834.

86. Svedstrom E, Puhakka H, Kero P. How accurate is chest radiography in the diagnosis of tracheobronchial foreign bodies in children? Pediatr Radiol 1989;19:520.

87. Bai W, Zhou X, Gao X, et al. The value of chest CT in the diagnosis and management of tracheobronchial foreign bodies. Pediatr Int 2010. DOI:10.1111/j.1442-200X.2010.03299.x. [Epub ahead of print].

88. Hong SJ, Goo HW, Roh JL. Utility of spiral and cine CT scans in pediatric patients suspected of aspirating radiolucent foreign bodies. Otolaryngol Head Neck Surg 2008;138:576.

89. Kosucu P, Ahmetoglu A, Koramaz I, et al. Low-dose MDCT and virtual bronchoscopy in pediatric patients with foreign body aspiration. AJR Am J Roentgenol 2004;183:1771.

90. Carden KA, Boiselle PM, Waltz DA, et al. Tracheomalacia and tracheobronchomalacia in children and adults: an in-depth review. Chest 2005;127:984.

91. Lee EY, Tracy DA, Bastos M, et al. Expiratory volumetric MDCT evaluation of air trapping in pediatric patients with and without tracheomalacia. AJR Am J Roentgenol 2010;194:1210.

Pneumonia in Normal and Immunocompromised Children: An Overview and Update

Hedieh K. Eslamy, MD, Beverley Newman, MD*

KEYWORDS

• Pneumonia • Children • Imaging • Complicated pneumonia

Pneumonia is an infection of the lower respiratory tract, involving the lung parenchyma. The World Health Organization estimates that there are 150.7 million cases of pulmonary infection each year in children younger than 5 years, with as many as 20 million cases severe enough to require hospital admission.[1] In North America and Europe, the annual incidence of pneumonia in children younger than 5 years is estimated to be 34 to 40 cases per 1000, and decreases to 7 cases per 1000 in adolescents 12 to 15 years of age.[2,3] The mortality in pediatric patients caused by pneumonia in developed countries is currently low (<1 per 1000 per year).[3] However, pneumonia is still the number one cause of childhood mortality in developing countries.[1,4] The overarching goal of this article is to review cause, current role of imaging, imaging techniques, and the spectrum of acute and chronic pneumonias in children. Pneumonia in the neonate and immunocompromised host is also discussed.

CAUSE OF PNEUMONIA

Infectious agents causing pneumonia in children include viruses, bacteria, mycobacteria, mycoplasmas, fungi, protozoa, and helminths. Etiologic diagnoses of pneumonia are not so easy to determine or so accurate as is sometimes implied. In addition, proof of the cause of pneumonia is not obtained in most cases. There is a great deal of overlap in the radiographic appearance of pneumonias caused by different organisms. Imaging is usually poor at predicting the broad category (eg, bacterial vs viral) of infectious agent, let alone the specific agent. Preexisting lung disease may not only predispose to pulmonary infection but also modify the appearance of pulmonary consolidation. Furthermore, because the lungs can respond to a diverse disease processes in only a limited number of ways, it is common for the radiographic features of both acute and chronic infectious pneumonia to overlap considerably with many noninfectious lung diseases. Such noninfectious lung diseases are identified as pneumonia mimics in this article.

Viral pneumonia is rare in the neonatal period, because of conferred maternal antibody protection, whereas bacterial pneumonia is most frequently caused by pathogens acquired during labor and delivery, and is more prevalent in premature babies. With decreasing maternal antibody levels, viral pneumonia occurs at a peak between 2 months to 2 years of age. Bacterial infections become relatively more common in older children from 2 years to 18 years of age.[5] The lung response to an infective antigen seems to be more age-specific than antigen-dependent (ie, bacteria vs viral). Therefore, lobar and alveolar lung opacities

The authors have nothing to disclose.

Department of Radiology, Lucile Packard Children's Hospital, Stanford University School of Medicine, 725 Welch Road, Stanford, CA 94305, USA

* Corresponding author.

E-mail address: bevn@stanford.edu

Radiol Clin N Am 49 (2011) 895–920

doi:10.1016/j.rcl.2011.06.007

are more common in older children and are more frequently caused by bacterial infections, whereas interstitial opacities are seen in all age groups, and are relatively nonspecific as to the type of causative organism.[6,7]

ROLE OF IMAGING AND IMAGING TECHNIQUES

The role of imaging, including chest radiographs, ultrasound (US) and computed tomography (CT), is to detect the presence of pneumonia, determine its location and extent, exclude other thoracic causes of respiratory symptoms, and show complications such as parapneumonic effusion/empyema and suppurative lung complications.[5] Although magnetic resonance (MR) imaging is not routinely used for evaluating pneumonia in children, it is a promising imaging modality particularly for children with chronic lung conditions who require repeat imaging studies.

Frontal and lateral chest radiographs are the mainstay, and often the only, imaging needed in pediatric pulmonary infection. This imaging can be supplemented with other views such as lateral decubitus or other imaging modalities as the circumstances warrant. Decubitus views are not useful when an entire hemithorax is opacified because layering fluid cannot be identified without any adjacent air. The main use of US is to identify, quantify, and characterize a parapneumonic effusion/empyema, as well as provide image guidance for drainage and identify residual collections after treatment.[8,9] Operator availability and expertise are important factors in making US a useful tool for evaluating pulmonary infection. Although intrapulmonary fluid-filled cavities and even lung abscesses within consolidated lung can be identified on US, CT provides a more global view of the disease process. CT is often used to further evaluate: (1) suppurative lung complications and to differentiate these from parapneumonic effusion/empyema; (2) patients with recurrent or chronic pneumonia and concern for an underlying lesion; and (3) immunocompromised children with noncontributory or confusing chest radiographs and clinical findings that could be secondary to lung infection.[5]

Close attention to CT technique is crucial for imaging evaluation of pneumonia in pediatric patients. CT with low radiation dose technique should be carefully performed in all cases. Eighty to 120 kVp with weight-based low milliampere-seconds coupled with radiation dose modulation techniques is appropriate in most children for evaluation of pneumonia. Multiple CT image acquisitions are usually not needed and the scan field of view should be tailored to the area of interest (especially if following a specific lesion serially over time) to further decrease the overall radiation dose.[10] Occasionally, it may be useful to acquire additional expiratory scans to assess air trapping, which is an early imaging finding associated with small airway disease. In this situation, often at least 1 or both CT acquisitions can be obtained using a high-resolution CT (HRCT) gap technique. To obtain optimal CT imaging at peak inspiration and close to expiratory residual volume, controlled ventilation (CViCT) in infants and young children ($\leq$5 years old) or spirometer-controlled CT in older children may be needed.[11] Young children have little intrinsic tissue contrast. Therefore, intravenous contrast is almost always needed for CT imaging of infection especially if mediastinal delineation is required. The exception is when HRCT is used only for evaluating lung parenchymal and airway disease. Breath-holding is usually desirable but can be adapted on a case-by-case basis depending on the needs of the study and the ability of the child to cooperate. However, for the study to be interpretable, gross patient motion should be absent. Sedation or anesthesia may be required in infants, young children, or children with intellectual disability. Delays between induction of anesthesia and scanning need to be minimized to prevent the potential for lung atelectasis with anesthesia. The anesthesiologist needs to pay close attention to techniques for preventing atelectasis or recruiting lung before the CT imaging.[12]

Peltola and colleagues[13] recently published their experience with MR imaging of lung infections in children using free-breathing T2-weighted, short tau inversion recovery, and T1-weighted with fat saturation precontrast and postcontrast sequences. Their study showed that lung parenchymal, pleural, and lymph node inflammatory abnormalities can be characterized by MR imaging in children with lung infection. Therefore, MR imaging might potentially be used to further evaluate suspected, acute complications of pneumonia.[13] Children with chronic lung conditions and recurrent infection, such as cystic fibrosis, who are often subjected to substantial radiation exposure from repeated CT studies, would benefit the most from MR imaging evaluation of the lungs instead of CT. Although MR imaging may not provide as much detail compared with CT especially with early, small or subtle changes (**Fig. 1**), there are promising indications of a role for MR imaging in pulmonary infection.[13–15]

RADIOGRAPHIC CHANGES IN RESPIRATORY INFECTION

There are several different descriptions of basic patterns of lung diseases on chest radiographs.

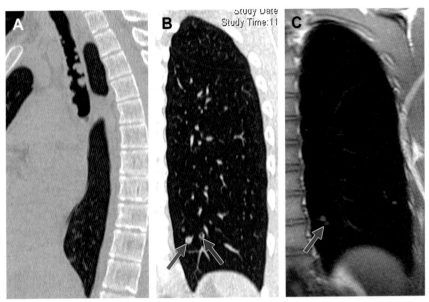

Fig. 1. Chronic lung nodules in respiratory papillomatosis in a 17-year-old male. *(A)* Sagittal contrast-enhanced (CE) CT image shows multiple intraluminal, multilobulated, nodular lesions in the trachea. *(B)* Coronal lung window CT image shows several solid parenchymal nodules *(red arrow)* in the left lower lobe. Cavitation is seen in one of the nodules *(blue arrow)*. *(C)* Follow-up, coronal double-inversion recovery, MR imaging 7 weeks after CT shows the same nodules although only the larger nodule *(arrow)* seen on previous CT could be appreciated on MR imaging.

In this review article, we adopt the one described by Hansell and colleagues.[16] Almost all of these are seen as part of the spectrum of infectious lung disease (**Table 1**).

BRONCHIOLITIS VERSUS PNEUMONIA

Pneumonia and bronchiolitis are both common in infants and have overlapping clinical and imaging features. Many studies, particularly those in the developing world, use the term acute lower respiratory tract illness and make no attempt to differentiate pneumonia from bronchiolitis.[17]

Bronchiolitis occurs in children less than 2 years of age, who typically present with cough, coryza, and wheezing. Bronchiolitis is a major cause of morbidity and mortality in infants.[18] Respiratory syncytial virus (RSV) is the most common cause

---

Table 1
Radiographic changes in respiratory infection

Radiographic Pattern	Examples of Radiographic Pattern in Specific Pneumonias
Airspace opacities	Lobar pneumonia, round pneumonia, and bronchopneumonia
Atelectasis (collapse)	Lobar, patchy, subsegmental, linear, or discoid atelectasis may be associated with bronchiolitis and interstitial pneumonia
Linear and bandlike opacities	Bronchial/peribronchial thickening in bronchiolitis; discoid atelectasis
Cysts and bullae	Pneumatoceles, cavitary necrosis, lung abscess
Nodules and masses (solitary and multiple)	Fungal infections, septic emboli
Diffuse nodular and reticulonodular opacities	
1. Diffuse bilateral small nodular opacities	Tuberculous and nontuberculous infections
2. Diffuse bilateral reticular or reticulonodular opacities	Interstitial pneumonia
3. Diffuse ground-glass opacities	Noncardiogenic pulmonary edema (ARDS) related to sepsis or diffuse pneumonias such as pneumocystis in the immunocompromised host

of bronchiolitis, followed by rhinovirus. Other less common causes of bronchiolitis include parainfluenza virus, human metapneumovirus, adenovirus, influenza virus, coronaviruses, and human bocavirus. Chest radiographs usually show hyperinflation, perihilar opacities, peribronchial thickening, and patchy, often mobile, atelectasis (**Fig. 2**). Such imaging findings are related to diffuse airway inflammation and partial (air trapping) or complete (atelectasis) airway obstruction.[19] Similar changes are seen in older children (>2 years of age) with bronchitis although the features of diffuse small airway obstruction are less common in these older children with larger airways.

SPECTRUM OF PNEUMONIA

Pneumonia can be divided into several syndromes based on clinical presentation, imaging appearance, underlying predisposition, and cause. Pneumonia syndromes that are discussed in this article include acute focal pneumonia, atypical pneumonia, miliary or nodular pneumonia, progressive or fulminant pneumonia, aspiration pneumonias, pulmonary infiltrates with eosinophilia (PIE), and chronic or recurrent pneumonia.[20] Neonatal pneumonia is briefly highlighted separately. Pneumonia in immunosuppressed individuals is included in the general discussion of pneumonia syndromes and then specifically reviewed with regard to the different infections associated with various types of immunodeficiency. Acute and chronic complications of pneumonia are also reviewed.

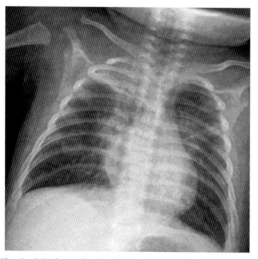

Fig. 2. RSV bronchiolitis in a 6- week-old boy. Frontal chest radiograph shows perihilar streaky opacities, peribronchial thickening, hyperinflation, and patchy atelectasis.

Acute Focal Pneumonia

Characteristics that are typical for acute focal pneumonia include fever more than 38.8°C (102°F), a toxic appearance, and a focal opacity on chest radiographs. Pleuritic chest pain in lower-lobe pneumonia is sometimes referred to the abdomen and may be mistaken clinically for an acute abdominal condition. Acute focal pneumonia is most often caused by bacterial infection with streptococcus pneumonia. Other causes of acute focal pneumonia are summarized in **Box 1**. The chest radiograph of acute focal pneumonia usually shows a dense, typically more peripheral airspace opacity, which may appear segmental, lobar, or spherical (**Figs. 3** and **4**).[21–23] In a febrile child with a spherical density on a chest radiograph, the most likely diagnosis is a round pneumonia but the possibility of an underlying neoplasm may be considered. Round pneumonias tend to be solitary, have well-defined borders, and are often located in the perihilar region or posteriorly in the lungs. The radiograph should be carefully scrutinized for features of consolidation such as air bronchograms as opposed to those of a mass such as vascular/airway displacement or bony erosion. A second view such as a lateral radiograph may be helpful because a round pneumonia

---

Box 1
Causes of acute focal pneumonia in children

Usual

Streptococcus pneumonia

Uncommon

Bacteria: *Hemophilus influenzae* type B, nontypable *H influenza*, *Staphylococcus aureus*, group A streptococcus, *Mycoplasma pneumoniae*, *Chlamydia pneumoniae*

Rare

Bacteria and mycobacteria: *Francisella tularensis*, *Mycobacterium tuberculosis*, *Meningococcus*, enteric bacteria

Viruses (usually lobular): RSV, parainfluenza, adenovirus, human metapneumo virus

Fungi: *Histoplasma*, other systemic fungi

Data from Fisher RG, Boyce TG. Pneumonia syndromes. In: Fisher RG, Boyce TG, editors. Moffet's pediatric infectious diseases: a problem-oriented approach. 4th edition. Philadelphia: Lippincott Williams & Wilkins; 2005. p. 174–221; and Brodzinski H, Ruddy RM. Review of new and newly discovered respiratory tract viruses in children. Pediatr Emerg Care 2009;25(5): 352–60.

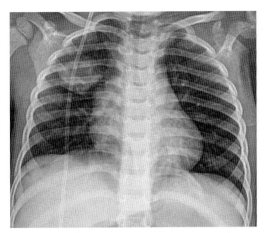

Fig. 3. Acute focal pneumonia (ie, round pneumonia) in a 3-year-old boy. Frontal chest radiograph shows a spherical consolidation in the right upper lobe. Follow-up chest radiograph after treatment showed interval resolution of this spherical consolidation.

is often less masslike in appearance on an orthogonal view. This is one of the few scenarios in which radiologic follow-up after about 2 weeks may be useful to document interval resolution of acute pneumonia.[22] Acute respiratory distress may be secondary to an intrathoracic mass causing airway or lung compression, especially when there is complete opacification of a hemithorax on radiographs (**Fig. 5**). Intrapulmonary masses including both benign and malignant entities may present clinically with acute superinfection. In addition, other conditions or anatomic variants may be mistaken for pneumonia when a chest radiograph is obtained in a child with a fever and respiratory symptoms.

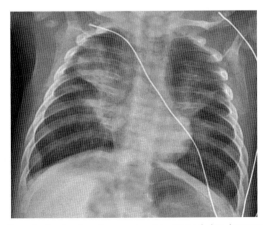

Fig. 4. Acute focal pneumonia caused by human metapneumovirus in a 3-month-old boy. Frontal chest radiograph shows multiple focal pulmonary consolidations bilaterally.

Atypical Pneumonia

Atypical features in pneumonia include prominent extrapulmonary features (eg, headache, sore throat, and pharyngeal exudates), minimal or disparate chest signs on physical examination, subacute onset, nonfocal lung opacity on chest radiographs, lack of clinical response to antibiotics, lack of substantial leukocytosis, and a slow disease course. Common infectious causes of atypical pneumonia are summarized in **Box 2**. On chest radiographs, the pulmonary opacity is seen as either airspace, reticular (linear), or bandlike opacities in a nonfocal, patchy, or mottled distribution, with various degrees of density, usually without a single dense area of consolidation (**Fig. 6**). Most patients with atypical pneumonia can be classified into one of the following subgroups or a combination of two of them based on findings on chest radiographs:[20]

Acute interstitial pneumonia

Chest radiographs show a patchy, nonfocal reticular pattern. Causes of acute interstitial pneumonia include self-limited viral infections and other pathogens.

Subacute minimal patchy pneumonia

Chest radiographs show 1 or more patches of minimal foci of airspace opacity. The most common causes of subacute minimal patchy pneumonia are *Mycoplasma pneumoniae*, *Chlamydia pneumoniae,* and adenoviruses.

Subacute dense focal pneumonia

Chest radiographs show a dense focal airspace opacity that is segmental or subsegmental. Most of the other features of acute focal pneumonia are absent. Tuberculosis needs to be excluded in these patients.

Most children exposed to *Mycobacterium tuberculosis* do not develop active disease but can have latent foci that may reactivate at a later date particularly if they become immunosuppressed or debilitated. Primary infection of *Mycobacterium tuberculosis* is more likely in infants with local spread from the initial parenchymal/lymph node complex to form larger single or multifocal parenchymal lesions, typically with prominent hilar and mediastinal lymph node involvement (**Fig. 7**) and occasional pleural or pericardial disease. The primary focus as well as involved nodes may cavitate with liquefaction of the caseous material and ultimately calcification (see **Fig. 7**). Enlarged lymph nodes may encroach on adjacent bronchi and cause bronchial narrowing with resultant air trapping or collapse in the distal lung (**Fig. 8**). Distant spread to other organs may occur either via

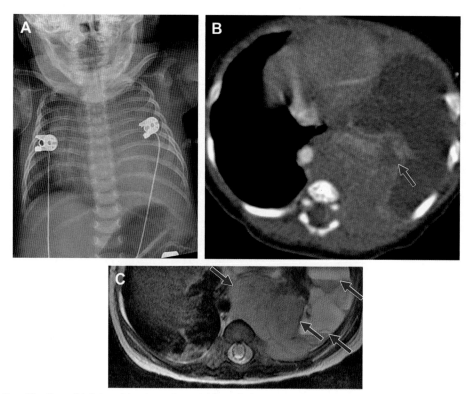

Fig. 5. Opacification of left hemithorax and respiratory distress caused by ruptured paraspinal neuroblastoma in a 5-week-old-boy. (*A*) Frontal chest radiograph shows complete opacification of the left hemithorax with contralateral mediastinal shift, which was initially believed to represent pneumonia with large pleural effusion. (*B*) Axial contrast-enhanced CT shows a left paraspinal mass (*blue arrow*) with intraspinal extension associated with a large pleural effusion, compressive atelectasis of the left lung, and contralateral mediastinal shift. (*C*) Axial T2-weighted MR image shows the left paraspinal mass (*blue arrows*) and a complex left pleural effusion with multiple loculations and fluid-debris levels (*red arrows*).

lymphatics or hematogenously (including miliary lung involvement).[24,25]

Infections with more than 1 organism may cause the atypical pneumonia pattern, resulting in confusing persistence of the illness or prominent findings in another organ system. An example of this situation is influenza infection with superimposed typical or atypical pneumonia (see **Fig. 6**B). The more common mimics that simulate the appearance of atypical pneumonia syndromes are summarized in **Box 3**.

Miliary or Nodular Pneumonia

Miliary or nodular pneumonia is characterized by chest radiographic findings of multiple miliary or larger nodular opacities. Miliary pneumonia in pediatric patients is seen most commonly in tuberculous and fungal infections (**Fig. 9**). Nodular pneumonia (including reticular and reticulonodular patterns) in pediatric patients is seen in septic emboli, viral pneumonia, lymphocytic interstitial pneumonia associated with Epstein-Barr virus (EBV) infection with underlying human immunodeficiency virus (HIV) infection, and some fungal and bacterial infections (**Box 4**; **Figs. 10** and **11**).[25,26] Septic pulmonary emboli usually occur secondary to a focal *Staphylococcus aureus* infection (eg, right-sided bacterial endocarditis, septic thrombophlebitis, osteomyelitis, soft tissue

---

Box 2
Common infectious causes of atypical pneumonia syndrome in children

Viruses: RSV (<5 years), adenoviruses, parainfluenza viruses, influenza virus (in epidemics), cytomegalovirus (CMV), varicella zoster virus (immunosuppressed)

Bacteria: *Chlamydia trachomatis* (<4 months), *Mycoplasma pneumoniae* (>5 years), *Chlamydia pneumoniae* (>5 years), *Bordatella pertussis*

Data from Fisher RG, Boyce TG. Pneumonia syndromes. In: Fisher RG, Boyce TG, editors. Moffet's pediatric infectious diseases: a problem-oriented approach. 4th edition. Philadelphia: Lippincott Williams & Wilkins; 2005. p. 174–221.

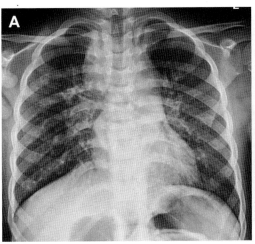 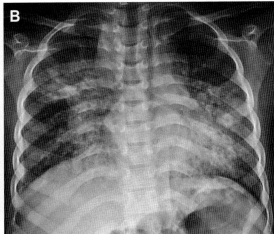

Fig. 6. Atypical pneumonia caused by influenza virus A subtype H1N1 with superimposed hospital-acquired pneumonia in an 8-year-old boy with history of renal transplant. *(A)* Frontal chest radiograph shows bilateral parahilar streaky opacities. *(B)* Patient developed respiratory distress while on Tamiflu. Frontal chest radiograph 4 days after initial chest radiograph *(A)* shows multifocal consolidations suggestive of superimposed hospital-acquired pneumonia.

infection, or urinary tract infection). The pulmonary nodules in septic emboli may cavitate (see **Fig. 11**).[27] Mimics of the pattern of miliary or nodular pneumonia are summarized in **Box 5**.

Progressive or Fulminant Pneumonia

Pneumonia is deemed progressive when it becomes radiologically and clinically worse despite antibiotic therapy that should be effective against the presumed cause. In this situation, the cause is often nonbacterial pathogens and mimics should also be carefully considered. Fulminant pneumonia is defined as a severe bilateral

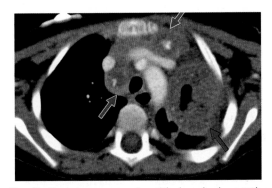

Fig. 7. Chronic pneumonia with lymphadenopathy caused by disseminated *Mycobacterium tuberculosis* in a 2-year-old boy. Axial contrast-enhanced CT shows mediastinal (*blue arrows*) and hilar (*not shown*) lymphadenopathy with central low attenuation, peripheral rim enhancement, and calcification. A left upper lobe mass with cavitation and punctuate calcification is consistent with a cavitating tuberculoma (*red arrow*).

pneumonia with an unusually rapid progression clinically or radiologically, over 24 to 48 hours after initial presentation. A common cause of progressive or fulminant pneumonia is the influenza virus during an epidemic. Uncommon infectious causes of this pattern and mimics are summarized in **Boxes 6** and **7**, respectively (**Fig. 12**).[20]

Aspiration Pneumonia

Aspiration pneumonia refers to the pulmonary consequences of abnormal entry of fluid, particulate matter, or endogenous secretions into the lower airways. Aspirated material can be relatively inert, toxic, or oropharyngeal secretions. The most commonly aspirated materials in children include oropharyngeal secretions, gastric contents, water, hydrocarbon, lipid, and foreign bodies. Radiographic pulmonary opacities related to aspiration may have an upper rather than lower lobe distribution when the child aspirates in the supine position.

Bacterial aspiration pneumonia is an infectious process caused by the inhalation of oropharyngeal secretions that are colonized by pathogenic bacteria. The basic defect leading to bacterial aspiration pneumonia is failure of the normal oropharyngeal defense mechanisms. The patient typically has a depressed state of consciousness, abnormal swallowing, a neuromuscular defect that prevents adequate coughing, or an abnormal connection between the airway and esophagus (such as an H-type tracheoesophageal fistula).

Acute lung aspiration (Mendelson syndrome) is an acute chemical injury caused by inhalation of gastric contents. In neurologically normal children,

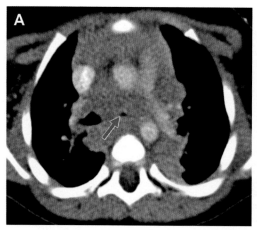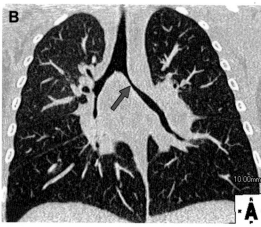

Fig. 8. *Mycobacterium tuberculosis* in an 11-month-old boy with 1.5-month history of intermittent stridor. *(A)* Axial contrast-enhanced CT shows low attenuation mediastinal and hilar lymphadenopathy with compression of the left mainstem bronchus *(arrow)*. *(B)* Curved oblique multiplanar reformation (MPR) shows the extent and degree of left mainstem bronchial narrowing *(arrow)*.

gastric aspiration usually occurs as a complication of anesthesia. The diagnosis of acute aspiration is mainly clinical and usually involves witnessed inhalation of vomitus or tracheal suctioning of gastric contents.[28,29]

Chronic lung aspiration (CLA) is repeated passage of food, gastric reflux, or saliva into the subglottic airways that causes chronic or recurrent respiratory symptoms. CLA may present with chronic cough, wheeze, noisy breathing, choking during feeding, recurrent episodes of pneumonia or bronchitis, and failure to thrive. Chronic aspiration often results in progressive lung disease, recurrent pneumonia, chronic airway inflammation, bronchiectasis, and respiratory failure. It is

a major cause of death in children with severe neurologic disorders (**Fig. 13**). Pulmonary aspiration may occur as a result of swallowing dysfunction, gastroesophageal reflux, and inability to adequately protect the airway from oral secretions or a combination of these. Anatomic conditions that predispose to aspiration lung disease include esophageal stricture or obstruction (eg, vascular ring, foreign body, achalasia), cleft palate, tracheoesophageal fistula (**Fig. 14**), laryngeal cleft, and bronchobiliary fistula.[28,29]

Aspiration related to near-drowning occurs when fluid enters the lungs without being prevented by laryngospasm. It typically manifests as pulmonary edema radiographically.[30] In a recent series of 83 children, secondary infections from aspiration related to near-drowning were rare.[31]

Box 3
Mimics of atypical pneumonia pattern

Congestive heart failure

Hypersensitivity pneumonitis

Drug hypersensitivity

Collagen vascular diseases (rheumatic fever, rheumatoid arthritis)

Pulmonary infarction or embolism (uncommon in children)

Airway and lung injury from toxic fume inhalation (silo filler diseases and other occupational inhalants)

Data from Fisher RG, Boyce TG. Pneumonia syndromes. In: Fisher RG, Boyce TG, editors. Moffet's pediatric infectious diseases: a problem-oriented approach. 4th edition. Philadelphia: Lippincott Williams & Wilkins; 2005. p. 174–221.

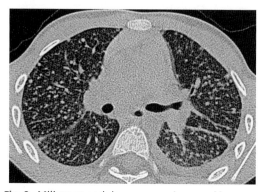

Fig. 9. Miliary or nodular pneumonia caused by recurrent *Mycobacterium avium-intracellulare* in an 8-year-old boy with immunodeficiency (interferon γ receptor 2 deficiency). Axial CT shows multiple, diffuse 2-mm to 3-mm nodules in bilateral lungs.

Hydrocarbon pneumonia is an acute, intense chemical pneumonitis after unintentional aspiration of volatile hydrocarbon compounds. Most cases of hydrocarbon pneumonia occur in children. Chest radiographs typically show bilateral, scattered pulmonary densities with middle and lower zone predominance. Such densities may become confluent and progress to acute respiratory distress syndrome (ARDS) and respiratory failure. They typically worsen over the first 72 hours and then clear over the next few days. However, occasionally radiographic changes may take weeks to months to be cleared. Obstructive emphysema, pneumatoceles, subsegmental, or segmental atelectasis may also be seen.[32]

Lipoid pneumonia is a rare form of pneumonia caused by inhalation or aspiration of a fatty substance. Oral administration of various oils is a common cultural practice, including mineral oil, olive oil, shark liver oil, cod liver oil, coconut oil, and ghee. Such oily materials can readily slide into the airway even in normal infants and young children without eliciting a cough reflex and are poorly removed by cilia. Lipoid pneumonias are typified by mild, subacute, or chronic clinical findings with accompanying marked radiographic changes. Chest radiographs of children with lipoid pneumonia typically show bilateral parahilar ill-defined, airspace opacities. In a series of 7 pediatric patients, CT showed dense consolidation surrounded by ground-glass opacity with a geographic lobular distribution.[33] Within the dense consolidations, areas with relatively low attenuation were identified in only 1 patient. Therefore, low-density consolidation in the posterior lungs is an infrequent CT finding in the diagnosis of lipoid pneumonia in children (**Fig. 15**). Interlobular septal thickening in areas of ground-glass opacity (ie, crazy paving pattern) has also been described in children with lipoid pneumonia.[33] Lipoid pneumonias may be complicated by superimposed infection especially with atypical mycobacteria. Slow recovery usually takes place with cessation of the oil administration. There may be residual scarring/fibrosis especially with animal rather than vegetable oils.[34,35]

Foreign body aspiration can also result in pneumonia. Accidental aspiration of both organic and nonorganic foreign bodies is a cause of childhood morbidity and mortality, requiring prompt recognition and early treatment to minimize the potentially serious and sometimes fatal consequence. Eating is the most common circumstance during which it occurs, with small food items being

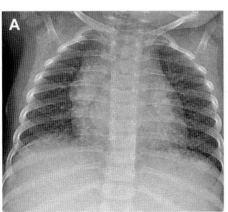
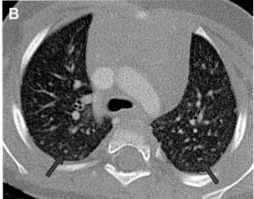

Fig. 10. Miliary or nodular pneumonia caused by lymphocytic interstitial pneumonia in a 19-month-old boy with HIV. *(A)* Frontal chest radiograph shows diffuse reticulonodular pattern. *(B)* Axial chest CT shows multiple bilateral 2-mm to 3-mm nodules *(arrows)*.

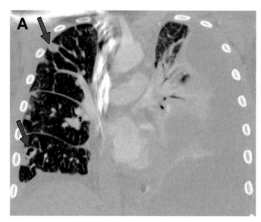
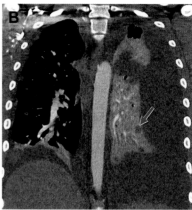

Fig. 11. Nodular pneumonia caused by septic emboli in an 18-year-old male with L3 vertebral body osteomyelitis and an epidural abscess. *(A, B)* Coronal contrast-enhanced CT reformats in lung and soft tissue windows show a large left pleural effusion and compressive atelectasis of the left lung. There are multiple, predominantly peripheral, solid and cavitating nodules in bilateral lungs *(arrows)* consistent with septic emboli. Left lung septic emboli are seen as hypoattenuating rounded lesions in the atelectatic lung; some are cavitating.

the most common foreign bodies aspirated. Coughing, choking, acute dyspnea, and sudden onset of wheezing are the most common symptoms. Clinical signs of foreign body aspiration have low positive predictive values. Chest radiographs are the initial imaging modality for patients with clinically suspected tracheobronchial aspiration of a foreign body. Chest radiographs may show air trapping, atelectasis, a radiopaque foreign body (rare), or be normal **(Fig. 16)**.[36] When the routine inspiratory chest radiograph is unhelpful or confusing, inspiratory and expiratory radiographs (in a cooperative child) or bilateral decubitus views (in a younger child unable to follow breathing instruction) are useful in confirming focal or unilateral air trapping. In selected cases, CT (possibly integrated with virtual bronchoscopy) may be considered to exclude a foreign body. CT evaluation may avoid bronchoscopy or provide the exact location and postobstructive complications of the foreign body before bronchoscopy.[37] An underlying chronic unrecognized airway foreign body should be considered among other causes of recurrent or chronic pneumonia, particularly in the pediatric population (see **Fig. 16**).

Box 5
Mimics of acute miliary and nodular pattern (including reticular and reticulonodular patterns)

Miliary: pulmonary edema; airway and lung injury from toxic fume inhalation (constrictive bronchiolitis)

Nodular: Wegener granulomatosis, recurrent aspirations

Bilateral reticular or reticulonodular pattern: Langerhans cell histiocytosis, hypersensitivity pneumonitis, lipoid pneumonia (bilateral airspace opacities in most cases)

Pulmonary alveolar proteinosis produces variable patterns including airspace, nodular, miliary, and scattered linear densities

Data from Fisher RG, Boyce TG. Pneumonia syndromes. In: Fisher RG, Boyce TG, editors. Moffet's pediatric infectious diseases: a problem-oriented approach. 4th edition. Philadelphia: Lippincott Williams & Wilkins; 2005. p. 174–221.

Box 6
Uncommon infectious causes of progressive or fulminant pneumonia in children

Viruses: measles virus, varicella zoster virus, adenovirus, hantavirus, Nipah virus (exposure to pigs in Malaysia and Singapore), Hendra virus (exposure to horses in Australia), severe acute respiratory syndrome coronavirus

Bacteria: *Bordetella pertussis, Mycoplasma pneumonia, Chlamydia psittaci, Listeria monocytogenes* (in newborn), *Legionella pneumophila, Coxiella burnetti*, group A streptococcus, group C streptococcus, Rocky Mountain spotted fever, ehrlichosis

Data from Fisher RG, Boyce TG. Pneumonia syndromes. In: Fisher RG, Boyce TG, editors. Moffet's pediatric infectious diseases: a problem-oriented approach. 4th edition. Philadelphia: Lippincott Williams & Wilkins; 2005. p. 174–221.

Pulmonary Infiltrates with Eosinophilic Pneumonia

PIE syndrome comprises a group of heterogeneous disorders having the common findings of lung disease and eosinophilia in the peripheral blood, bronchoalveolar lavage fluid, or pulmonary interstitium. PIE syndrome is rare in children. A subclassification for the PIE syndromes in children is summarized in **Box 8**.[38,39] Infectious causes of PIE syndrome are uncommon and include *Chlamydia trachomatis* (especially in infants less than 3 months of age), allergic bronchopulmonary aspergillosis (in asthmatics and cystic fibrosis), parasitic larvae in lungs (*Toxocara*, *Ascaris*, and others), and fungi (eg, *Cryptococcus*, *Candida* species).[20]

The radiographic findings in PIE syndromes tend to be nonspecific. Chest radiographs may show interstitial, alveolar, or mixed (interstitial and alveolar) infiltrates, which tend to be bilateral and diffuse. Certain PIE syndromes may be associated with more specific findings. The classic radiographic appearance of chronic eosinophilic pneumonia is characterized by peripheral infiltrates with sparing of the central lung zones. This radiographic appearance has been described as the "photographic negative of pulmonary edema."[40] Bronchiectasis with mucoid impaction is generally present on chest radiographs or CT in patients with allergic bronchopulmonary aspergillosis (**Fig. 17**).[41] Acute eosinophilic pneumonia is frequently associated with small bilateral pleural effusions. Imaging is often helpful in determining the extent of disease, localizing the potential sites for lung biopsy, and in assessing response to therapy once treatment has begun.[38]

Chronic or Recurrent Pneumonia

Chronic pneumonia is defined as a pulmonary opacity that does not improve within 1 month. It is best classified from the anatomic pattern, as focal, interstitial, with hilar lymphadenopathy, or with cysts, cavities, or spherical masses. Spherical masses, with or without cavitations, are often features of an infectious cause. Infectious causes and mimics of this pattern are summarized in **Boxes 9** and **10** (see **Fig. 16**; **Figs. 18–20**).[42] Obstructive atelectasis may both mimic and predispose to chronic pneumonia. It may have many underlying causes, including foreign body, mucoid impaction, narrowed bronchus, and extrinsic bronchial compression by cardiovascular anomalies, lymphadenopathy, tumor, or postpneumonic inflammatory changes. Anomalies of the lung, mediastinum, and diaphragm that may mimic an acute or chronic pneumonia pattern include atypical thymus, diaphragmatic eventration and hernia, tracheal bronchus, lung hypoplasia, and congenital bronchopulmonary malformations (BPMs).[20] Several of these lesions, such as the BPMs, predispose to recurrent or chronic infection but differentiating an infected from uninfected lesion may be difficult or impossible on imaging. Sometimes having previous imaging for comparison is helpful in terms of features such as the new presence of fluid in a previously air-filled cavity or perilesional consolidation.

Recurrent pneumonia is defined as more than 1 episode within a 1-year period or more than 3 episodes in a lifetime. Many children with a chronic pulmonary lesion (especially a congenital anomaly) are believed to have recurrent pneumonias if chest radiographs are taken only during a febrile illness. Recurrent pneumonias may be either focal or interstitial (linear). Underlying abnormalities that may

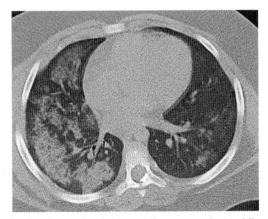

Fig. 12. Acute alveolar hemorrhage secondary to idiopathic pulmonary vasculitis in a 4-year-old child mimicking progressive or fulminant pneumonia. Axial contrast-enhanced CT shows multifocal consolidation, with sparing of the peripheral bilateral lungs.

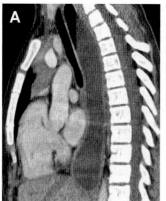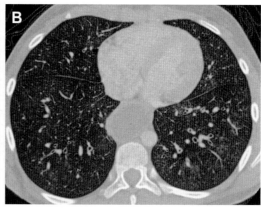

Fig. 13. Chronic lung aspiration secondary to lower esophageal stricture in an 11-year-old girl with history of gastroesophageal surgery at the age of 3 years in Mexico. *(A)* Sagittal contrast-enhanced CT reformation shows marked dilatation of the fluid-filled esophagus. *(B)* Axial contrast-enhanced CT shows bilateral diffuse centrilobular lung nodules and peripheral tree-in-bud pattern.

predispose to recurrent focal pneumonia include chronic aspiration (see section on aspiration pneumonia), congenital heart disease, bronchopulmonary foregut malformations (including BPMs with enteric-respiratory tract fistula), airway abnormalities (foreign body, stenosis, bronchiectasis, cystic fibrosis, immotile cilia disease), paralysis or eventration of the diaphragm, and congenital, acquired, and iatrogenic immune deficiencies.[43,44] Recurrent

interstitial pneumonia may be secondary to asthma, hypersensitivity pneumonitis, or pneumonias in children with AIDS (including *Pneumocystis jiroveci* pneumonia, lymphoid interstitial pneumonitis, and recurrent *Streptococcus pneumoniae* infection) (see **Fig. 10**).[20]

NEONATAL PNEUMONIA

Neonatal lung infections can be generally classified into 3 types depending on the initial source of neonatal infection: transplacental, perinatal, and postnatal (including nosocomial) infections.

Transplacental infections enter the fetus hematogenously via the umbilical cord. Most infants affected with transplacental infections typically

Fig. 14. Recurrent aspiration caused by tracheoesophageal fistula without esophageal atresia in a 6-day-old girl who presented with recurrent episodes of apnea, cyanosis, and choking desaturations. Barium esophagram shows an oblique connection (*red arrow*) coursing anterosuperiorly from the esophagus to the trachea at the level of the thoracic inlet. Contrast has opacified the central tracheobronchial airways. Inferior to the fistula, there is a focal mild narrowing of the esophagus (*blue arrow*), raising concern for a congenital esophageal stricture.

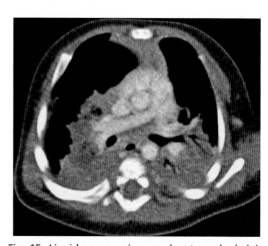

Fig. 15. Lipoid pneumonia secondary to oral administration of olive oil in a 3-month-old infant who presented with mild chronic cough and marked persistent opacities on chest radiographs. Axial contrast-enhanced CT shows bilateral airspace opacities in the posterior lungs with low density (−60 Hounsfield units).

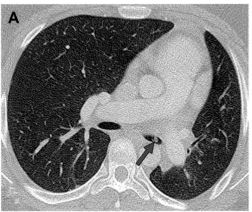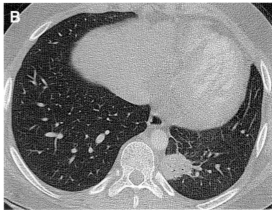

Fig. 16. Chronic pneumonia caused by foreign body in left mainstem bronchus in a 13-year-old boy. *(A, B)* Axial contrast-enhanced CT shows the foreign body (a piece of plastic) in the left mainstem bronchus *(arrow)*, mediastinal shift to the left, and focal consolidation in the left lower lobe.

manifest systemic and multiorgan disease rather than a primary lung infection. The most common transplacental infection is caused by CMV, which manifests as a diffuse reticulonodular pattern.[45] Other less common, transplacentally acquired pneumonias include rubella, syphilis, *Listeria monocytogenes*, and tuberculosis.

Perinatal infections can be acquired via ascending infection from the vaginal tract (most commonly group B *Streptococcus* or *Escherichia coli*), transvaginally during the birth process, or nosocomially in the neonatal period.[46] Radiographic findings in neonatal pneumonia are nonspecific in differentiating between various etiologic pathogens, as well as differentiating pneumonia from other causes of respiratory distress (eg, transient tachypnea of the newborn, surfactant deficiency

disease, and meconium aspiration). The most common radiographic manifestation of neonatal pneumonia is bilateral coarse perihilar reticular densities with possible scattered airspace opacities (**Fig. 21**). Solitary lobar consolidations are uncommon.[47] There is an association between group B streptococcal pneumonia and an ipsilateral diaphragmatic hernia.[48] Chest radiographs in group B streptococcal sepsis can mimic the diffuse ground-glass opacity seen in surfactant deficiency disease. However, the presence of this finding in a full-term infant or the presence of cardiomegaly or pleural effusions may help to differentiate group B streptococcal infection from surfactant deficiency disease.[49]

Pneumonia caused by *Chlamydia trachomatis* occurs in about 10% of infants born to women who carry this organism in their genital tract and becomes symptomatic more than 2 to 3 weeks after birth. Chlamydia pneumonia is characterized

---

Box 8
PIE syndromes: subclassification

Simple pulmonary eosinophilia (Loeffler syndrome)

Chronic eosinophilic pneumonia (rare in children)

Acute eosinophilic pneumonia

Allergic granulomatosis (Churg-Strauss syndrome)

Allergic bronchopulmonary aspergillosis (in asthmatics, cystic fibrosis)

Parasite-induced eosinophilia (*Strongyloides*, *Ascaris*, *Toxocara*, and *Ancylostoma*)

Drug reaction

Idiopathic hypereosinophilic syndrome (rare in children)

Infant pulmonary eosinophilia

Data from Refs.[20,38,39]

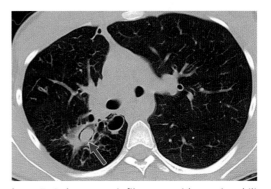

Fig. 17. Pulmonary infiltrates with eosinophilia caused by allergic bronchopulmonary aspergillosis in a 12-year-old girl with cystic fibrosis. Axial contrast-enhanced CT shows central bronchiectasis with intraluminal mucoid impaction/mycetomas *(arrow)*.

Box 9
Infectious causes of chronic pneumonia syndrome

1. *Chronic focal pulmonary disease*
   a. Untreated or undertreated acute pneumonia
      i. *Bacteria and Mycobacteria: Mycobacterium tuberculosis*, nontuberculous mycobacteria (especially in children with defective cell-mediated immunity)
      ii. *Systemic fungi:* histoplasmosis, coccidioidomycosis, blastomycosis cryptococcosis, sporotrichosis
      iii. *Parasites: Paragonimiasis*
2. *Chronic interstitial pulmonary disease*
   a. *Bacteria: Chlamydia trachomatis*
   b. *Viruses:* CMV, late-onset congenital rubella syndrome, LIP (in HIV infection)
   c. *Fungi: Pneumocystis jiroveci*
3. *Chronic pneumonia with hilar lymphadenopathy*
   a. Common
      i. *Bacteria and Mycobacteria: Mycobacterium tuberculosis, Mycoplasma pneumonia, Chlamydia pneumonia; Fungi:* histoplasmosis
   b. Uncommon
      i. *Bacteria:* nontuberculous mycobacteria, *Actinomyces, Francisella tularensis, Bacillus anthracis*
      ii. *Fungi:* coccidioidomycosis, blastomycosis
      iii. *Lung abscess*
4. *Chronic cavitary, cystic, or nodular pneumonias*
   a. Lung abscess, necrotizing bacterial pneumonia
      i. *Bacteria and Mycobacteria:* tuberculosis, actinomycosis, nocardiosis; *Nocardia* and *Rhodococcus equi* in immunocompromised patients
      ii. *Fungi: Aspergillus, Pneumocystis jiroveci* and other systemic fungi in immunocompromised patients
      iii. *Viruses:* atypical measles, papillomatosis of lung
      iv. *Protozoa and helminths:* paragonimiasis, *Entamoeba histolytica, Ecchinococcus, Dirofilaria immitis*

Data from Fisher RG, Boyce TG. Pneumonia syndromes. In: Fisher RG, Boyce TG, editors. Moffet's pediatric infectious diseases: a problem-oriented approach. 4th edition. Philadelphia: Lippincott Williams & Wilkins; 2005. p. 174–221; and Kawanami T, Bowen A. Juvenile laryngeal papillomatosis with pulmonary parenchymal spread. Case report and review of the literature. Pediatr Radiol 1985;15(2):102–4.

---

by hyperinflation and bilateral diffuse reticular perihilar densities that are disparate with relatively mild clinical symptoms.[50] Concomitant conjunctivitis, which used to be a useful clue to the cause, is prevented by the routine instillation of antibacterial eye drops at birth. Neonates with chlamydia pneumonia frequently have accompanying eosinophilia.

Bordetella pertussis has recently resurfaced to produce epidemics of infection, probably related to waning community immunity. The clinical presentation of pertussis in the newborn may lack some features (characteristic whooping cough and fever) typical of the disease in older children. The clinical presentation of the most severely affected newborns may be dominated by marked respiratory distress, cyanosis, and apnea. Mortality caused by pertussis usually results from secondary pneumonia, encephalopathy, cardiac failure, or pulmonary hypertension. A suggested mechanism for pulmonary hypertension that may develop in newborns with *Bordetella pertussis* infection is formation of leukocyte thrombi in pulmonary venules secondary to hyperleukocytosis.[51,52] The classic radiographic appearance in pertussis is the shaggy heart with diffuse peribronchial cuffing related to airway inflammation. However, chest radiographic findings such as hyperaeration, atelectasis, segmental

Box 10
Mimics of chronic pneumonia pattern

1. *Chronic focal pulmonary disease pattern*

   a. Malignancy (neuroblastoma)

   b. Obstructive atelectasis

   c. Foreign body, mucous plug, or endobronchial tumor

   d. Congenital anomalies of lung, thymus, or mediastinum

   e. Vascular rings

   f. Eventration of diaphragm

   g. Inflammatory pseudotumor of lung

2. *Chronic interstitial pulmonary disease pattern*

   a. Bronchopulmonary dysplasia

   b. Congestive heart failure

   c. Pulmonary sarcoidosis

   d. Collagen vascular diseases

   e. Idiopathic interstitial pneumonia

   f. Pulmonary hemosiderosis

   g. Constrictive bronchiolitis

   h. Histiocytosis (including Langerhans cell histiocytosis)

   i. Pulmonary alveolar proteinosis

3. *Chronic pneumonia pattern with hilar lymphadenopathy*

   a. Benign lymphoproliferative disorders and lymphoma

   b. Other neoplasms

4. *Chronic cavitary, cystic, or nodular pneumonia pattern*

   a. Congenital anomalies

   b. Malignancy (lymphoma and metastases)

   c. Traumatic pneumatocele

   d. Hyper-IgE syndrome

   e. α_1-antitrypsin deficiency

   f. Langerhans cell histiocytosis

   g. Pulmonary sarcoidosis

   h. Bronchopulmonary dysplasia

   i. Cystic bronchiectasis

   j. Wegener granulomatosis

Data from Fisher RG, Boyce TG. Pneumonia syndromes. In: Fisher RG, Boyce TG, editors. Moffet's pediatric infectious diseases: a problem-oriented approach. 4th edition. Philadelphia: Lippincott Williams & Wilkins; 2005. p. 174–221.

consolidation, and lymphadenopathy are usually nonspecific.

Recurrent pulmonary infection, with bacterial, viral, or occasionally fungal pathogens, are frequent problems in neonates undergoing prolonged hospitalization and complex treatments, especially in premature infants with chronic lung disease. Radiographic alterations caused by infection may be subtle when superimposed on chronic lung changes.[47]

PNEUMONIA IN IMMUNOCOMPROMISED HOSTS

Pneumonia is a common disease in the immunocompromised host. Immunocompromise may be congenital (congenital immunodeficiencies), acquired (HIV/AIDS, malnutrition) or iatrogenic (during chemotherapy for cancer or after tissue transplantation). Immunodeficient states can result in: (1) humoral immunodeficiency (hypogammaglobulinemia, functional B-lymphocyte deficiency accompanying HIV infection); (2) cellular immunodeficiency (severe malnutrition, late stages of AIDS, some congenital immunodeficiencies such as DiGeorge syndrome); and (3) neutrophil dysfunction and neutropenia (chronic granulomatous disease, pure neutropenia). Iatrogenic immunodeficiencies may be a combination of neutropenia or neutrophil dysfunction, innate or drug-induced defective lymphocyte function, and drug-induced breaks in the oral and intestinal mucosal barriers.[53]

The causes of pneumonia in the immunocompromised host consist not only of the same agents that cause pneumonia in the normal host but also of several opportunistic agents depending on the type and severity of immunodeficiency as well as temporal pattern after chemotherapy or transplant.

In an immunocompromised child with a noncontributory chest radiograph and clinical findings that could be attributed to a lung infection, chest CT is often required for evaluation of a possible lung infection. In this situation, there are 4 major advantages of chest CT over chest radiographs. First, the presence, pattern, and extent of the disease process are better visualized. Second, more than 1 pattern of abnormality may be detected, suggesting dual pathologic entities. Third, invasive diagnostic procedures (eg, bronchoscopy or needle aspiration) can be more precisely planned. Fourth, CT also allows for increased sensitivity in assessment of the response to treatment.[54,55]

Although the radiographic or CT appearance might not be specific for a pathogen, knowledge of the clinical setting in combination with the

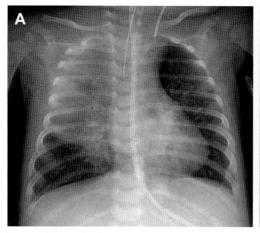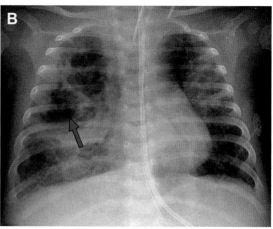

Fig. 18. Chronic focal pneumonia caused by persistent pulmonary coccidioidomycosis in a 3-month-old girl who presented with a 5-week history of pneumonia unresponsive to antibacterial agents. *(A)* Frontal chest radiograph shows consolidation of the right upper and middle lobes in addition to diffuse bilateral reticulonodular opacities. *(B)* Frontal chest radiograph obtained 8 days after initial chest radiograph *(A)*, shows development of multiple cavities *(arrow)* bilaterally superimposed on reticulonodular opacities.

type and severity of immunodeficiency and imaging pattern may narrow the differential diagnosis. A commonly encountered clinical issue is the possibility of fungal infection in immunocompromised children. The hallmark CT finding of fungal infections is the presence of pulmonary nodules. Such pulmonary nodules are often clustered peripherally and can show poorly defined margins, cavitation, or a surrounding halo of ground-glass opacity (CT halo sign) **(Fig. 22)**. The CT halo sign is a nonspecific finding and represents either hemorrhage around a nodule or neoplastic or inflammatory infiltration of the lung parenchyma. In the immunocompromised host, the CT halo sign can be seen most commonly with fungal infections (eg, aspergillosis, mucormycosis, or *Candida*) but also in viral infections (eg, CMV infection, herpes infection), organizing pneumonia, and pulmonary hemorrhage.[54,56–61] Microorganisms associated with severe pneumonia in immunodeficiency states are summarized in **Box 11**.

LIP is a form of subacute pneumonia seen in several states of immunologic dysregulation, particularly in children with HIV infection. LIP is characterized by micronodules of proliferating lymphoid tissue associated with infection by EBV. Chest radiographs in LIP show a characteristic diffuse, bilateral nodular, or reticulonodular pattern

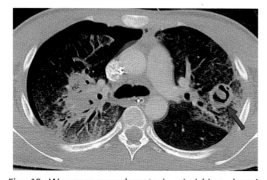

Fig. 19. Wegener granulomatosis mimicking chronic cavitary pneumonia in a 15-year-old male who presented with hemoptysis and respiratory distress. Initial chest radiograph showed bilateral confluent airspace opacities secondary to diffuse pulmonary hemorrhage *(not shown)*. contrast-enhanced CT obtained 9 days after initial presentation shows multifocal consolidation with cavitation *(arrow)*, ground-glass opacities, and a right pneumothorax.

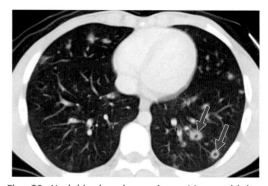

Fig. 20. Hodgkin lymphoma in a 14-year-old boy mimicking chronic cavitary pneumonia. Axial contrast-enhanced CT shows multiple bilateral cavitating lung nodules *(arrows)*. Mediastinal and bilateral hilar lymphadenopathy was also present *(not shown)*.

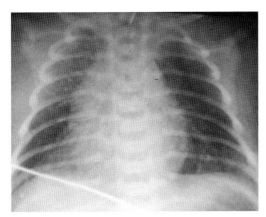

Fig. 21. Neonatal pneumonia caused by group B *Streptococcus* in a newborn infant. Frontal chest radiograph shows bilateral coarse perihilar reticular densities with scattered airspace opacities.

(see **Fig. 10**). Other recognized associated imaging findings of LIP include consolidation, mediastinal adenopathy, and bronchiectasis.[26,58,62] Radiologic features in common HIV-associated infections in pediatric patients are summarized in **Table 2**.

In pediatric patients with iatrogenic deficiencies of the immune system, pneumonia is commonly caused by opportunistic bacteria and fungi, acquired nosocomially or from resident mucosal flora (**Fig. 23**). In addition, after solid-organ transplantation although total immunoglobulin levels are normal, children and adolescents may be susceptible to encapsulated bacteria (eg, *Streptococcus pneumoniae*, *Haemophilus influenzae*). Viruses that commonly cause pneumonia in healthy hosts (eg, RSV, influenza, parainfluenza viruses, human

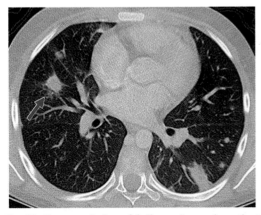

Fig. 22. Pneumonia in a febrile neutropenic patient caused by angioinvasive aspergillosis in a 7-year-old boy. Axial contrast-enhanced CT shows multiple bilateral pulmonary nodules, some have rims of ground-glass opacity (*arrow*), which is also known as the CT halo sign.

Box 11

Microorganisms associated with severe pneumonia in immunodeficiency states in pediatric patients

Humoral immunodeficiency

Viruses: enteroviruses

Pyogenic bacteria: *Streptococcus pneumonia*, *Haemophilus influenza*

Cellular immunodeficiency

Viruses: varicella zoster virus, rubeola virus, herpes simplex virus, CMV, adenovirus, RSV, parainfluenza virus, human metapneumovirus

Pyogenic bacteria: *Listeria monocytogenes*, *Pseudomonas aeruginosa*, *Stenotrophomonas* spp, *Burkholderia* spp, *Legionella* spp, *Nocardia* spp, other opportunistic bacteria

Mycobacteria: *Mycobacterium avium- intracellulare*, *Mycobacterium fortuitum*, Calmette-Guérin bacillus, other opportunistic mycobacteria

Fungi: *Pneumocystis jirovecii*, *Candida albicans*, *Cryptococcus neoformans*

Neutrophil dysfunction and neutropenia

Pyogenic bacteria: *Staphylococcus aureus*, *Burkholderia cepacia*, *Serratia marcescens*, *Nocardia* spp, *Pseudomonas aeruginosa*, *Stenotrophomonas* spp, *Burkholderia* spp, other opportunistic bacteria

Mycobacteria: Calmette-Guérin bacillus, nontuberculous mycobacteria

Fungi: *Aspergillus* spp, *Candida* spp, *Pseudallescheria boydii*, agents of mucormycosis

Iatrogenic immunodeficiency

Pyogenic bacteria: *Pseudomonas aeruginosa* and *Stenotrophomonas maltophilia*, α-hemolytic streptococci and other oral bacteria, *Nocardia*, *Streptococcus pneumoniae*, *Haemophilus influenza*

Mycobacteria: *Mycobacterium tuberculosis*

Viruses: CMV, varicella zoster virus, herpes simplex virus, human herpesvirus 6, RSV, influenza, parainfluenza viruses, human metapneumovirus, and adenovirus

Fungi: *Candida*, *Aspergillus* spp, and other fungi

Data from McIntosh K, Harper M, Murray M. Pneumonia in the immunocompromised host. In: Long SS, Pickering LK, Prober CG, editors. Principles and practice of pediatric infectious diseases revised reprint. 3rd edition. Philadelphia: Saunders; 2009. p. 265–9.

Table 2
Radiologic features in common HIV-associated infections in pediatric patients

Organism/Disease	Alveolar	Interstitial	LN	Cavities/Cysts
Bacteria	++			+
Mycobacterium tuberculosis	++	+	++	+
Atypical mycobacteria	+	++	+	+
Pneumocystis jiroveci	+	++		+(cysts)
Cryptococcus neoformans	+	+	+	
Invasive aspergillosis	+	+		++
RSV	+			
CMV	+	++	+	+
Measles	+	++		
Varicella	+	++		
Herpes simplex		+		

Abbreviations: Alveolar, focal of diffuse alveolar pattern; interstitial, focal or diffuse interstitial pattern; LN, lymphadenopathy; + and ++, refer to relative frequency of radiographic finding with each organism/disease.
Data from George R, Andronikou S, Theron S, et al. Pulmonary infections in HIV-positive children. Pediatr Radiol 2009;39(6):545–54.

metapneumovirus, and adenovirus) display greater virulence in both children and adults after solid-organ or human stem cell transplantation, particularly when cellular immunity is profoundly suppressed. In the posttransplant setting, EBV can cause progressive pulmonary disease in the form of posttransplantation lymphoproliferative disease.[53] In 2 studies of HRCT in bone marrow transplant recipients, the most useful distinguishing feature was the presence of large nodules and visualization of the halo sign, suggestive of fungal infection.[63,64]

After solid-organ transplantation, nosocomially acquired bacteria predominate as a cause of pneumonia in the first month. Later, viruses, especially

CMV and adenovirus, as well as *Listeria*, *Nocardia*, and *Aspergillus*, may be the cause. After more than 6 months after solid-organ transplantation, community-associated bacterial pneumonia becomes more common.[53]

A variety of noninfectious pulmonary processes can present with acute or subacute clinical findings mimicking pulmonary infection.[54] These findings include alveolar hemorrhage, pulmonary edema, drug reaction, idiopathic interstitial pneumonia, benign and malignant lymphoproliferative disorders, constrictive bronchiolitis, bronchiolitis obliterans with organizing pneumonia, and chronic graft-versus-host disease. The CT findings of many of these entities are nonspecific.[54,57–61]

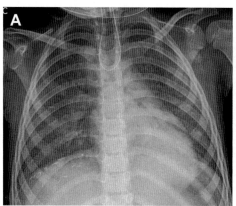 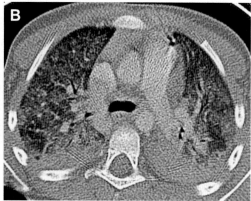

Fig. 23. *Pneumocystis jiroveci* pneumonia in a 4-year-old girl 2 years after liver transplant with known posttransplant lymphoproliferative disorder. *(A)* Frontal chest radiograph shows diffuse bilateral ground-glass opacities and malpositioned nasogastric tube coiled in the esophagus. *(B)* Axial contrast-enhanced CT shows bilateral diffuse ground-glass opacities and dependent atelectasis.

ACUTE COMPLICATIONS OF PNEUMONIA

Acute complications of pneumonia can be categorized as suppurative lung parenchymal complications and pleural complications.

Suppurative Lung Parenchymal Complications

Suppurative lung parenchymal complications span a spectrum of abnormalities and include cavitary necrosis, lung abscess, pneumatocele, bronchopleural fistula (BPF), and pulmonary gangrene. The name given to the suppurative process depends on several factors including the severity and distribution of the process, condition of the adjacent lung parenchyma, and temporal relationship with disease resolution.[65,66]

Cavitary necrosis

Cavitary necrosis represents a dominant area of lung necrosis associated with a variable number of thin-walled cysts. Characteristic findings on CT for cavitary necrosis include loss of normal lung architecture, poor parenchymal enhancement, loss of the lung-pleural margin, and multiple thin-walled fluid-filled or air-filled cavities (**Fig. 24**). Cavitary necrosis is seen earlier in chest US or CT compared with chest radiography because these cavities need to be filled with air to be visible on chest radiographs. Such cavities filled with air are accomplished only after communication with bronchial airways. Most pediatric patients can be managed successfully with conservative treatment. Follow-up chest radiographs typically show complete or near-complete resolution of the cavitary necrosis (see **Fig. 24**).[65,66]

Lung abscess

Lung abscess is a severe complication of pneumonia in children, mostly occurring in the presence of predisposing factors, such as congenital or acquired lung abnormalities, or immunodeficiency. Lung abscess represents a dominant focus of suppuration surrounded by a well-formed fibrous wall. The predominant pathogens isolated from primary lung abscesses in children include streptococcal species, *Staphylococcus aureus* and *Klebsiella pneumoniae*. Children with a lung abscess have a significantly better prognosis than adults with the same

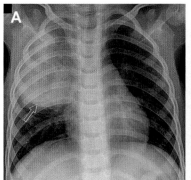
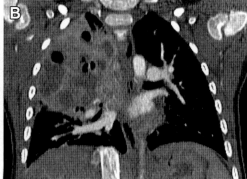
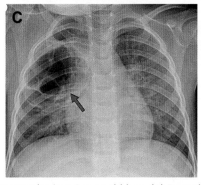

Fig. 24. Cavitary necrosis and pneumatoceles in a 2-year-old boy. *(A)* Frontal chest radiograph shows consolidation of the right upper lobe with an inferiorly bulging minor fissure *(arrow)* and multiple lucencies suggestive of underlying cavitation. *(B)* Coronal contrast-enhanced CT obtained 1 day after initial chest radiograph *(A)* shows consolidation of the right upper lobe and multiple thin-walled cavities with air-fluid levels. *(C)* Frontal chest radiograph obtained 1.5 months after initial chest radiograph *(A)* shows evolution of the cavitary necrosis into thin-walled air-filled cysts (ie, pneumatoceles; *arrow*). These cysts subsequently resolved on chest radiographs obtained at 3.5 months after presentation, with no significant lung scarring *(not shown)*.

condition.[67] Lung abscesses are uncommon in immunocompetent children. On contrast-enhanced CT, a lung abscess appears as a fluid-filled or air-filled cavity with a thick definable, enhancing wall (**Fig. 25**).[65,66,68] Although lung abscess in children has been managed successfully for many years with prolonged courses of intravenous antibiotics, the evolution of interventional radiology has seen the accelerated use of percutaneously placed pigtail drainage catheters using US and CT guidance.[67]

Pneumatocele

Pneumatocele is a term given to thin, smooth-walled air-filled cysts seen at imaging and may represent a later or less severe stage of resolving or healing lung necrosis (see **Fig. 24**). Pneumatoceles are most often caused by severe lung infection from staphylococcal pneumonia. However, they may be seen with other bacterial infections including streptococcus pneumonia and after hydrocarbon aspiration. On CT, thin-walled small or large cysts containing air with or without fluid are identified. The wall of a pneumatocele does not enhance. The surrounding lung may be opacified but does not typically show findings of lung necrosis.[65,66] Pneumatoceles usually resolve spontaneously over time although pneumatoceles may be atypically persistent in children with hyper-IGE syndrome. Large pneumatoceles containing fluid can be a source of ongoing infection and may occasionally require drainage.

Bronchopleural fistula

BPF is defined as a communication between the lung parenchyma or airways and the pleural space. Central BPFs (ie, main or lobar bronchi communicating with the pleural cavity) most often develop after traumatic injury to large airways or leak from the bronchial stump after pneumonectomy or lobectomy. The main causes for peripheral BPFs (ie, segmental or more distal airways or lung parenchyma communicating with the pleural cavity) are necrotizing pulmonary infection (ie, cavitary necrosis), trauma, lung surgery, and malignancy.[69,70] Presence of air in the pleural space before aspiration or drainage attempts is suggestive of either a peripheral BPF or infection with a gas-producing organism. Multidetector CT with thin-section axial and multiplanar reformation images may show a fistulous tract between the pleural space and peripheral airway or lung parenchyma in peripherally located BPFs (**Fig. 26**).[70]

Pulmonary gangrene

Pulmonary gangrene is a rare complication of severe lung infection with devitalization of lung parenchyma and secondary infection.[71] The primary feature that distinguishes pulmonary gangrene from necrotizing pneumonia and lung abscess is the extent of necrosis and the fact that thrombosis of large vessels plays a prominent role in the pathogenesis. Chest imaging shows lobar consolidation with bulging fissures and is followed by tissue breakdown to form many small cavities, which subsequently coalesce into a single large cavity occupying the entire lobe. Such a large cavity is filled with fluid and irregular pieces of sloughed lung parenchyma. However, these findings are not invariably present. Surgical resection of necrotic tissue is often necessary for proper management of children with pulmonary gangrene.[71–74]

The differential diagnosis of suppurative lung complications includes an underlying cystic

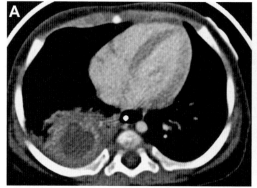
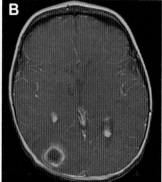

Fig. 25. Lung abscess in immunocompromised host caused by angioinvasive aspergillosis in a 6-month-old girl with acute myelogenous leukemia on induction chemotherapy. *(A)* Axial contrast-enhanced CT shows an air-filled cavity with a thick, definable enhancing wall in the right lower lobe and surrounding consolidation. *(B)* Axial contrast-enhanced T1-weighted MR image of the brain shows a rim-enhancing brain abscess in the right occipital lobe. The patient underwent right lower lobectomy and craniotomy for resection of these lesions.

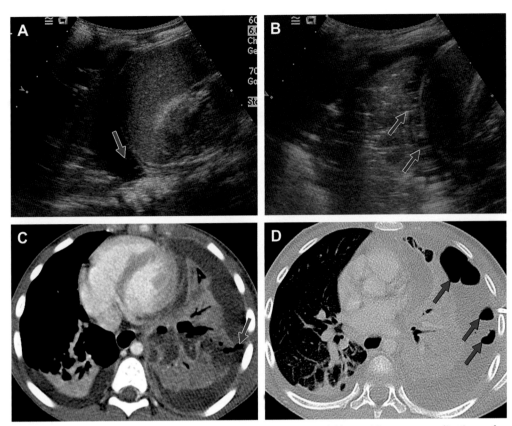

Fig. 26. Cavitary necrosis, peripheral BPF, and empyema in a 7-year-old boy with acute complications of pneumonia. *(A, B)* US shows fibrinous strands in the left pleural effusion (*red arrow*) and multiple, small cavities in the left lower lobe (*blue arrows*). Left lung is consolidated with echogenic air bronchograms. *(C)* Axial contrast-enhanced CT soft tissue window, performed 2 days after US, shows consolidation of the left lung with multiple thin-walled cavities with air-fluid levels. There is an abnormal communication between the peripheral airways and the pleural space (*arrow*) consistent with a BPF. *(D)* Axial contrast-enhanced CT image located at a higher level to *(C)* on bone window image reconstruction shows a multiloculated left pleural fluid collection with multiple air-fluid levels (*arrows*). The drained fluid was mucopurulent consistent with an empyema.

congenital BPM that has become secondarily infected. Prior and follow-up imaging may aid in the distinction. The presence of large, well-defined cysts early in the course of the illness or a systemic arterial supply to the lung may be helpful in suggesting an underlying BPM, although a chronic inflammatory process in the lower lobe can acquire some systemic vascular supply from diaphragmatic vessels.

Pleural Complications of Acute Pneumonia

Pleural complications from acute pneumonia include parapneumonic effusion and empyema. Parapneumonic effusion is defined as a pleural effusion in the setting of a known pneumonia. It may be simple or complicated based on the absence or presence of the infecting organism within the pleural space, respectively.[75] Empyema is defined as thick purulent pleural effusion. It may

be free-flowing or loculated. Progression of a pleural effusion to empyema occurs through 3 stages: exudative, fibrinopurulent, and organization. Parapneumonic effusions complicate pneumonia in 36% to 56% of cases in pediatric patients.[76] Empyema complicates an estimated 0.6% of all childhood pneumonias.[77]

Chest radiographs can often detect a parapneumonic collection, although some fluid, especially in a subpulmonic location, may not be visible and is often seen better on a decubitus film. In cases with complete or almost complete opacification of a hemithorax with or without contralateral mediastinal shift, additional erect or decubitus views are unhelpful in defining the quantity or nature of the pleural fluid. US is most helpful in this situation because it can readily distinguish a parapneumonic collection from extensive consolidation or an underlying mass. The US determination of the echogenicity of the pleural collection (anechoic or echogenic) and showing fibrin strands, septations, loculations, or fibrinous pleural rind is helpful in determining appropriate therapy (see **Fig. 26**). Treatment options for parapneumonic effusions/empyemas include antibiotics alone, simple tube drainage, chest drain insertion with fibrinolytics, or surgery (eg, video-assisted thoracoscopic surgery or open thoracotomy with decortication). Although imaging techniques are used as a guideline, they do not always accurately stage empyema, predict outcome, or guide decisions regarding surgical versus medical management.[75]

CT provides a more global overview of pleural and pulmonary abnormality from acute pneumonia, but is poor at differentiating parapneumonic effusion from empyema in pediatric patients. Findings on CT, in patients with parapneumonic effusion/empyema, include: (1) enhancement and thickening of visceral and parietal pleura; (2) thickening and increased density of extrapleural subcostal tissues; and (3) increased attenuation of extrapleural subcostal fat.[78] Loculation can be inferred by the presence of a lenticular fluid collection or nondependent air. Septations are usually not appreciated on CT (see **Fig. 26**).

Pleuropulmonary infection may occasionally spread to involve the chest wall, including soft tissues and adjacent bones. *Mycobacterium tuberculosis*, *Aspergillus*, and *Actinomyces* are the most common organisms in this scenario.

CHRONIC COMPLICATIONS OF PNEUMONIA

Chronic complications or consequences of pneumonia include parenchymal scarring, bronchial wall thickening, bronchiectasis, a predisposition to asthma, constrictive bronchiolitis, fibrothorax and a trapped lung, fibrosing mediastinitis, constrictive pericarditis, and pleural thickening. For practical purposes, bronchiectasis, constrictive bronchiolitis, fibrothorax and trapped lung, and fibrosing mediastinitis are discussed in the following sections.

Bronchiectasis

Bronchiectasis is defined by the presence of permanent and abnormal dilation of the bronchi. This condition usually occurs in the context of chronic airway infection causing inflammation. Bronchiectasis is nearly always diagnosed using HRCT. The main diagnostic features of bronchiectasis on HRCT are: (1) internal diameter of a bronchus that is wider than its adjacent pulmonary artery; (2) failure of the bronchus to taper peripherally; and (3) visualization of bronchi in the outer 1 to 2 cm of the lung zones (see **Fig. 17**; **Figs. 27 and 28**). A wide variety of factors predisposing to the development of bronchiectasis have been identified, including hereditary (cystic fibrosis, ciliary dyskinesia), infective, immunodeficiency (antibody deficiency), obstructive (intrabronchial foreign body), and systemic causes. Causes most

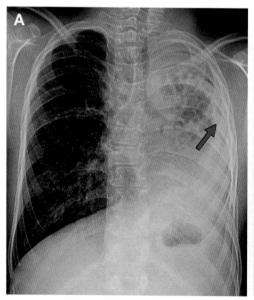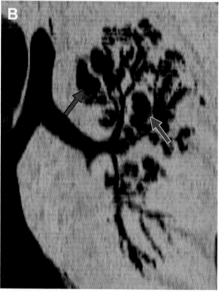

Fig. 27. Bronchiectasis secondary to recurrent infections, fibrothorax, and trapped left upper lobe in a 12-year-old boy with history of left lower lobectomy. *(A)* Frontal chest radiograph shows contraction of the left hemithorax with ipsilateral mediastinal shift and elevation of the left hemidiaphragm. Bronchiectasis of the left upper lobe and severe pleural thickening *(arrow)* are also seen. *(B)* Coronal minimum intensity projection (MinIP) image shows varicose and cystic bronchiectasis *(arrows)*.

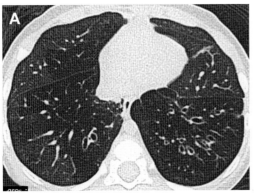 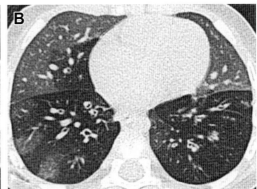

Fig. 28. Constrictive bronchiolitis in a 1-year-old boy. Chest CViCT scans were obtained at 30 and 0 cm H_2O pressures after intubation and lung recruitment maneuvers. Inspiratory *(A)* and expiratory *(B)* axial CT images of the lower lung zone show cylindrical bronchiectasis and mosaic attenuation pattern; patchy air trapping is more apparent in expiration.

commonly associated with bronchiectasis are childhood infections, including pneumonia, pertussis, complicated measles, and tuberculosis (eg, *Mycobacterium tuberculosis* and *Mycobacterium avium* complex).[79–81]

Constrictive Bronchiolitis (Bronchiolitis Obliterans)

Constrictive bronchiolitis (bronchiolitis obliterans) is characterized by the presence of concentric narrowing or obliteration of the bronchioles caused by submucosal and peribronchiolar fibrosis. A common cause of constrictive bronchiolitis is previous childhood infection, resulting in the so-called Swyer-James syndrome, identifiable as asymmetric hyperlucent lung on chest radiographs. Whereas the process may appear unilateral on chest radiographs, there is usually bilateral but asymmetric abnormality on CT (see **Fig. 28**). Central bronchiectasis and a characteristic mosaic appearance with patchy expiratory air trapping are seen on HRCT. Causes and associations of constrictive bronchiolitis include previous infections (viral including adenovirus, RSV, influenza, parainfluenza; mycoplasma and pertussis), collagen vascular diseases, previous transplant, toxic fume exposure, ingested toxins, drugs, and cryptogenic constrictive bronchiolitis.[82]

Fibrothorax and Trapped Lung

Pleural fibrosis can result from a variety of inflammatory processes (**Box 12**). The development of pleural fibrosis follows severe pleural inflammation, which is usually associated with an exudative pleural effusion. Fibrothorax and trapped lung are 2 uncommon consequences of pleural fibrosis (see **Fig. 27**).[83]

Fibrothorax represents the most severe form of pleural fibrosis. With a fibrothorax, there is dense fibrosis of the visceral and parietal pleural surfaces, leading to fusion of these membranes, contracture of the involved hemithorax (and ipsilateral mediastinal shift), and reduced mobility of the lung and thoracic cage (see **Fig. 27**). Decortication is the only potentially effective treatment of fibrothorax in patients with severe respiratory compromise.[83,84]

A trapped lung is characterized by the inability of the lung to expand and fill the thoracic cavity because of a restrictive, fibrous, visceral pleural peel (see **Fig. 27**). Restriction of lung parenchymal expansion and subsequent negative pressure in the pleural space result in filling of the pleural space with pleural fluid (usually a transudate). The diagnosis of a trapped lung implies chronicity, stability over time, and a purely mechanical cause for the persistence of a fluid-filled pleural space. Patients with a trapped lung usually do not

---

Box 12
Noninfectious causes of pleural fibrosis

Immunologic diseases such as rheumatoid pleurisy

Asbestos exposure

Malignancy

Improperly drained hemothorax

Postcoronary artery bypass graft surgery

Medications

Uremic pleurisy

Data from Jantz MA, Antony VB. Pleural fibrosis. Clin Chest Med 2006;27(2):181–91.

experience improvement in dyspnea after thoracentesis. In symptomatic patients, decortication should be considered. The underlying lung parenchyma should be assessed before decortication. If the trapped lung is severely diseased and fibrotic, decortication is unlikely to result in lung reexpansion and the procedure does not provide symptomatic benefit. In contrast, lung entrapment is the result of an active inflammatory process or malignancy in the pleural space, leading to a restricted pleural space. Pleural fluid from lung entrapment is an exudate, and symptoms in patients with lung entrapment typically improve after thoracentesis.[83,85]

Fibrosing Mediastinitis

Fibrosing mediastinitis is a rare condition characterized by proliferation of fibrous tissue within the mediastinum. Symptoms are related to compression of the central airways, superior vena cava, pulmonary veins, pulmonary arteries, and esophagus. The most common cause of this disorder is fungal infection, especially *Histoplasma capsulatum* in the United States.[86]

SUMMARY

Pneumonia is an infection of the lung parenchyma caused by a wide variety of organisms in pediatric patients. Imaging evaluation plays an important role in children with pneumonia by detecting the presence of pneumonia and determining its location and extent, excluding other thoracic causes of respiratory symptoms, and showing complications such as effusion/empyema and suppurative lung changes. Clear understanding of the underlying potential cause, current role of imaging, proper imaging techniques, and characteristic imaging appearances of acute and chronic pneumonias can guide optimal management of pediatric patients with pneumonia.

REFERENCES

1. Rudan I, Tomaskovic L, Boschi-Pinto C, et al. WHO Child Health Epidemiology Reference Group. Global estimate of the incidence of clinical pneumonia among children under five years of age. Bull World Health Organ 2004;82(12):895–903.
2. Murphy TF, Henderson FW, Clyde WA Jr, et al. Pneumonia: an eleven-year study in a pediatric practice. Am J Epidemiol 1981;113(1):12–21.
3. Jokinen C, Heiskanen L, Juvonen H, et al. Incidence of community-acquired pneumonia in the population of four municipalities in eastern Finland. Am J Epidemiol 1993;137(9):977–88.
4. Wardlaw T, Salama P, Johansson EW, et al. Pneumonia: the leading killer of children. Lancet 2006; 368(9541):1048–50.
5. Westra SJ, Choy G. What imaging should we perform for the diagnosis and management of pulmonary infections? Pediatr Radiol 2009;39(Suppl 2):S178–83.
6. Virkki R, Juven T, Rikalainen H, et al. Differentiation of bacterial and viral pneumonia in children. Thorax 2002;57(5):438–41.
7. Korppi M, Heiskanen-Kosma T, Jalonen E, et al. Aetiology of community-acquired pneumonia in children treated in hospital. Eur J Pediatr 1993;152(1):24–30.
8. Riccabona M. Ultrasound of the chest in children (mediastinum excluded). Eur Radiol 2008;18(2): 390–9.
9. Kim OH, Kim WS, Kim MJ, et al. US in the diagnosis of pediatric chest diseases. Radiographics 2000; 20(3):653–71.
10. Nievelstein RA, van Dam IM, van der Molen AJ. Multidetector CT in children: current concepts and dose reduction strategies. Pediatr Radiol 2010;40(8):1324–44.
11. Robinson TE. Computed tomography scanning techniques for the evaluation of cystic fibrosis lung disease. Proc Am Thorac Soc 2007;4(4):310–5.
12. Sargent MA, Jamieson DH, McEachern AM, et al. Increased inspiratory pressure for reduction of atelectasis in children anesthetized for CT scan. Pediatr Radiol 2002;32(5):344–7.
13. Peltola V, Ruuskanen O, Svedström E. Magnetic resonance imaging of lung infections in children. Pediatr Radiol 2008;38(11):1225–31.
14. Hebestreit A, Schultz G, Trusen A, et al. Follow-up of acute pulmonary complications in cystic fibrosis by magnetic resonance imaging. Acta Paediatr 2004; 93:414–6.
15. Puderbach M, Eichinger M. The role of advanced imaging techniques in cystic fibrosis follow-up: is there a place for MRI? Pediatr Radiol 2010;40(6):844–9.
16. Hansell DM, Lynch DA, McAdams HP, et al. Basic patterns in lung disease. In: Hansell DM, Lynch DA, McAdams HP, et al, editors. Imaging of diseases of the chest. 5th edition. Philadelphia: Mosby; 2010. p. 89, 139–43.
17. Selwyn BJ. The epidemiology of acute respiratory tract infection in young children: comparison of findings from several developing countries. Rev Infect Dis 1990;12(Suppl 8):S870–88.
18. Vicencio AG. Susceptibility to bronchiolitis in infants. Curr Opin Pediatr 2010;22(3):302–6.
19. Dawson KP, Long A, Kennedy J, et al. The chest radiograph in acute bronchiolitis. J Paediatr Child Health 1990;26(4):209–11.
20. Fisher RG, Boyce TG. Pneumonia syndromes. In: Fisher RG, Boyce TG, editors. Moffet's pediatric infectious diseases: a problem-oriented approach. 4th edition. Philadelphia: Lippincott Williams & Wilkins; 2005. p. 174–221.

21. Kantor HG. The many radiologic facies of pneumococcal pneumonia. AJR Am J Roentgenol 1981; 137(6):1213–20.

22. Kim YW, Donnelly LF. Round pneumonia: imaging findings in a large series of children. Pediatr Radiol 2007;37(12):1235–40.

23. Brodzinski H, Ruddy RM. Review of new and newly discovered respiratory tract viruses in children. Pediatr Emerg Care 2009;25(5):352–60.

24. Powell DA, Hunt WG. Tuberculosis in children: an update. Adv Pediatr 2006;53:279–322.

25. Inselman LS. Tuberculosis in children: an update. Pediatr Pulmonol 1996;21(2):101–20.

26. Pitcher RD, Beningfield SJ, Zar HJ. Chest radiographic features of lymphocytic interstitial pneumonitis in HIV-infected children. Clin Radiol 2010;65(2): 150–4.

27. Wong KS, Lin TY, Huang YC, et al. Clinical and radiographic spectrum of septic pulmonary embolism. Arch Dis Child 2002;87(4):312–5.

28. de Benedictis FM, Carnielli VP, de Benedictis D. Aspiration lung disease. Pediatr Clin North Am 2009;56(1):173–90.

29. Lodha R, Puranik M, Natchu UCM, et al. Recurrent pneumonia in children: clinical profile and underlying causes. Acta Paediatr 2002;91(11):1170–3.

30. Wunderlich P, Rupprecht E, Trefftz F, et al. Chest radiographs of near-drowned children. Pediatr Radiol 1985;15(5):297–9.

31. Forler J, Carsin A, Arlaud K, et al. Respiratory complications of accidental drownings in children. Arch Pediatr 2010;17(1):14–8.

32. Eade NR, Taussig LM, Marks MI. Hydrocarbon pneumonitis. Pediatrics 1974;54(3):351–7.

33. Lee KH, Kim WS, Cheon JE, et al. Squalene aspiration pneumonia in children: radiographic and CT findings as the first clue to diagnosis. Pediatr Radiol 2005;35(6):619–23.

34. Zanetti G, Marchiori E, Gasparetto TD, et al. Lipoid pneumonia in children following aspiration of mineral oil used in the treatment of constipation: high-resolution CT findings in 17 patients. Pediatr Radiol 2007;37(11):1135–9.

35. Hadda V, Khilnani GC, Bhalla AS, et al. Lipoid pneumonia presenting as non resolving community acquired pneumonia: a case report. Cases J 2009; 16(2):9332.

36. Passàli D, Lauriello M, Bellussi L, et al. Foreign body inhalation in children: an update. Acta Otorhinolaryngol Ital 2010;30(1):27–32.

37. Adaletli I, Kurugoglu S, Ulus S, et al. Utilization of low dose multidetector CT and virtual bronchoscopy in children with suspected foreign body aspiration. Pediatr Radiol 2007;37:33–40.

38. Oermann CM, Panesar KS, Langston C, et al. Pulmonary infiltrates with eosinophilia syndromes in children. J Pediatr 2000;136(3):351–8.

39. Chitkara RK, Krishna G. Parasitic pulmonary eosinophilia. Semin Respir Crit Care Med 2006;27(2):171–84.

40. Gaensler EA, Carrington CB. Peripheral opacities in chronic eosinophilic pneumonia: the photographic negative of pulmonary edema. AJR Am J Roentgenol 1977;128:1–13.

41. Allen JN, Davis WB. Eosinophilic lung diseases: state of the art. Am J Respir Crit Care Med 1994; 150:1423–38.

42. Kawanami T, Bowen A. Juvenile laryngeal papillomatosis with pulmonary parenchymal spread. Case report and review of the literature. Pediatr Radiol 1985;15(2):102–4.

43. Kaplan KA, Beierle EA, Faro A, et al. Recurrent pneumonia in children: a case report and approach to diagnosis. Clin Pediatr (Phila) 2006;45(1):15–22.

44. Couriel J. Assessment of the child with recurrent chest infections. Br Med Bull 2002;61(1):115–32.

45. Manson D. Diagnostic imaging of neonatal pneumonia. In: Donoghue VK, editor. Radiological imaging of the neonatal chest. 2nd edition. Berlin: Springer; 2007. p. 102.

46. Belady PH, Farkouh LJ, Gibbs RS. Intra-amniotic infection and premature rupture of the membranes. Clin Perinatol 1997;24(1):43–57.

47. Newman B. Imaging of medical disease of the newborn lung. Radiol Clin North Am 1999;37(6):1049–65.

48. Potter B, Philipps AF, Bierny JP, et al. Neonatal radiology. Acquired diaphragmatic hernia with group B streptococcal pneumonia. J Perinatol 1995;15(2): 160–2.

49. Leonidas JC, Hall RT, Beatty EC, et al. Radiographic findings in early onset neonatal group b streptococcal septicemia. Pediatrics 1977;59(Suppl[6 Pt 2]): 1006–11.

50. Hammerschlag MR. Chlamydia trachomatis in children. Pediatr Ann 1994;23(7):349–53.

51. Soares S, Rocha G, Pissarra S, et al. Pertussis with severe pulmonary hypertension in a newborn with good outcome–case report. Rev Port Pneumol 2008; 14(5):687–92.

52. Kundrat SL, Wolek TL, Rowe-Telow M. Malignant pertussis in the pediatric intensive care unit. Dimens Crit Care Nurs 2010;29(1):1–5.

53. McIntosh K, Harper M, Murray M. Pneumonia in the immunocompromised host. In: Long SS, Pickering LK, Prober CG, editors. Principles and practice of pediatric infectious diseases revised reprint. 3rd edition. Philadelphia: Saunders; 2009. p. 265–9.

54. Mori M, Galvin JR, Barloon TJ, et al. Fungal pulmonary infections after bone marrow transplantation: evaluation with radiography and CT. Radiology 1991;178(3):721–6.

55. Wilson S, Grundy R, Vyas H. Investigation and management of a child who is immunocompromised and neutropoenic with pulmonary infiltrates. Arch Dis Child Educ Pract Ed 2009;94:129–37.

56. Lee YR, Choi YW, Lee KJ, et al. CT halo sign: the spectrum of pulmonary diseases. Br J Radiol 2005; 78(933):862–5.

57. McAdams HP, Rosado-de-Christenson ML, Templeton PA, et al. Thoracic mycoses from opportunistic fungi: radiologic-pathologic correlation. Radiographics 1995; 15(2):271–86.

58. Marks MJ, Haney PJ, McDermott MP, et al. Thoracic disease in children with AIDS. Radiographics 1996; 16(6):1349–62.

59. Winer-Muram HT, Rubin SA, Fletcher BD, et al. Childhood leukemia: diagnostic accuracy of bedside chest radiography for severe pulmonary complications. Radiology 1994;193(1):127–33.

60. Brown MJ, Miller RR, Müller NL. Acute lung disease in the immunocompromised host: CT and pathologic examination findings. Radiology 1994;190(1):247–54.

61. Kang EY, Patz EF Jr, Müller NL. Cytomegalovirus pneumonia in transplant patients: CT findings. J Comput Assist Tomogr 1996;20(2):295–9.

62. George R, Andronikou S, Theron S, et al. Pulmonary infections in HIV-positive children. Pediatr Radiol 2009;39(6):545–54.

63. Escuissato DL, Gasparetto EL, Marchiori E, et al. Pulmonary infections after bone marrow transplantation: high-resolution CT findings in 111 patients. AJR Am J Roentgenol 2005;185(3):608–15.

64. Gasparetto TD, Escuissato DL, Marchiori E. Pulmonary infections following bone marrow transplantation: high-resolution CT findings in 35 paediatric patients. Eur J Radiol 2008;66(1):117–21.

65. Donnelly LF, Klosterman LA. Pneumonia in children: decreased parenchymal contrast enhancement–CT sign of intense illness and impending cavitary necrosis. Radiology 1997;205(3):817–20.

66. Donnelly LF, Klosterman LA. Cavitary necrosis complicating pneumonia in children: sequential findings on chest radiography. AJR Am J Roentgenol 1998;171(1):253–6.

67. Patradoon-Ho P, Fitzgerald DA. Lung abscess in children. Paediatr Respir Rev 2007;8(1):77–84.

68. Leonardi S, del Giudice MM, Spicuzza L, et al. Lung abscess in a child with Mycoplasma pneumoniae infection. Eur J Pediatr 2010;169(11):1413–5.

69. Westcott JL, Volpe JP. Peripheral bronchopleural fistula: CT evaluation in 20 patients with pneumonia, empyema, or postoperative air leak. Radiology 1995;196:175–81.

70. Seo H, Kim TJ, Jin KN, et al. Multi-detector row computed tomographic evaluation of bronchopleural fistula: correlation with clinical, bronchoscopic, and surgical findings. J Comput Assist Tomogr 2010; 34(1):13–8.

71. Refaely Y, Weissberg D. Gangrene of the lung: treatment in two stages. Ann Thorac Surg 1997;64(4): 970–3.

72. Danner PK, McFarland DR, Felson B. Massive pulmonary gangrene. Am J Roentgenol Radium Ther Nucl Med 1968;103(3):548–54.

73. Penner C, Maycher B, Long R. Pulmonary gangrene. A complication of bacterial pneumonia. Chest 1994; 105(2):567–73.

74. Kothari PR, Jiwane A, Kulkarni B. Pulmonary gangrene complicating bacterial pneumonia. Indian Pediatr 2003;40(8):784–5.

75. Calder A, Owens CM. Imaging of parapneumonic pleural effusions and empyema in children. Pediatr Radiol 2009;39(6):527–37.

76. Kurt BA, Winterhalter KM, Connors RH, et al. Therapy of parapneumonic effusions in children: video-assisted thoracoscopic surgery versus conventional thoracostomy drainage. Pediatrics 2006;118: e547–53.

77. Jaffe A, Balfour-Lynn IM. Management of empyema in children. Pediatr Pulmonol 2005;40:148–56.

78. Donnelly LF, Klosterman LA. CT appearance of parapneumonic effusions in children: findings are not specific for empyema. AJR Am J Roentgenol 1997; 169(1):179–82.

79. Pasteur MC, Helliwell SM, Houghton SJ, et al. An investigation into causative factors in patients with bronchiectasis. Am J Respir Crit Care Med 2000; 162(4 Pt 1):1277–84.

80. King PT. The pathophysiology of bronchiectasis. Int J Chron Obstruct Pulmon Dis 2009;4:411–9.

81. Pappalettera M, Aliberti S, Castellotti P, et al. Bronchiectasis: an update. Clin Respir J 2009;3(3):126–34.

82. Devakonda A, Raoof S, Sung A, et al. Bronchiolar disorders: a clinical-radiological diagnostic algorithm. Chest 2010;137(4):938–51.

83. Jantz MA, Antony VB. Pleural fibrosis. Clin Chest Med 2006;27(2):181–91.

84. Morton JR, Boushy SF, Guinn GA. Physiological evaluation of results of pulmonary decortication. Ann Thorac Surg 1970;9:321–6.

85. Doelken P, Sahn SA. Trapped lung. Semin Respir Crit Care Med 2001;22:631–5.

86. Miyata T, Takahama M, Yamamoto R, et al. Sclerosing mediastinitis mimicking anterior mediastinal tumor. Ann Thorac Surg 2009;88(1):293–5.

Congenital Pulmonary Malformations in Pediatric Patients: Review and Update on Etiology, Classification, and Imaging Findings

Edward Y. Lee, MD, MPH[a],*, Henry Dorkin, MD[b],
Sara O. Vargas, MD[c]

KEYWORDS
- Congenital pulmonary malformations • Parenchymal lesions
- Combined parenchyma and vascular lesions
- Pediatric patients

Congenital pulmonary malformations represent a heterogeneous group of developmental disorders affecting the lung parenchyma, the arterial supply to the lung, and the lung's venous drainage. At present, the estimated annual incidence of congenital pulmonary malformations ranges from 30 to 42 cases per 100,000 population.[1,2] The advent of prenatal imaging and the advancement of postnatal imaging have lead to an increase in the number of diagnoses, especially in the past decade.[3–7] In addition, they have also increasingly enhanced our understanding of the onset, timing, natural history, and etiologic associations of congenital pulmonary malformations.[3–10]

Congenital pulmonary malformations may be detected by prenatal imaging evaluation or remain undiagnosed in asymptomatic children. However, they can also present as acute respiratory distress in the newborn period or as recurrent infections in older children.[11,12] In both asymptomatic and symptomatic pediatric patients with congenital pulmonary malformations, the diagnosis of such malformations usually requires imaging evaluation, particularly in cases of surgical lesions for preoperative assessment.[11–13] Understanding proper imaging techniques and characteristic imaging appearances of congenital pulmonary malformations in pediatric patients is important because it can lead to early and correct diagnosis, which in turn can result in optimal patient management.

In this article the authors first briefly discuss complexities and uncertainties regarding the etiology of congenital pulmonary malformations. The current imaging techniques for evaluating congenital pulmonary malformations and their characteristic imaging findings, which can allow differentiation among various congenital pulmonary malformations, are reviewed. The correlation of imaging findings with gross pathologic and histologic findings in several of the more commonly

[a] Division of Thoracic Imaging, Departments of Radiology and Medicine, Pulmonary Division, Children's Hospital Boston and Harvard Medical School, 330 Longwood Avenue, Boston, MA 02115, USA
[b] Division of Respiratory Diseases, Department of Medicine, Children's Hospital Boston and Harvard Medical School, 330 Longwood Avenue, Boston, MA 02115, USA
[c] Department of Pathology, Children's Hospital Boston and Harvard Medical School, 300 Longwood Avenue, Boston, MA 02115, USA
* Corresponding author.
E-mail address: Edward.Lee@childrens.harvard.edu

Radiol Clin N Am 49 (2011) 921–948
doi:10.1016/j.rcl.2011.06.009
0033-8389/11/$ – see front matter © 2011 Elsevier Inc. All rights reserved.

encountered surgical lesions is highlighted to enhance the understanding of often complex underlying anatomic structures of these pulmonary malformations.

COMPLEXITIES AND UNCERTAINTIES REGARDING THE ETIOLOGY OF CONGENITAL PULMONARY MALFORMATIONS

Understanding congenital pulmonary malformations is often difficult and confusing, primarily because the etiology of these malformations has not been clearly established. Among many potential etiologic factors proposed so far for the development of congenital pulmonary malformations, there are 4 main theories: (1) defective foregut budding, differentiation, and separation[13–25]; (2) airway obstruction[26,27]; (3) vascular abnormality[13]; and (4) genetic cause.[28–30] These proposed mechanisms may act alone or in combination.

According to one long-held theory, some investigators believe that the defective budding, differentiation, and separation of the primitive foregut, which occur during early tracheobronchial tree development between days 24 and 36 of gestation, may be the most frequent cause of the congenital pulmonary malformations.[13–25] Another proposed origin of congenital pulmonary malformations is airway obstruction with subsequent secondary pulmonary dysplastic changes.[26,27] Such a theory has an advantage because variability in the timing, location, and severity of airway obstruction may account for the occurrence of various pathologic and imaging appearances of hybrid or overlapping lesions.[3,6] A recent report suggesting that the airway obstruction in utero is the underlying cause of congenital pulmonary malformations further supports this theory.[27] Vascular abnormality has also been frequently suggested as the underlying cause of congenital pulmonary malformations.[13] Such a theory may explain various primarily vascular abnormalities associated with congenital pulmonary malformations, including absent pulmonary artery associated with pulmonary agenesis. However, it does not explain the focal lung parenchymal lesions without associated vascular anomalies. In recent years, a genetic cause has been proposed by some researchers as an underlying mechanism of developing congenital pulmonary malformations. These investigators[28–30] believe that common congenital pulmonary malformation such as congenital pulmonary airway malformation (CPAM) are potentially caused by an aberration in the signaling pathways responsible for controlling airway development.

Although there are several potential etiologic factors proposed to explain the development of congenital pulmonary malformations, as stated, it is also important to recognize that perhaps these theories may not be mutually exclusive. The ultimate development of congenital pulmonary malformations may be due to a combination of different factors interacting with one another at various time periods of lung development.

IMAGING ALGORITHM AND TECHNIQUES

A detailed discussion of imaging techniques for the currently available imaging modalities in the evaluation of congenital pulmonary malformations is beyond the scope of this article. The focus here is on reviewing practical imaging algorithms and basic techniques for evaluating congenital pulmonary malformations in pediatric patients.

Congenital pulmonary malformations are increasingly being detected with prenatal ultrasonography (US), often supplemented by magnetic resonance (MR) imaging.[3–7] In asymptomatic infants with prenatal imaging findings suspicious for congenital pulmonary malformations as well as symptomatic infants and children, 2-view chest radiographs (ie, posteroanterior and lateral views) are the initial imaging modality of choice. For young infants (≤6 months old) in whom the lateral chest radiograph cannot be easily obtained, an anteroposterior view may suffice. The chest radiographic findings that may provide clues to the presence of congenital pulmonary malformations include: (1) focal hyperlucency; (2) focal cystic or solid pulmonary or mediastinal mass; (3) vascular abnormality; (4) airway abnormality; and (5) thoracic asymmetry.[31,32] The findings seen on chest radiographs often provide not only valuable information for the diagnosis but also guidance for advanced imaging studies such as US, computed tomography (CT), and MR imaging for confirmation and further characterization of abnormalities.

US is a practical imaging modality, due to its widespread availability, relative ease of performance, and lack of ionizing radiation exposure. It is useful for assessing focal congenital pulmonary malformations such as foregut duplication cysts or pulmonary sequestration in neonates and young infants.[33,34] However, the utility of US for completely evaluating congenital pulmonary malformations is more limited in older children, who do not have favorable sonographic acoustic windows. To achieve optimal sonographic imaging evaluation in neonates and young infants, a high-resolution 10- to 15-MHz linear-array transducer in a transsternal, parasternal, or intercostal approach can be used.[33,34] In characterizing the lesions, imaging in at least 2 planes is recommended, and color flow may aid in demonstrating associated anomalous vessels.[33,34]

In recent years, multidetector CT (MDCT) employing a CT angiography protocol has assumed a greater role as a diagnostic imaging modality of choice for a thorough assessment of congenital pulmonary malformations in pediatric patients.[6,11,35–37] The combination of fast acquisition times, high spatial resolution, and the superb imaging quality of multiplanar reformation (MPR) and 3-dimensional (3D) reconstructions make MDCT an ideal noninvasive method for evaluating congenital pulmonary malformations in children.[11,35] Although technical parameters vary somewhat based on the type of MDCT scanners and specific types of congenital pulmonary malformations, accurate CT evaluation of congenital pulmonary malformations depends on basic CT parameters, including tube current or milliamperage, kilovoltage peak, table speed, detector collimation, and reconstruction thickness. The guideline for tube current and kilovoltage is shown in **Table 1**. Other basic MDCT parameters include fast table speed (<1 second), thin detector collimation (<1 mm), and a 1- to 2-mm reconstruction interval with the goal of obtaining approximately 50% of overlap for high image quality multiplanar 2-dimensional (2D) and 3D reconstruction images.[11] Once an axial CT data set is obtained, 3D images of the airway, lung, and vascular structures can be subsequently reconstructed at an interactive 2D/3D workstation for detailed anatomic assessment of congenital pulmonary malformations. The use of intravenous contrast is essential for assessing anomalous vessels often associated with congenital pulmonary malformations. The usual recommended contrast material dose is 1.5 to 2 mL per kilogram of patient body weight (not to exceed 3 mL/kg or 125 mL). Contrast material can be administered by means of manual injection or mechanical injection depending on the size, location, and stability of the angiocatheter.[11] The guideline for the contrast amount and injection rate is shown in **Table 2**. In general, mechanical injection of contrast material is the preferred method because it provides more homogeneous and reproducible contrast enhancement within the vascular structures, which is particularly helpful for subsequent 3D reconstruction.[11] The typical anatomic coverage is from the thoracic inlet level to the level of the diaphragm. However, in the setting of pulmonary sequestration, inclusion of the upper abdomen is important because the anomalous arterial vessels associated with pulmonary sequestration may arise from the proximal abdominal aorta and/or its major branches, particularly in the case of extralobar sequestration, which may occur in a subdiaphragmatic location.[11] Due to the greater radiosensitivity in pediatric patients, close adherence of ALARA (As Low As Reasonably Achievable) principles for radiation exposure during MDCT examination is paramount.[38,39]

MR imaging is an excellent modality for evaluating solid and vascular components of congenital pulmonary malformations. MR imaging is a particularly useful modality in pediatric patients because it is not associated with ionizing radiation exposure. However, complete evaluation of congenital pulmonary malformation is limited using MR imaging, due to its limited capability to accurately assess the lung parenchymal abnormality often associated with congenital pulmonary malformations. The basic MR imaging protocol for evaluating nonvascular congenital pulmonary malformations consists of axial fast relaxation fast spin echo (FRFSE) T2 fast saturation, axial T1 or double inversion recovery (DIR), coronal FRFSE T2 fat saturation, coronal 3D MR angiography, spoiled

| Table 1 |
| Guideline for the tube current and kilovoltage by patient weight |

Weight (kg)	Tube Current (mA)	Kilovoltage (kVp)
<10	40	80
10–14	50	80
15–24	60	80
25–34	70	80
35–44	80	80
45–54	90	90
55–70	100–120	100–120

| Table 2 |
| Guideline for the contrast amount and injection rate by patient weight |

Patient Weight (kg)	Amount of Contrast (mL)	Injection Rate[a] (mL/s)	Intravenous Catheter Size (g) (Preferred)
<10	<15	0.5–1	24
10–19	15–29	1	24
20–29	30–44	1.5–2	22
30–39	45–59	2.5–3	20
40–69	60–100	3–3.5	18–20
>70	>100	3–5	18

[a] Rates can vary ±0.5 mL based on intravenous catheter size and stability.

gradient-recalled echo (SPGR) with gadolinium, and axial and coronal T1 fat saturation (after gadolinium) typically using 8-channel cardiac coils. For vascular congenital pulmonary malformation evaluation, the typical MR imaging protocol includes axial, sagittal, and coronal oblique fast spin echo (FSE) DIR as well as sagittal 3D MR angiography SPGR with gadolinium. Ideally, a breath-hold/respiratory trigger should be used for FRFSE sequence. In sedated and intubated infants and young children, a breath-hold sequence may be used without requiring patient cooperation. Electrocardiography gating and breath-hold are necessary for a DIR sequence.

SPECTRUM OF CONGENITAL PULMONARY MALFORMATIONS IN PEDIATRIC PATIENTS

Classification of congenital pulmonary malformations is both challenging and often controversial from embryologic, radiologic, pathologic, and clinical viewpoints. There have been several ways of classifying congenital pulmonary malformations in the past.[40,41] Some investigators used embryology as their base and classified congenital pulmonary malformations according to the stage of intrauterine development in which the event giving rise to the malformation occurs.[41] Other investigators classified congenital pulmonary malformations based on a morphologic-radiological basis and divided them into two groups: whole lung malformations (eg, lung hypoplasia) and focal malformations (eg, bronchial atresia).[41,42] The authors' approach groups congenital pulmonary malformations according to morphology-radiology-pathology, with emphasis on considering them as a continuum ranging from pure pulmonary parenchymal anomalies to isolated vascular anomalies, with an intermediate group in which both pulmonary and vascular components are intertwined.[11,13] Such a morphology-radiology-pathology–based classification has the advantage of allowing for clear classification, relatively easy differentiation on imaging studies, and preoperative assessment of surgical lesions. Based on this classification system, congenital pulmonary malformations can be classified into 3 groups: parenchymal lesions (ie, abnormal lung and normal vasculature), vascular lesions (ie, normal lung and abnormal vasculature), and a combination of both (ie, abnormal lung and abnormal vasculature) (Fig. 1).[11,13] However, it is also important to recognize that some of these lesions may exhibit more than one component (ie, hybrid lesions) and specific terminology for these congenial pulmonary malformations may be controversial and occasionally confusing.[11,31]

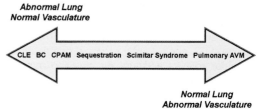

Fig. 1. Continuum of congenital pulmonary malformations. The 6 main congenital pulmonary malformations can be considered to span a continuum, ranging from an abnormal lung containing normal vessels to a normal lung containing abnormal vessels. Although many cases of congenital pulmonary malformations have the classic features of a single anomaly, other cases may have features common to 2 or more anomalies (ie, hybrid lesions). AVM, arteriovenous malformation; BC, bronchogenic cyst; CLE, congenital lobar emphysema. (*From* Panicek DM, Heitzman ER, Randall PA, et al. The continuum of pulmonary developmental anomalies. Radiographics 1987;7(4):748; with permission.)

Parenchymal Lesions (Nonvascular Lesions)

Bronchial atresia

Bronchial atresia, also known as bronchial mucocele, results from focal obliteration or stenosis of a segmental, subsegmental, or lobar bronchus at or near its origin.[3,11,43,44] The bronchus distal to the obliteration or stenosis dilates and eventually accumulates a variable amount of mucus (Fig. 2). Such a process may occur in utero or later in life. The congenital form is considered here. The constellation of features associated with congenital bronchial atresia includes postobstructive

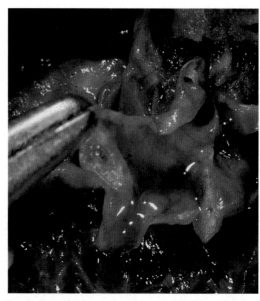

Fig. 2. Bronchial atresia. Gross surgical specimen of bronchial atresia demonstrates intraluminal mucus accumulation.

mucus retention (also known as mucocele), congenital lobar emphysema/overinflation, CPAM, and intralobar sequestration.[27] The former 3 conditions are all associated with a type of maldevelopment described histologically as "CCAM-like changes."[27] Riedlinger and colleagues[27] recently found bronchial atresia in 100% of extralobar pulmonary sequestration, 82% of intralobar pulmonary sequestration, 70% of CPAM, and 50% of congenital lobar emphysema using microdissection techniques. Such findings raise the possibility that bronchial atresia and other congenital pulmonary malformations (eg, pulmonary sequestration, CPAM, and congenital lobar emphysema) may have the same etiopathogenesis with anatomic differences accounted for by aberrant genetic programs or other insults, perhaps modified by time of onset or duration. Although affected patients may present with recurrent infections or respiratory compromise depending in large part on the size and the severity of the associated parenchymal disease, the majority of bronchial atresia is incidentally detected on chest radiographs or CT obtained for other indications in the past. However, bronchial atresia has been diagnosed more frequently in recent years, particularly on prenatal imaging studies.[26,27,45]

At prenatal imaging, bronchial atresia typically presents as a focal area of increased echogenicity on US and homogenously high signal intensity on T2-weighted images on MR.[46] The area of impacted mucus in the bronchus usually presents as a round or oval-shaped opacity in the apical or apicoposterior segment of the upper lobes on chest radiographs. A dilated tubular-shaped opacity with adjacent segmental hyperattenuation due to air trapping and decreased vascularity is a characteristic CT imaging finding, which can help in confirming the diagnosis of bronchial atresia (**Fig. 3**). Hyperinflation is usually seen within the lung parenchyma adjacent to the bronchial atresia, which is believed to be caused by the collateral air drift via the interstitium and pores of Kohn.[11,26,47] It has been reported that MDCT 2D and 3D reconstructions are valuable for identifying the atretic bronchus and the "bronchocele/mucocele", imaging feature that is unique to bronchial atresia.[6] The current management of choice for bronchial atresia is usually surgical resection, even in asymptomatic patients, because of the increased risk of infection.

Bronchogenic cysts
Bronchogenic cysts are developmental anomalies, which most likely result from defective ventral budding or branching of the tracheobronchial tree, between the 26th and 40th days of fetal life.[48–50] These cysts are a part of the spectrum

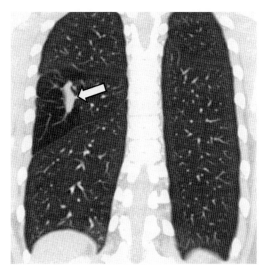

Fig. 3. Bronchial atresia in a 16-year-old girl with an abnormal chest radiograph obtained for recurrent cough. Coronal lung window CT image shows a dilated tubular-shaped opacity (*arrow*) in the right upper lobe with adjacent segmental hypoattenuation due to air trapping.

of foregut duplication cysts that include bronchogenic cysts, enteric cysts, and neurenteric cysts. In practice this distinction proves to be artificial, as cysts attached to the esophagus may contain respiratory epithelium, cysts attached to the tracheobronchial tree may contain squamous epithelium, and a majority of the foregut cysts in these locations show features of more than one foregut-derived structure (**Fig. 4**). Although bronchogenic cysts are typically located within the mediastinum (70%) near the subcarinal, hilar, or right paratracheal locations, they can also occur

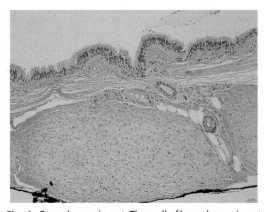

Fig. 4. Bronchogenic cyst. The wall of bronchogenic cyst consists of duplicated foregut structures predominantly recapitulating the airway. Ciliated respiratory epithelium, mucosal glands, and cartilage are shown here (hematoxylin-eosin; original magnification ×200).

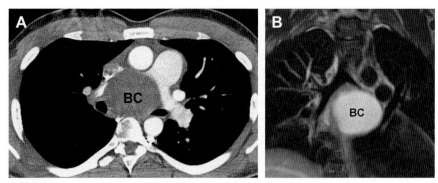

Fig. 5. Bronchogenic cyst in an 18-year-old man with respiratory distress. (*A*) Enhanced axial CT image shows a well-circumscribed round mass (BC) located in the subcarinal region. Due to the increased internal proteinaceous-mucoid material within the bronchogenic cyst, CT attenuation of this lesion is higher than water. (*B*) Coronal T2-weighted MR image demonstrates high signal intensity of the mass (BC), confirming the fluid-filled lesion.

within the lung parenchyma, with the majority of cases located in the lower lobes.[51–54] Other rare locations of bronchogenic cysts include neck, pericardium, or abdominal cavity.[52–55] Mediastinal bronchogenic cysts usually do not communicate with the adjacent bronchial tree. By contrast, intrapulmonary bronchogenic cysts often communicate with the adjacent bronchial tree. Such a connection may be responsible for recurrent infections in patients with intrapulmonary bronchogenic cysts. Infected bronchogenic cysts are more often seen in older children.[32] Affected patients can also present with symptoms such as chest pain, respiratory distress, and dysphagia if the lesions are large enough to result in a mass effect on adjacent mediastinal structures such as airways and esophagus.[11,32]

On chest radiographs, bronchogenic cysts typically present as a well-circumscribed round or oval mass in the middle mediastinal compartment,[11,52–54] and are hypoechoic lesions on US. Bronchogenic cysts usually present as well-defined hypoattenuating lesions with uniform fluid attenuation (0–20 Hounsfield units) in approximately 50% of cases on CT (**Fig. 5**).[11,50,54,56] Due to the increased internal proteinaceous-mucoid material within the bronchogenic cysts or complication by intracyst hemorrhage, CT attenuation of the lesions may be higher than water and may mimic solid masses. In this situation, MR imaging can be used as a problem solver, because bronchogenic cysts always demonstrate high signal intensity on T2-weighted images, whereas on T1-weighted images the signal intensity ranges from low to high depending on the cyst contents (see **Fig. 5**).[57,58] On both postcontrast CT and MR images, no internal contrast enhancement is seen within bronchogenic cysts. The presence of

air-fluid level, thick enhancing wall, and surrounding inflammatory changes are clues to diagnosing infected bronchogenic cysts (**Fig. 6**). The current treatment options for bronchogenic cysts, particularly in symptomatic pediatric patients, include percutaneous or transbronchial needle aspirations and complete or partial resection by thoracoscopic or open surgery.

Congenital lobar emphysema

Congenital lobar emphysema, also known as infantile lobar emphysema or congenital lobar hyperinflation, is a condition characterized by the overinflation and distension of one or more pulmonary lobes.[49,52,56,59–63] The cause of congenital lobar emphysema can be either intrinsic or extrinsic bronchial narrowing with subsequent air

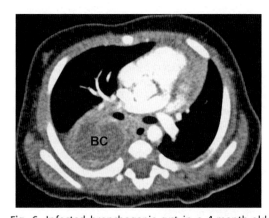

Fig. 6. Infected bronchogenic cyst in a 4-month-old girl who presented with fever and respiratory distress. Enhanced axial CT image shows a round mass (BC) with thick enhancing wall and surrounding inflammatory changes located posterior to the right main stem bronchus.

trapping. Whereas intrinsic narrowing can result from the weakness or absence of underlying bronchial cartilage, extrinsic narrowing may develop from the mass effect on the bronchus from adjacent mediastinal masses or enlarged vessels. There are two types of congenital lobar emphysema, distinguished histologically based on the number of alveoli: hypoalveolar type (fewer than expected number of alveoli) and polyalveolar type (> expected number of alveoli).[11,64] Whereas there are decreased numbers of alveoli that are overdistended in patients with the hypoalveolar type of congenital lobar emphysema, there are more alveoli (threefold to fivefold) than expected in a more recently described polyalveolar type of congenital lobar emphysema (Fig. 7).[64] In the polyalveolar type of congenital lobar emphysema, hyperinflation of the lobe is due to the sheer increase in number of normally inflated air spaces. Affected patients typically present with respiratory distress within the first 6 months of life.[32] The symptoms primarily depend on the size of the affected lobe as well as the degree of compression on adjacent normal lung tissues and mediastinal structures.

On chest radiographs the lung involved by congenital lobar emphysema may initially appear opaque, due to the underlying retention of fetal lung fluid after birth (Fig. 8).[32] As fetal lung fluid is cleared by the tracheobronchial system, lymphatics, and capillary network, the affected lobe usually shows hyperlucency with increase in size and subsequent mass effect on the adjacent, nonaffected lobes and mediastinal structures. The left upper lobe is the most frequently affected (42%), followed by right middle (35%) and right upper lobe (21%).[65] Rarely, congenital lobar emphysema may show bilateral or multifocal involvement.[66] The characteristic CT finding of congenital lobar emphysema is a hyperinflated lobe with attenuated pulmonary vessels (Fig. 9).[11] Recognizing attenuated lung markings within the overinflated lobe can be helpful for differentiating congenital lobar emphysema from a pneumothorax. CT is also useful for diagnosing multilobar involvement and excluding secondary causes of lobar overinflation due to vascular rings or mediastinal masses. The current management options for congenital lobar emphysema primarily depend on the clinical presentation of patients.[62,63] Asymptomatic children or those with only mild symptoms may benefit from conservative management because the previous studies showed gradual reduction in size of the congenital lobar emphysema in such patient groups. However, lobectomy by open or thoracoscopic approach is the current management of choice in symptomatic patients with severe and progressively worsening respiratory distress.[62,63]

Congenital pulmonary airway malformations

CPAMs, also previously known as congenital cystic adenomatoid malformations (CCAMs), are a heterogeneous group of congenital cystic and noncystic lung masses characterized by extensive overgrowth of the primary bronchioles, which are in communication with the abnormal bronchial tree lacking cartilage (Figs. 10 and 11).[49,52,56,67–69] In the majority of CPAMs, blood supply is from the pulmonary artery and venous drainage is into the pulmonary vein.[11] Affected patients usually present with respiratory difficulty or infection between the neonatal period and 2 years of age unless previously detected by prenatal imaging studies. Our understanding of CPAM has recently been advanced with the recognition of its association with bronchial atresia.[27,45,70,71] It is becoming well accepted that the histologic changes of CPAM may be secondary to intrauterine obstruction of the airway.

There has been considerable controversy over classification and nomenclature regarding these pulmonary malformations. Recently, the new term CPAM has been recommended instead of the previous term CCAM, for two main reasons. First, the lesions are cystic in only 3 (type 1, 2, and 4) of the 5 types of these pulmonary malformations. Second, only one type (type 3) is characterized by adenomatoid proliferation on histopathological evaluation. The most updated classification by Stocker[69] consists of 5 types (0–4), based on the

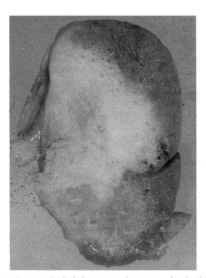

Fig. 7. Congenital lobar emphysema (polyalveolar type). Partial pneumonectomy specimen shows polyalveolar type lobar emphysema, which appears as a pale area predominately located in the right upper lobe.

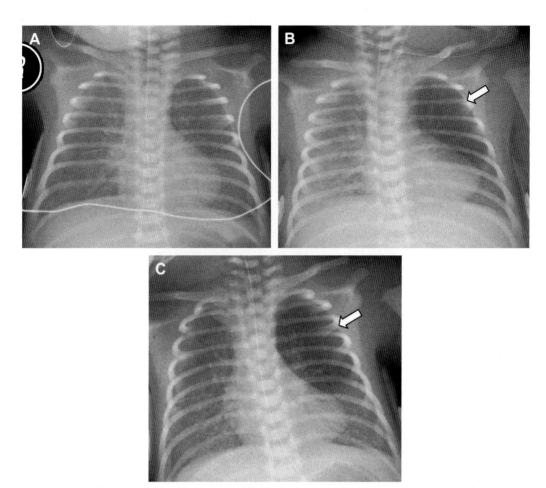

Fig. 8. Congenital lobar emphysema in a 2-day-old girl who presented with progressively worsening respiratory distress. (*A*) Initial frontal chest radiograph obtained at birth is unremarkable. (*B*) Frontal chest radiograph obtained 4 hours after birth demonstrates interval development of hyperlucency (*arrow*) in the left upper lobe. (*C*) Frontal chest radiograph obtained 7 hours after birth shows increased hyperlucency (*arrow*) of the left upper lobe.

cyst size and histologic resemblance to segments of the developing bronchial tree and airspaces. This new classification of CPAMs by Stocker is an extension of his original classification (3 types).[68] Type 0 CPAM is characterized by acinar dysgenesis or dysplasia of the large airways such as trachea or bronchus involving all lung lobes.[6,12,69] Type 0 CPAM is incompatible with life. Type 1 CPAM is characterized by single or multiple cysts (>2 cm) of bronchial or bronchiolar origin.[6,12,69] Type 2 CPAM is characterized by single or multiple cysts (≤2 cm) of bronchiolar origin.[6,12,69] Type 3 CPAM is a predominantly solid lesion, with small cysts (<0.5 cm) of bronchiolar-alveolar duct origin.[6,12,69] Type 4 CPAM is characterized by large air-filled cysts of distal acinar origin.[6,12,69] Unfortunately, this classification scheme can be difficult to apply in clinical practice.

Imaging findings of CPAMs often correlate with underlying histopathological characteristics, and appear as one or more, air-filled "cystic" structures. Solid areas may be present. The typical imaging appearance of Type 1 CPAM is one or more large, air-filled cystic structures (**Fig. 12**).[12] Type 2 CPAM usually presents as an air-filled multicystic mass or focal area of consolidation (**Fig. 13**).[12] Type 3 CPAM appears solid at imaging due to microscopic cysts that can be identified only at histologic evaluation (**Fig. 14**).[12] Type 4 CPAM (**Fig. 15**) usually presents as a large cyst at imaging, and has been reported to be radiographically indistinguishable from a predominantly cystic pleuropulmonary blastoma (Type 1) (**Fig. 16**).[12,72,73] Patients with Type 0 CPAM is incompatible with life; therefore, imaging studies are not usually performed. In patients with infected CPAMs, associated findings of internal air-fluid level and enhancing thick wall are often seen.

The current management of choice for CPAMs in symptomatic pediatric patients is surgical resection by either lobectomy or segmentectomy.

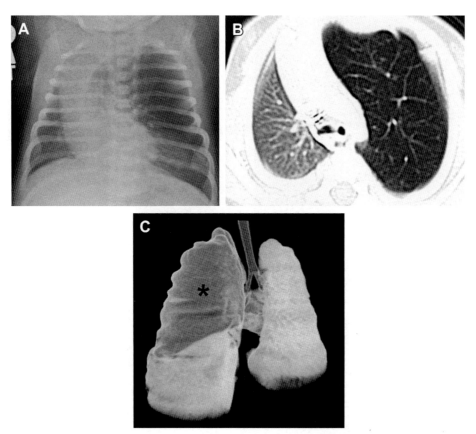

Fig. 9. Congenital lobar emphysema in a 3-day-old boy who presented with respiratory distress. (*A*) Frontal chest radiograph shows a marked hyperinflation of the left upper lobe. (*B*) Axial lung window CT image demonstrates a hyperinflated left upper lobe with attenuated lung markings and mediastinal shift to the right side. (*C*) Posterior view of 3-dimensional (3D) volume-rendered image of the lungs shows a hyperinflated left upper lobe (*asterisk*).

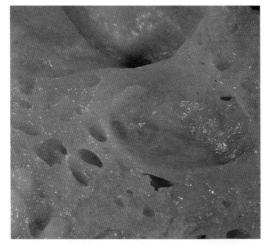

Fig. 10. Congenital pulmonary airway malformation. A gross surgical specimen of congenital pulmonary malformation (previously termed as congenital pulmonary adenomatoid malformation) shows the "cystic" structure interconnected to an adjacent smaller-caliber airway-like structure.

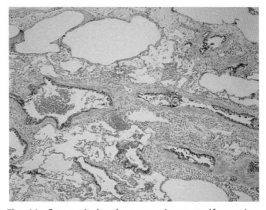

Fig. 11. Congenital pulmonary airway malformation. The malformed tissue consists of frequent airway-like structures lined by smooth muscle and respiratory epithelium, surrounded by enlarged alveoli (H&E; original magnification ×100).

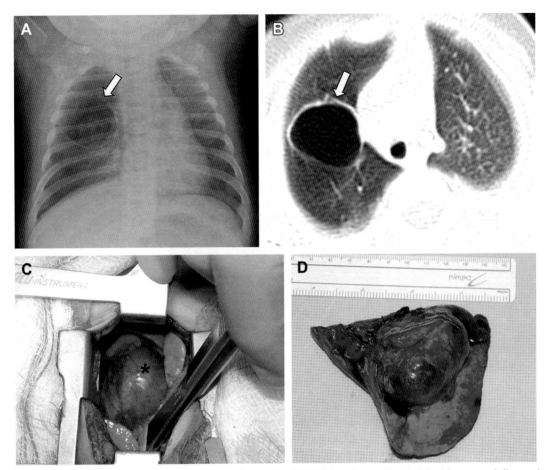

Fig. 12. Type 1 congenital pulmonary airway malformation (CPAM) in a 2-month-old girl with prenatal diagnosis of a lung mass. Surgical pathology was consistent with the diagnosis of CPAM. (*A*) Frontal chest radiograph show a large cystic mass (*arrow*) located in the right upper lung zone. (*B*) Axial lung window CT image demonstrates a large cystic mass (*arrow*) with thin wall located in the right upper lobe. (*C*) Intraoperative image show a large cystic mass (*asterisk*). (*D*) Gross surgical specimen of type 1 CPAM. (*Courtesy of* Carl-Christian Jackson, MD.)

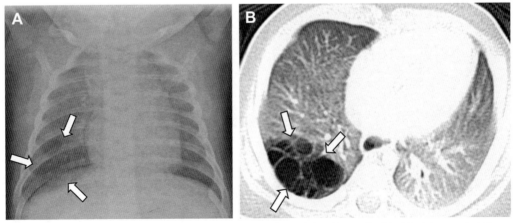

Fig. 13. Type 2 congenital pulmonary airway malformation (CPAM) in a 2-month-old girl with prenatal diagnosis of a lung mass. Surgical pathology confirmed the diagnosis of CPAM. (*A*) Frontal chest radiograph shows an area (*arrows*) of hyperlucency in the right lower lobe. (*B*) Axial lung window CT image demonstrates an air-filled multicystic mass (*arrows*).

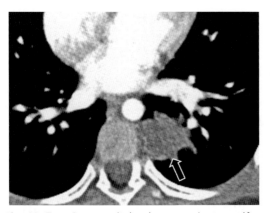

Fig. 14. Type 3 congenital pulmonary airway malformation (CPAM) in a 3-year-old girl with recurrent left lower lobe pneumonia. Enhanced axial CT image shows a solid mass (*arrow*) located in the left lower lobe without the presence of associated anomalous artery or vein. Surgical pathology was consistent with the diagnosis of type 3 CPAM.

Although the necessity for surgical resection of CPAMs in asymptomatic infants and children is somewhat controversial, potential recurrent infection, pneumothorax, and hemorrhage have been the main reasons for advocating elective surgical resection of CPAMs.[11] Others have advocated surgical resection, due to the inability to distinguish CPAM radiologically from type 1 or 2 cystic pleuropulmonary blastoma, which is a very rare primary lung neoplasm in children.[11,74] The recent discovery of the genetic defect for pleuropulmonary blastoma may prove to be of further help in guiding surgical decision making.[75]

Vascular Lesions

Anomalies of pulmonary artery
Pulmonary agenesis, aplasia, and hypoplasia Lung underdevelopment can be classified into 3 groups: (1) lung agenesis (total absence of the lung,

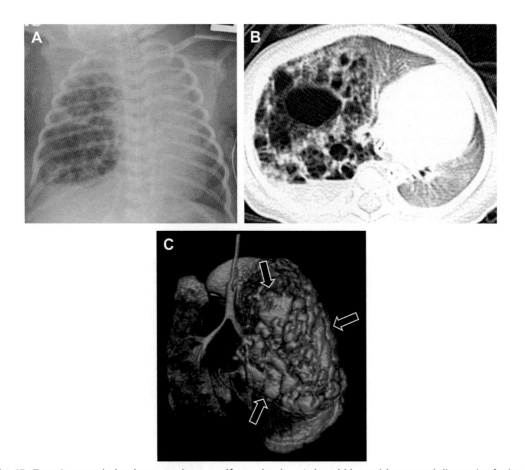

Fig. 15. Type 4 congenital pulmonary airway malformation in a 1-day-old boy with prenatal diagnosis of a lung mass. (*A*) Frontal chest radiograph shows a large multicystic mass occupying the entire right hemithorax with mediastinal shift to the contralateral side. (*B*) Axial lung window CT image demonstrates a large mass containing cysts with varying size. Again noted is the mediastinal shift to the left side. (*C*) Posterior view of 3D volume-rendered image of the lungs shows multiple cysts (*arrows*) occupying the entire right lung.

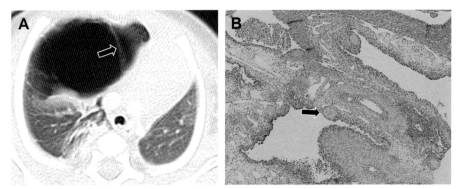

Fig. 16. Cystic (type 1) pleuropulmonary blastoma (PPB) in a 2-month-old boy who presented with an abnormal breathing pattern. (A) Axial lung window CT image shows a large cystic mass located in the right upper lung with a thin septation (arrow) and mediastinal shift to the left side. (B) Surgical resection specimen demonstrates epithelium-lined cysts with septa containing cellular stroma and occasional nodules (arrow) of developing cartilage (H&E; original magnification ×100).

bronchus, and pulmonary artery) (Fig. 17); (2) lung aplasia (total absence of the lung and pulmonary artery with a rudimentary main bronchus) (Fig. 18); and (3) lung hypoplasia (hypoplastic bronchus and pulmonary artery and an associated variable amount of lung tissue) (Fig. 19).[11,41,49,52] The underlying etiology of lung agenesis or aplasia is currently unknown; however, genetic, teratogenic, and mechanical factors have all been postulated to play a role. By contrast, lung hypoplasia can be primary with no identifiable cause of underdevelopment, or secondary to the limitation of normal fetal lung development by various causes including maternal oligohydramnios, thoracic dystrophies, large diaphragmatic hernias, and congenital lung masses. Bilateral pulmonary agenesis is incompatible with life.[11] However,

patients with pulmonary agenesis, aplasia, and hypoplasia either may be asymptomatic or may present with various degrees of respiratory distress depending on the severity of lung underdevelopment. In asymptomatic pediatric patients, lung agenesis, aplasia, or hypoplasia is often an incidental finding. Lung agenesis is associated with other congenital anomalies including vertebral anomalies, cardiovascular defects, anorectal malformations, esophageal atresia, tracheoesophageal fistula, and genitourinary anomalies.[76,77]

The chest radiographic findings of lung agenesis and aplasia are often similar. The frontal chest radiograph typically shows a small, opaque hemithorax, mediastinal shift to the ipsilateral side, and elevation of the hemidiaphragm on the affected side.[11,32] On the lateral view an increased lucency

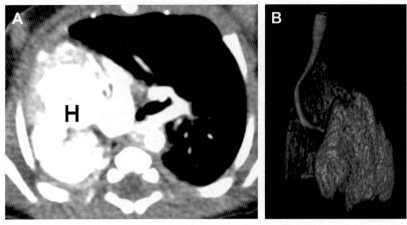

Fig. 17. Lung agenesis in a 5-day-old girl who presented with respiratory distress and abnormal chest radiograph. (A) Enhanced axial CT image shows a complete absence of the right lung. Mediastinal structures including heart (H) are located in the right hemithorax. (B) Anterior view of 3D volume-rendered image of the central airway and lungs shows a complete absence of the right bronchus and lung.

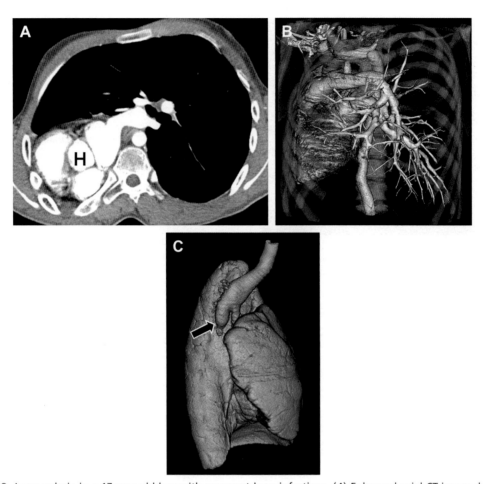

Fig. 18. Lung aplasia in a 17-year-old boy with recurrent lung infections. (*A*) Enhanced axial CT image demonstrates a complete absence of the lung and right pulmonary artery. Mediastinal structures including heart (H) are located in the right hemithorax. (*B*) Anterior view of 3D volume-rendered image of the vascular structures shows an absent right pulmonary artery and compensatory hypertrophy of left pulmonary artery. (*C*) Anterior oblique view of 3D volume-rendered image of the central airway and lungs demonstrates a rudimentary right main stem bronchus (*arrow*).

is located behind the sternum, representing compensatory overinflation and herniation of the contralateral lung, while mediastinal structures are displaced posteriorly. The chest radiographic findings of pulmonary hypoplasia depend on the severity of underling lung hypoplasia. Variable degrees of decreased lung volume associated with ipsilateral cardiomediastinal shift and diaphragmatic elevation are seen in patients with unilateral lung hypoplasia. Although MR imaging can accurately define vascular anomalies associated with lung agenesis, lung aplasia, and lung hypoplasia, evaluation of lung parenchyma and airways is limited with MR imaging. The current imaging modality of choice for a complete assessment of congenital underdevelopment of lung is MDCT.[11,78–82] MDCT with 2D/3D reconstructions of the vascular structures, airways, and

lung parenchyma can accurately detect all thoracic abnormalities and helps in differentiating between lung agenesis, lung aplasia, and lung hypoplasia (see **Figs. 17–19**). The prognosis of pediatric patients with underdevelopment of lung depends on the degree of underdevelopment and the severity of any associated congenital anomalies.

Proximal interruption of the pulmonary artery Proximal interruption of the pulmonary artery is characterized by the absence of the proximal portion of the pulmonary artery.[11,31,83–87] This congenital vascular anomaly occurs when the proximal portion of the main pulmonary artery, which arises from the primitive proximal sixth aortic arch, fails to appear during embryologic development.[11,31,83–87] Although the proximal portion of the main pulmonary artery is absent in

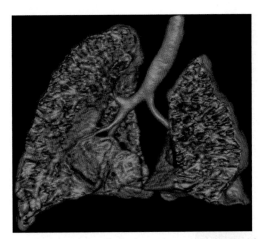

Fig. 19. Lung hypoplasia in a 1-year-old boy with multiple congenital anomalies. Anterior view of 3D volume-rendered image of the central airways and lungs shows hypoplastic left main stem bronchus and left lung.

this condition, the pulmonary artery in the hilar region and distal pulmonary arteries are almost always present[31]; this may be explained by the different embryologic origins of the proximal and distal pulmonary artery branches. While the primitive proximal sixth aortic arch gives rise to the proximal portion of the pulmonary artery, the primitive distal sixth aortic arch becomes the ductus. In the case of proximal interruption of the proximal pulmonary artery, the pulmonary artery in the hilar region and the distal pulmonary artery branches are still developed by the blood supply from the ductus originating either from the base of the right innominate artery or occasionally from an aberrant right subclavian artery.[31,84,85] Therefore, a residual ductus bump is often seen in this location in patients with proximal interruption of the pulmonary artery.[31] Subsequently, blood supply to the affected side of the lung is from the collateral vessels such as bronchial and intercostal arteries. For the lower lobes in these patients, collateral vessels may also arise directly from the aorta. Although proximal interruption of the pulmonary artery can affect either the right or left pulmonary artery, it is more common on the right side. It has been reported that when this condition occurs on the left, which is the opposite side of the normal left aortic arch, it is often associated with other congenital heart disease including right aortic arch, tetralogy of Fallot, patent ductus arteriosus, and septal defects.[31] Although asymptomatic patients with this condition may be detected incidentally, some patients can present with symptoms including recurrent pulmonary infection, hemoptysis, and pulmonary hypertension.[84,86]

Typical chest radiographic findings of proximal interruption of pulmonary artery include: (1) a hypoplastic lung on the same side as the absent pulmonary artery; (2) small or absent hilar shadow; (3) mediastinal shift to the affected lung side; and (4) a reticular network of vascular markings in the peripheral portion of the affected lung, which represent the collateral arterial supply (Fig. 20A).[31,32,83] Cross-sectional imaging studies such as CT and MR imaging can better demonstrate the affected pulmonary artery, which usually terminates within 1 cm of its origin from the main pulmonary artery (see Fig. 20B, C).[11,88] MDCT with 3D reconstructions is particularly valuable for a complete assessment of the proximal interruption of the pulmonary artery by displaying the affected pulmonary artery, the enlarged contralateral-side pulmonary artery, multiple collateral vessel formation, and central airway anomalies.[11] Early and correct diagnosis of this condition is important because early surgical reanastomosis or graft reattachment of the main and hilar pulmonary arteries may provide adequate blood supply to the affected lung. Such early revascularization of the affected lung may result in improved lung and pulmonary artery growth.[31,87] Embolization of the large collateral vessels may be indicated in pediatric patients with proximal interruption of pulmonary artery who present with recurrent hemoptysis or pulmonary hypertension.

Pulmonary artery sling Pulmonary artery sling is a rare congenital mediastinal vascular anomaly. In this condition, a pulmonary sling is created by an anomalous origin of the left pulmonary artery, which arises from the posterior aspect of the right pulmonary artery and courses between the trachea and esophagus toward the left hemithorax.[3,11,49,52,78,80,89] The term "sling" refers to the looping appearance of the anomalous left pulmonary artery around the central airways. Embryologically, pulmonary artery sling results from obliteration of the primitive left sixth aortic arch.[11,43] The concomitant presence of the ligamentum arteriosus results in a complete vascular ring that encircles the trachea but spares the esophagus. There are two main types of pulmonary artery sling: type 1 and type 2.[11,90] In type 1 pulmonary artery sling, the position of the carina is usually normal, at the T4-T5 level.[11,90] The anomalous left pulmonary artery usually compresses the posterior aspect of the trachea, lateral aspect of the right main stem bronchus, and anterior aspect of the esophagus. By contrast, type 2 pulmonary artery sling is characterized by the low position of the carina, typically at the T6 level.[11,90] Long-segment tracheal stenosis due to

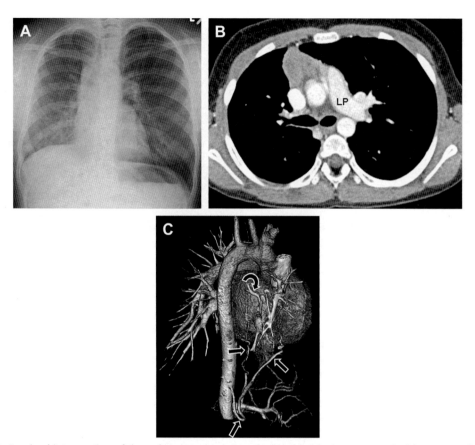

Fig. 20. Proximal interruption of the pulmonary artery in a 6-year-old girl who presented with recurrent hemoptysis and abnormal chest radiograph. (*A*) Frontal chest radiograph shows an absent right hilar vascular marking, small right hemithorax, and elevated right hemidiaphragm. (*B*) Enhanced axial CT image demonstrates a complete absence of the proximal portion of the right main pulmonary artery. Bilateral main stem bronchi are symmetric and normal in size. Right hemithorax is smaller than left hemithorax. LP, left pulmonary artery. (*C*) Posterior oblique view of 3D volume-rendered image of the vascular structures shows the collateral vessels (*straight arrows*) arising directly from the aorta and supplying blood to the right lower lobe. Also noted is a hypoplastic segment of the hilar portion of the right pulmonary artery (*curved arrow*).

complete cartilaginous rings, T-shaped carina (ie, a horizontal course of the main bronchi), and a bridging bronchus are often seen in patients with type 2 pulmonary artery sling. Other congenital anomalies of the large airways associated with pulmonary artery sling include tracheal bronchus and tracheomalacia.[11,90,91] Affected patients usually present with respiratory symptoms including stridor, apneic spells, and hypoxia during the neonatal period. However, this anomaly also may be incidentally discovered in asymptomatic older children.

Imaging findings of pulmonary artery sling depend on its type and other associated congenital anomalies. On chest radiographs, a hyperinflated right lung due to the compression of the right main stem bronchus from the anomalous left pulmonary artery may be seen.[11,80–82] Currently, MDCT with 3D reconstructions is the imaging modality of choice for a complete assessment of pulmonary artery sling (**Fig. 21**).[11,78,80–82] The origin, size, and entire course of the anomalous left pulmonary artery with associated central airway anomalies can be accurately displayed on MDCT 3D reconstruction images. Furthermore, the recently developed paired inspiratory-expiratory MDCT technique can now accurately assess the concomitant tracheomalacia often associated with pulmonary artery sling.[80,92,93] The current management of choice for pulmonary artery sling is the surgical reimplantation of the anomalous left pulmonary artery with tracheal reconstruction in cases of concomitant tracheal stenosis.[94] Surgical resection with end-to-end anastomosis is usually performed for short-segment tracheal stenosis, whereas tracheoplasty may be required for long-segment tracheal stenosis.[94,95]

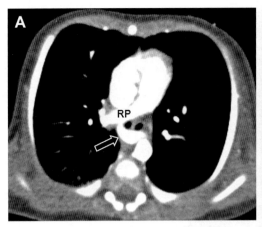
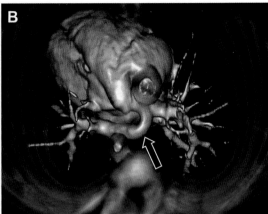

Fig. 21. Pulmonary artery sling in a 3-day-old boy who presented with respiratory distress. (*A*) Enhanced axial CT image shows an anomalous left pulmonary artery (*arrow*) arising from the right pulmonary artery (RP) and courses behind the main stem bronchi. (*B*) Superior view of the 3D volume-rendered image of the vascular structures demonstrates an entire course of the anomalous left pulmonary artery (*arrow*).

Anomalies of pulmonary vein

Pulmonary vein stenosis Pulmonary vein stenosis is a rare condition in which there is a narrowing or obstruction in the pulmonary vein.[11,96,97] It can be either congenital or acquired.[97] The congenital form of pulmonary vein stenosis without history of prior surgery or catheterization is currently believed to be attributable to uncontrolled growth of fibroblastic cells that cause thickening and narrowing of the pulmonary vein (**Fig. 22**).[11] Findings can be isolated or may follow repair of other congenital anomalies such as congenital heart disease and partial or total anomalous pulmonary venous return. Affected patients usually present with cyanosis, shortness of breath, and fatigue.[11,96] Such symptoms may progress rapidly, especially in pediatric patients with an isolated form of congenital pulmonary vein stenosis.

Chest radiographic findings of congenital pulmonary vein stenosis include increased reticular opacities with thickened septal lines due to poor venous drainage in the affected lung. CT is currently the diagnostic imaging modality of choice for evaluating congenital pulmonary vein stenosis. Characteristic CT imaging findings of pulmonary vein stenosis include pulmonary vein narrowing associated with thickening of the vein wall and pleural thickening (**Fig. 23**).[11] Although pulmonary vein stenosis typically occurs at the pulmonary venous and left atrial junction, extension into the intraparenchymal segment of the pulmonary vein resulting in long-segment narrowing can be seen in patients with advanced disease.[96–98] CT is also helpful for accurately detecting the presence and extent of lung abnormalities often associated with pulmonary vein stenosis.[11,97] There are several treatment options currently available for pediatric patients with congenital pulmonary vein stenosis. Short-segment pulmonary vein stenosis may be amenable to a balloon dilatation procedure sometimes followed by stent placement.[98–100] However, in patients with severe long-segment pulmonary vein stenosis, particularly involving bilateral pulmonary veins, lung transplant may be the final treatment option.[98–100] Trials using antiproliferation therapy are under way to evaluate whether chemotherapy might affect growth of the fibroblastic cells in patients with congenital pulmonary vein stenosis.

Pulmonary varix Congenital pulmonary varix is a rare congenital vascular anomaly, which is characterized by an aneurysmal dilatation of a segment of pulmonary vein that has a normal connection to the left atrium.[43,97,100–105] Although the majority of pulmonary varices are congenital, they can be also acquired. Acquired pulmonary varices usually occur in patients who have underlying pathologies

Fig. 22. Pulmonary vein stenosis. A cross section of pulmonary vein shows fibrous luminal obliteration (H&E; original magnification ×100).

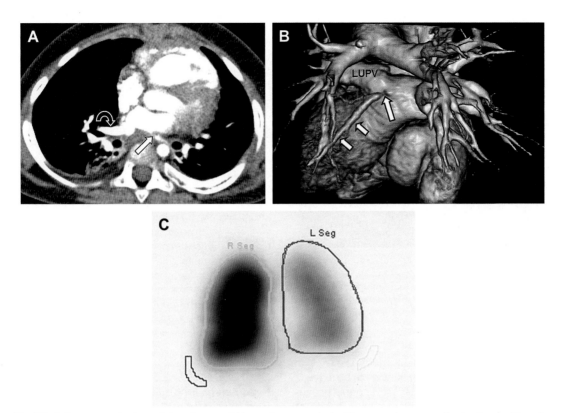

Fig. 23. Pulmonary vein stenosis in a 1-year-old boy who presented with worsening cyanosis, shortness of breath, and fatigue. Previously obtained echocardiogram suggested a narrowing of the left lower lobe pulmonary vein, and a CT angiogram was subsequently obtained for further evaluation. (A) Enhanced axial CT image shows a severe narrowing (*straight arrow*) of the left lower lobe pulmonary vein at the pulmonary venous and atrial junction. Patent and normal-sized right lower lobe pulmonary vein (*curved arrow*) is also seen. (B) Posterior view of the 3D volume-rendered image of the vascular structures and heart demonstrates a severe narrowing (*long arrow*) of the left lower lobe pulmonary vein. The distal portion of the left lower lobe pulmonary vein (*short arrows*) is also diffusely narrowed. Left upper lobe pulmonary vein (LUPV) is patent and normal in size. (C) Anterior view of the perfusion lung scan shows the differential pulmonary perfusion (23% left lung and 77% right lung). R seg, right lung; L seg, left lung.

that cause pulmonary venous hypertension, such as mitral valve stenosis and mitral valve insufficiency.[43,97] Most of patients with pulmonary varices are asymptomatic. In such patients, pulmonary varices are usually incidental findings. However, patients can be symptomatic, due to complications of pulmonary varices such as rupture and thromboembolism.[43,97,105]

On chest radiographs, pulmonary varices typically present as well-defined pulmonary or mediastinal masses near the heart borders. Although a pulmonary varix is a relatively benign lesion, it is important to differentiate it from other causes of mass lesions on chest radiographs in children, such as focal congenital lung anomaly, neoplasm, or infectious disease. In recent years, MDCT with 2D and 3D reconstructions has become a noninvasive imaging modality of choice for confirmation and characterization of pulmonary varix.[11,97,104] The characteristic CT imaging findings of pulmonary

varix include: (1) contiguity between the pulmonary varix and the adjacent pulmonary vein; (2) concurrent contrast material filling within these structures; and (3) absence of a feeding artery (Fig. 24).[11,97,102–105] 2D and 3D reconstruction MDCT images are particularly helpful for assessing tortuous pulmonary varix when accurate assessment cannot be made with axial CT images alone.[11] Treatment is usually not required in asymptomatic patients with small pulmonary varices that are detected incidentally. However, surgical resection may be necessary in symptomatic patients with large or complicated pulmonary varices.

Combined anomalies of pulmonary artery and vein

Pulmonary arteriovenous malformation Pulmonary arteriovenous malformation (AVM) is a vascular malformation characterized by a direct communication between a pulmonary artery and vein without

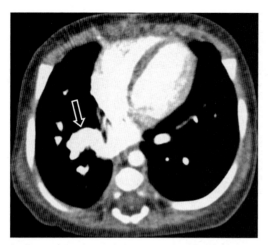

Fig. 24. Pulmonary varix in a 2-week-old girl who presented with respiratory distress and abnormal chest radiograph. Enhanced axial CT image shows an enlarged and tortuous right inferior pulmonary vein (*arrow*). There was an absence of anomalous feeding artery.

an intervening capillary network.[106–121] The origin of pulmonary AVM has been postulated to be a developmental defect in the formation of normal pulmonary capillaries.[11,97] It can be congenital or acquired. The acquired form of pulmonary AVM is usually seen in patients with prior congenital heart disease surgeries, chronic liver disease, or infections due to tuberculosis or actinomycosis.[11,43,97] Pulmonary AVM can be an isolated finding or can be associated with hereditary hemorrhagic telangiectasia (HHT), also known as Rendu-Osler-Weber syndrome.[106,107] The hereditary hemorrhagic telangiectasia is an autosomal dominant condition, which is characterized by the clinical triad of epistaxis, mucocutaneous or visceral telangiectasia, and family history of pulmonary AVM. Pulmonary AVM can be present in up to 35% of patients with HHT.[106,107] Therefore, family members with HHT should be screened for pulmonary AVM. Patients with small pulmonary AVM (<2 cm) may be asymptomatic, particularly during childhood.[11,106] However, large or multiple pulmonary AVMs can cause anatomic right-to-left shunts and result in desaturation, polycythemia, or paradoxic emboli.[32,106,107] Such patients usually present with dyspnea on exertion, cyanosis, chest pain, palpitations, and hemoptysis.

On chest radiographs, pulmonary AVM usually appears as a well-circumscribed serpiginous or lobulated opacity projecting over the either lungs or mediastinum.[11,32] Curvilinear opacities toward the hilum representing underlying feeding artery or draining vein may be seen on chest radiographs. In the past, pulmonary AVM was traditionally evaluated with conventional pulmonary angiography. However, in recent years MDCT has become the imaging modality of choice for a complete assessment of pulmonary AVM.[11] MDCT with 2D and 3D reconstruction can clearly demonstrate pulmonary AVM with its feeding artery and draining vein (**Figs. 25 and 26**).[11] Although the majority of pulmonary AVMs demonstrate a simple angioarchitecture consisting of a single feeding artery and draining vein, complex angioarchitecture with 2 or more feeding arteries and/or draining veins is seen in approximately 20% of cases.[122] MDCT with 2D and 3D reconstructions plays an important role in the preinterventional and posttreatment evaluation because it can clearly depict the number, size, extent, and angioarchitecture of the pulmonary AVM in detail.[11] In general, treatment is necessary for pulmonary AVMs with feeding arteries larger than 3 mm.[123–125] The current management choice of such pulmonary AVMs is endovascular coil embolization or balloon occlusion.

Combined Parenchymal and Vascular Lesions

Hypogenetic lung syndrome (scimitar syndrome)

Hypogenetic lung syndrome is a form of a partial anomalous pulmonary venous connection to the inferior vena cava and, less commonly, to portal or hepatic veins.[11,13,49,52,97] Other concomitantly associated anomalies of hypogenetic lung syndrome include hypoplastic right lung and pulmonary artery, cardiac dextroversion, and anomalous systemic arterial supply to the right lung.[11,24,52,97,126–128] This syndrome is also known as scimitar syndrome because the appearance of the anomalous pulmonary vein often resembles a scimitar, a curved Turkish sword (**Fig. 27**). Other congenital anomalies are seen in up to 25% of patients with hypogenetic lung syndrome, which include atrial and ventricular septal defects, patent ductus arteriosus, tetralogy of Fallot, diaphragmatic abnormalities, pulmonary sequestration, and horseshoe lung (**Fig. 28**).[11,24,52,97,126–128] Affected infants typically present with clinical signs and symptoms related to congestive heart failure that results from right heart volume overload. By contrast, hypogenetic lung syndrome may be incidental findings in older children, as with other congenital pulmonary malformations, or they can present with recurrent right basilar pulmonary infection.

The chest radiographs typically show a vertically oriented curvilinear opacity, which represents the scimitar vein, projecting over the right lower hemithorax in conjunction with a hypoplastic right lung

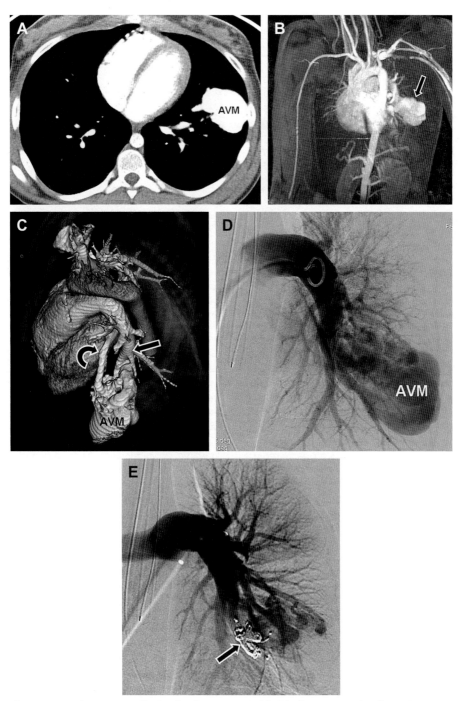

Fig. 25. Pulmonary arteriovenous malformation in a 13-year-old girl who presented to her primary care provider with progressively worsening fatigue and shortness of breath over the past 2 years. (*A*) Enhanced axial CT image shows a large vascular mass (AVM) located in the left hemithorax. (*B*) Coronal maximum-intensity projection MR image demonstrates a large enhancing mass (*arrow*). (*C*) Superior oblique view of the 3D volume-rendered image of the vascular structures shows a large vascular mass (AVM) with a feeding artery (*straight arrow*) from the left main pulmonary artery and a vein (*curved arrow*) draining into the left inferior pulmonary vein. (*D*) Pulmonary angiogram image demonstrates a large vascular mass (AVM), which correlates well with MR (*B*) and CT (*A* and *C*) imaging findings. (*E*) Pulmonary angiogram image after coil embolization (*arrow*) treatment shows interval obliteration of the large portion of the pulmonary arteriovenous malformation.

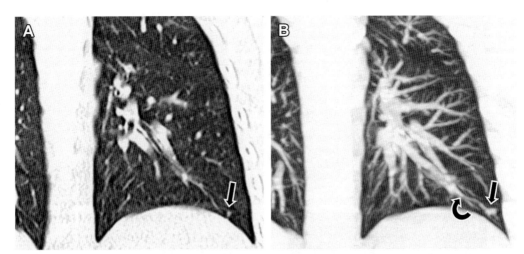

Fig. 26. Pulmonary arteriovenous malformation in a 6-year-old boy with shortness of breath and family history of hereditary hemorrhagic telangiectasia. (A) Coronal lung window CT image reformatted in a thin-section slice (1 mm) shows a small nodular lesion (arrow) in the left lower lobe. (B) Coronal maximum-intensity projection image reformatted in a slab thickness of 8 mm better demonstrates a small pulmonary arteriovenous malformation (arrow) by showing a feeding artery (curved arrow) than routine coronal lung window CT image reformatted in a thin-section slice (A).

(see **Fig. 27**A). Cross-sectional imaging studies such as CT or MR imaging are the current diagnostic imaging modalities of choice for confirming and characterizing hypogenetic lung syndrome in children. In recent years, 2D and 3D reconstructed images from MDCT have been reported as being particularly useful for displaying the entire course of the anomalous scimitar vein as a preprocedural or preoperative evaluation (see **Fig. 27**B, C).[11,24] Furthermore, they are also a helpful noninvasive imaging tool for evaluating postoperative complications including thrombosis or stenosis of reimplanted anomalous vein. In addition, abnormal lung parenchymal changes, abnormal lung lobulation, and anomalous bronchial branching patterns are often seen in patients with hypogenetic lung syndrome and can be also well evaluated with CT.[11,24] The absence of an ipsilateral inferior pulmonary vein is a helpful finding that supports diagnosis of hypogenetic lung syndrome on cross-sectional imaging studies. The current management choice for hypogenetic lung syndrome in symptomatic pediatric patients is surgical reconnection of the anomalous pulmonary vein into the left atrium and coil embolization of systemic arterial supply.[11,128,129]

Pulmonary sequestration

Pulmonary sequestration is a congenital pulmonary malformation that consists of a portion of nonfunctioning lung tissue that is not communicating with the adjacent tracheobronchial tree and receives systemic arterial blood supply.[3,6,11–13,31,52] Pulmonary sequestration has

been classified into two types: intralobar sequestration (75%) and extralobar sequestration (25%).[11–13,31,52] Intralobar sequestrations have been traditionally postulated to be acquired through recurrent infections, with subsequent bronchial obstruction and parasitized systemic arterial supply from the aorta. However, with the advent of prenatal imaging, an increasingly large number have been identified as congenital.[6]

Congenital intralobar pulmonary sequestration refers to a segment (or segments) of lung that has a systemic arterial supply and is invested by the same visceral pleura that covers the remainder of the lung. Most are located in the posterobasal segment of a lower lobe.[11–13,31,52] Recent advances in prenatal US and MR imaging have provided for the characterization of congenital intralobar pulmonary sequestration. The anomalous artery associated with intralobar pulmonary sequestration typically arises from the descending aorta while the anomalous vein drains into the left atrium via the inferior pulmonary vein (**Fig. 29**). Intralobar pulmonary sequestration is most often associated with an atretic bronchus.[26,27,71] The tissue contained in intralobar pulmonary sequestration usually grossly and microscopically resembles the cyst-like changes of CPAM. When such tissue is present, the maldevelopment may be considered a manifestation of "bronchial atresia sequence."[27] Affected children usually present with recurrent infections in the lower lobes, on the left side more often than the right side.[11,12] Intralobar pulmonary sequestration is seldom associated with other congenital anomalies.

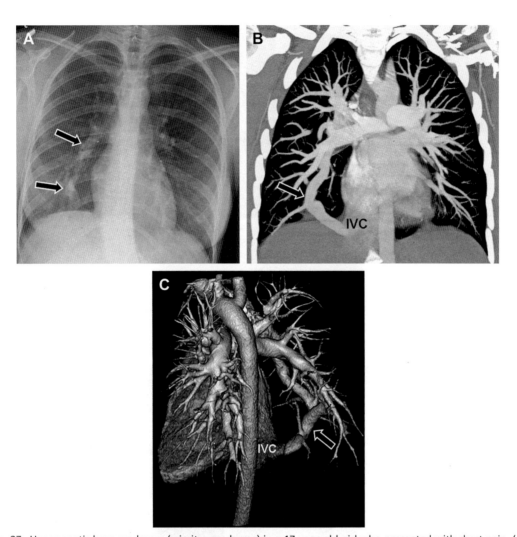

Fig. 27. Hypogenetic lung syndrome (scimitar syndrome) in a 17-year-old girl who presented with chest pain. (*A*) Frontal chest radiograph shows a vertically oriented curvilinear opacity (*arrows*) projecting over the right lower hemithorax. Also noted is hypoplastic right lung. (*B*) Coronal maximum-intensity projection image demonstrates a large scimitar vein (*arrow*) draining into inferior vena cava (IVC). (*C*) Posterior oblique view of the 3D volume-rendered image of the vascular structures clearly shows the size and course of the entire scimitar vein (*arrow*), which eventually drains into inferior vena cava (IVC). 3D imaging provides better "depth" information of vascular structure than maximum-intensity projection (*B*).

Extralobar pulmonary sequestration is a portion of lung tissue that is invested by its own visceral pleura, separate from the rest of the lung.[11,12] It has a systemic arterial supply and usually systemic venous drainage. Affected patients are usually infants who present during the neonatal period with focal lung masses, typically in the left lower thorax. Other less common locations of extralobar pulmonary sequestration include mediastinum, pericardium, and within or below the diaphragm.[3,6,11–13,31,52] The anomalous artery associated with extralobar pulmonary sequestration typically arises from the descending aorta or its branches such as the celiac axis, while the anomalous vein drains into various systemic veins (80%) including the azygous vein, the portal vein, the subclavian vein, or the internal mammary vein (**Fig. 30**).[3,6,11–13,31,52] Up to 50% of extralobar pulmonary sequestrations have been found to coexist with type 2 CPAM, also known as hybrid lesions (**Fig. 31**).[32,130] Unlike intralobar pulmonary sequestration, extralobar pulmonary sequestration is commonly associated with other congenital anomalies including congenital diaphragmatic defect and congenital heart disease.[11,32]

Imaging findings of pulmonary sequestration vary, mainly depending on the types, associated superimposed infection, and the concomitant

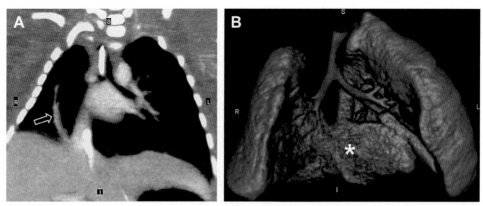

Fig. 28. Hypogenetic lung syndrome (scimitar syndrome) with horseshoe lung in a young child. (*A*) Enhanced coronal CT image shows a scimitar vein (*arrow*) and hypoplastic right lung. (*B*) Anterior view of 3D volume-rendered image of the central airway and lungs demonstrates a horseshoe lung. Inferior medial portions (*asterisk*) of both lungs are fused. (*Courtesy of* David Stringer, MD.)

presence of other congenital pulmonary malformations such as CPAM. It ranges from the heterogeneously enhancing solid mass to complex cystic mass with or without air-fluid level and/or internal

cavitation. US has sometimes been used for assessment of pulmonary sequestrations in infants or young children because pulmonary sequestrations and associated anomalous arteries

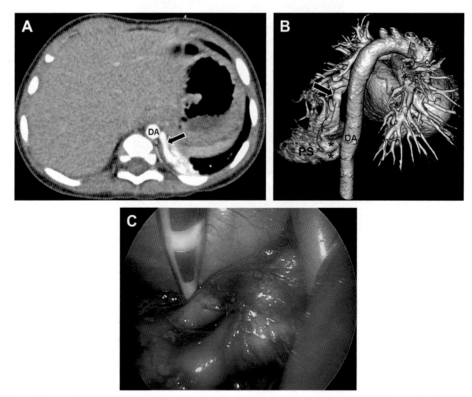

Fig. 29. Intralobar pulmonary sequestration in an 8-month-old boy with prenatal diagnosis of a lung mass. Surgical pathology confirmed the diagnosis of intralobar pulmonary sequestration. (*A*) Enhanced axial CT image shows an anomalous artery (*arrow*) arising from the descending aorta (DA). Just inferior to this level, there is also a second anomalous artery (not shown). (*B*) Posterior oblique view of the 3D volume-rendered image demonstrates a pulmonary sequestration (PS) with 2 large anomalous feeding arteries (*asterisks*) arising from the descending aorta (DA). Anomalous vein (*arrow*), which drains into the inferior pulmonary vein, is also seen. (*C*) Intraoperative image shows 2 large feeding arteries, which correspond well with imaging findings from the CT examination (*B*). (*Courtesy of* Terry L. Buchmiller, MD.)

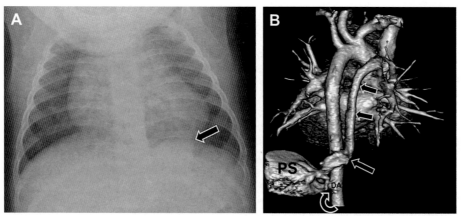

Fig. 30. Extralobar pulmonary sequestration in a 4-month-old boy who presented with respiratory distress. Surgical pathology was consistent with extralobar pulmonary sequestration. (*A*) Frontal chest radiograph shows a mass-like opacity (*arrow*) located within the inferior medial left hemithorax. (*B*) Posterior view of 3D volume-rendered image of the vascular structures demonstrates a large pulmonary sequestration (PS) with an anomalous feeding artery (*curved arrow*) arising from the descending aorta (DA), and a venous drainage via azygous (*long straight arrow*) and paraspinal (*short straight arrows*) veins.

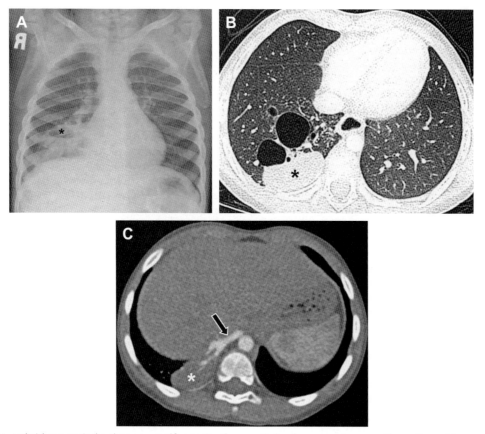

Fig. 31. Hybrid congenital pulmonary malformation (congenital pulmonary airway malformation with sequestration) in a 3-year-old boy with respiratory distress. Surgical specimen showed congenital pulmonary airway malformation with component of extralobar sequestration, which correlated with solid region seen on CT. (*A*) Frontal chest radiograph shows a large mass-like opacity with areas of lucency (*asterisk*) located in the right lower hemithorax. (*B*) Axial lung window CT image demonstrates a multicystic mass with solid component (*asterisk*). (*C*) Enhanced axial CT image demonstrates an anomalous feeding artery (*arrow*) arising from the descending aorta and supplying blood to the pulmonary sequestration portion (*asterisk*) of the hybrid congenital pulmonary malformation.

may be identified with this technique.[33,34] However, the current imaging modality of choice for evaluating pulmonary sequestration is MDCT.[6,11,12,35,36,80] MDCT with 2D and 3D reconstructions is helpful for making a correct diagnosis of pulmonary sequestration by accurately detecting not only anomalous artery but also anomalous vein associated with pulmonary sequestration.[11,35,36,80] The information regarding the venous drainage of the pulmonary sequestration is important for differentiating between intralobar and extralobar pulmonary sequestrations, because it may change the surgical approach. In cases of intralobar pulmonary sequestration, at least a segmentectomy of the involved lobe is performed while lobectomy can be performed in cases of extralobar sequestration, which has its own lung pleura.[11,35,36,80] A recent study in pediatric patients[131] demonstrated that the evaluation of anomalous veins associated with pulmonary sequestrations can benefit from using 2D and 3D reconstructed MDCT images. In this study, axial MDCT images allowed accurate diagnosis of the types, location, associated mass effect, and anomalous arteries of congenital pulmonary malformations, but supplemental 2D and 3D MDCT images added diagnostic value for the evaluation of congenital pulmonary malformations associated with anomalous veins. The investigators recommended that supplemental 2D and 3D MDCT images should be considered routinely, because such reconstructed images can enhance the evaluation of congenital pulmonary malformations associated with anomalous veins in children.[131] The complete and accurate preoperative assessment of anomalous vessels associated with pulmonary sequestration is paramount in avoiding accidental ligation of those vessels that can potentially lead to fatal hemorrhage. The current management of pulmonary sequestration is surgical resection, particularly for those presenting with recurrent infection. Alternative management of choice for pulmonary sequestrations in children is embolization of the feeding arterial vessels, which has been reportedly associated with a high success rate.[132,133]

SUMMARY

Congenital pulmonary malformations are a group of various anomalies involving lung parenchyma, pulmonary artery, and pulmonary vein, which can be the source for important morbidity and mortality in infants and children. The ability to diagnose congenital pulmonary malformations in children has advanced tremendously over the past decade. Traditional methods of chest radiographs, barium swallow study, bronchography, and conventional pulmonary angiography for evaluating these lesions are now being replaced or supplemented with MR and MDCT, which are noninvasive imaging techniques that provide superb imaging resolution in 2D and 3D viewing. Understanding proper imaging techniques, characteristic imaging findings, and underlying gross and histopathological structures of congenital pulmonary malformation can enhance the accurate diagnosis and proper management of pediatric patients with these often complex congenital pulmonary anomalies.

ACKNOWLEDGMENTS

The authors thank Harry Kozakewich, MD, for providing gross photographs of lungs demonstrating bronchial atresia.

REFERENCES

1. Sylvester KG, Albanese GT. Bronchopulmonary malformations. In: Ashcraft KW, Holcom GW, Murphy JP, editors. Ashcraft's pediatric surgery. Philadelphia: Saunders Elsevier; 2005. p. 276–89.
2. Costa Junior Ada S, Perfeito JA, Forte V. Surgical treatment of 60 patients with pulmonary malformations: what have we learned? J Bras Pneumol 2008; 34(9):661–6.
3. Biyyam DR, Chapman T, Ferguson MR, et al. Congenital lung abnormalities: embryologic features, prenatal diagnosis, and postnatal radiologic-pathologic correlation. Radiographics 2010;30(6):1721–38.
4. Liu YP, Chen CP, Shih SL, et al. Fetal cystic lung lesions: evaluation with magnetic resonance imaging. Pediatr Pulmonol 2010;45(6):592–600.
5. Santos XM, Papanna R, Johnson A, et al. The use of combined ultrasound and magnetic resonance imaging in the detection of fetal anomalies. Prenat Diagn 2010;30(5):402–7.
6. Epelman M, Kreiger PA, Servaes S, et al. Current imaging of prenatally diagnosed congenital lung lesions. Semin Ultrasound CT MR 2010;31(2): 141–57.
7. Pariente G, Aviram M, Landau D, et al. Prenatal diagnosis of congenital lobar emphysema: case report and review of the literature. J Ultrasound Med 2009;28(8):1081–4.
8. Correia-Pinto J, Gonzaga S, Huang Y, et al. Congenital lung lesions—underlying molecular mechanisms. Semin Pediatr Surg 2010;19(3):171–9.
9. Adzick NS. Management of fetal lung lesions. Clin Perinatol 2009;36:363–76.
10. Azizkhan RG, Crombleholme TM. Congenital cystic lung disease: contemporary antenatal and postnatal management. Pediatr Surg Int 2008;24:643–57.

11. Lee EY, Boiselle PM, Cleveland RH. Multidetector CT evaluation of congenital lung anomalies. Radiology 2008;247(3):632–48.

12. Yikilmaz A, Lee EY. CT imaging of mass-like nonvascular pulmonary lesions in children. Pediatr Radiol 2007;37(12):1253–63.

13. Panicek DM, Heitzman ER, Randall PA, et al. The continuum of pulmonary developmental anomalies. Radiographics 1987;7(4):747–72.

14. Demos NJ, Teresi A. Congenital lung malformations. A unified concept and a case report. J Thorac Cardiovasc Surg 1975;70:260–4.

15. Heithoff KB, Sane SM, Williams HJ, et al. Bronchopulmonary foregut malformations. A unifying etiological concept. AJR Am J Roentgenol 1976; 126(1):46–55.

16. Haller JA, Golladay ES, Pickard LR, et al. Surgical management of lung bud anomalies: lobar emphysema, bronchogenic cyst, cystic adenomatoid malformation, and intralobar pulmonary sequestration. Ann Thorac Surg 1979;28:33–43.

17. Keslar P, Newman B, Oh KS. Radiographic manifestations of anomalies of the lung. Radiol Clin North Am 1991;29:255–70.

18. Evrard V, Ceulemans J, Coosemans W, et al. Congenital parenchymatous malformations of the lung. World J Surg 1999;23:1123–32.

19. Luck SR, Reynolds M, Raffensperger JG. Congenital bronchopulmonary malformations. Curr Probl Surg 1986;23:251–314.

20. Buntain WL, Isaacs H, Payne VC, et al. Lobar emphysema, cystic adenomatoid malformation, pulmonary sequestration, and bronchogenic cyst in infancy and childhood: a clinical group. J Pediatr Surg 1974;9:85–93.

21. Restrepo S, Villamil MA, Rojas IC, et al. Association of two respiratory congenital anomalies: tracheal diverticulum and cystic adenomatoid malformation of the lung. Pediatr Radiol 2004;34:263–6.

22. Leithiser RE, Capitanio MA, Macpherson RI, et al. Communicating bronchopulmonary foregut malformations. AJR Am J Roentgenol 1986;146(2):227–31.

23. Bratu I, Flageole H, Chen MF, et al. The multiple facets of pulmonary sequestration. J Pediatr Surg 2001;36:784–90.

24. Konen E, Raviv-Zilka L, Cohen RA, et al. Congenital pulmonary venolobar syndrome: spectrum of helical CT findings with emphasis on computerized reformatting. Radiographics 2003;23:1175–84.

25. Johnson AM, Hubbard AM. Congenital anomalies of the fetal/neonatal chest. Semin Roentgenol 2004; 39:197–214.

26. Langston C. New concepts in the pathology of congenital lung malformations. Semin Pediatr Surg 2003;12:17–37.

27. Riedlinger WF, Vargas SO, Jennings RW, et al. Bronchial atresia is common to extralobar sequestration, intralobar sequestration, congenital cystic adenomatoid malformation, and lobar emphysema. Pediatr Dev Pathol 2006;9(5):361–73.

28. Volpe MV, Pham L, Lessin M, et al. Expression of Hoxb-5 during human lung development and in congenital lung malformations. Birth Defects Res A Clin Mol Teratol 2003;67:550–6.

29. Gonzaga S, Henriques-Coelho T, Davey M, et al. Cystic adenomatoid malformations are induced by localized FGF10 overexpression in fetal rat lung. Am J Respir Cell Mol Biol 2008;39:346–55.

30. Wagner AJ, Stumbaugh A, Tigue Z, et al. Genetic analysis of congenital cystic adenomatoid malformation reveals a novel pulmonary gene: fatty acid binding protein-7 (brain type). Pediatr Res 2008; 64:11–6.

31. Newman B. Congenital bronchopulmonary foregut malformations: concepts and controversies. Pediatr Radiol 2006;36:773–91.

32. Paterson A. Imaging evaluation of congenital lung abnormalities in infants and children. Radiol Clin North Am 2005;43:303–23.

33. Lee EY, Siegel MJ. Ultrasound evaluation of pediatric chest. In: Allan PL, Baxter G, Weston M, editors. Clinical ultrasound. 3rd edition. London: Elsevier; 2011. p. 1337–55.

34. Coley BD. Pediatric chest ultrasound. Radiol Clin North Am 2005;43(2):405–18.

35. Lee EY, Siegel MJ, Sierra LM, et al. Evaluation of angioarchitecture of pulmonary sequestration in pediatric patients using 3D MDCT angiography. AJR Am J Roentgenol 2004;183(1):183–8.

36. Lee EY, Dillon JE, Callahan MJ, et al. 3D multidetector CT angiographic evaluation of extralobar pulmonary sequestration with anomalous venous drainage into the left internal mammary vein in a paediatric patient. Br J Radiol 2006;79(945):e99–102.

37. Toma P, Rizzo F, Stagnaro N, et al. Multislice CT in congenital bronchopulmonary malformations in children. Radiol Med 2011;116(1):133–51.

38. Goske MJ, Applegate KE, Boyland J, et al. The image gently campaign: working together to change practice. AJR Am J Roentgenol 2008; 190(2):273–4.

39. Kim JE, Newman B. Evaluation of a radiation dose reduction strategy for pediatric chest CT. AJR Am J Roentgenol 2010;194(5):1188–93.

40. Clements BS, Warner JO. Pulmonary sequestration and related congenital bronchopulmonary-vascular malformations: nomenclature and classification based on anatomic and embryological considerations. Thorax 1987;42(6):401–8.

41. Mata JM, Caceres J. The dysmorphic lung: imaging findings. Eur Radiol 1996;6(4):403–14.

42. Mata JM, Caceres J, Lucaya J, et al. CT of congenital malformations of the lung. Radiographics 1990; 10(4):651–74.

43. Fraser R, Colman N, Muller NL, et al. Developmental and metabolic lung disease. In: Fraser R, Colman N, Muller NL, et al, editors. Synopsis of diseases of the chest. 3rd edition. Philadelphia: Elsevier Saunders; 2005. p. 188–221.

44. Webb W, Higgins CB. Congenital bronchopulmonary lesions. In: Webb WR, editor. Thoracic imaging: pulmonary and cardiovascular radiology. Philadelphia: Lippincott Williams & Wilkins; 2005. p. 1–29.

45. Kunisaki SM, Fauza DO, Nemes LP, et al. Bronchial atresia: the hidden pathology within a spectrum of prenatally diagnosed lung masses. J Pediatr Surg 2006;41:61–5.

46. Daltro P, Werner H, Gasparetto TD, et al. Congenital chest malformations: a multimodality approach with emphasis on fetal MR imaging. Radiographics 2010;30(2):385–95.

47. Talner LB, Gmelich JT, Liebow AA, et al. The syndrome of bronchial mucocele and regional hyperinflation of the lung. Am J Roentgenol Radium Ther Nucl Med 1970;110:675–86.

48. Chapman KR, Rebuck AS. Spontaneous disappearance of a chronic mediastinal mass. Chest 1985; 87:235–6.

49. Zylak CJ, Eyler WR, Spizarny DL, et al. Developmental lung anomalies in the adult: radiologic-pathologic correlation. Radiographics 2002; 22(Spec No):S25–43.

50. Aktgu S, Yuncu G, Halilocolar H, et al. Bronchogenic cysts: clinico-pathological presentation and treatment. Eur Respir J 1996;9:2017–21.

51. Nuchtern JG, Harberg FJ. Congenital lung cysts. Semin Pediatr Surg 1994;3:233–43.

52. Berrocal T, Madrid C, Novo S, et al. Congenital anomalies of the tracheobronchial tree, lung, and mediastinum: embryology, radiology, and pathology. Radiographics 2003;24:e17–62.

53. Winters WD, Effman EL. Congenital masses of the lung: prenatal and postnatal imaging evaluation. J Thorac Imaging 2001;16:196–206.

54. McAdams HP, Kirejczyk WM, Rosado-de-Christenson ML, et al. Bronchogenic cyst: imaging features with clinical and histopathologic correlation. Radiology 2000;217:441–6.

55. Kim YC, Goo JM, Han JK, et al. Subphrenic bronchogenic cyst mimicking a juxtahepatic solid lesion. Abdom Imaging 2003;28:354–6.

56. Williams HJ, Johnson KJ. Imaging of congenital cystic lung lesions. Paediatr Respir Rev 2002;3: 120–7.

57. Lee EY. Evaluation of non-vascular mediastinal masses in infants and children: an evidence-based practical approach. Pediatr Radiol 2009; 39(Suppl 2):S184–90.

58. Lee EY. Imaging evaluation of mediastinal masses in infants and children. In: Medina LS, Applegate KE, Blackmore CC, editors. Evidence-based imaging in pediatrics: optimizing imaging in pediatric patient care. New York: Springer-Verlag Science + Business Media, Inc; 2010. p. 381–400.

59. Karnak I, Senock ME, Ciftci AO, et al. Congenital lobar emphysema: diagnostic and therapeutic considerations. J Pediatr Surg 1999;34:1347–51.

60. Olutoye OO, Coleman BG, Hubbard AM, et al. Prenatal diagnosis and management of congenital lobar emphysema. J Pediatr Surg 2000;35:792–5.

61. Mei-Zahav M, Konen O, Monson D, et al. Is congenital lobar emphysema a surgical disease? J Pediatr Surg 2006;41:1058–61.

62. Ozcelik U, Gocmen A, Kiper N, et al. Congenital lobar emphysema: evaluation and long-term follow up of thirty cases at a single center. Pediatr Pulmonol 2003;35:384–91.

63. Nazem M, Hosseinpour M. Evaluation of early and late complications in patients with congenital lobar emphysema; a 12 year experience. Afr J Paediatr Surg 2010;7(3):144–6.

64. Cleveland RH, Weber B. Retained fetal lung liquid in congenital lobar emphysema: a possible predictor of polyalveolar lobe. Pediatr Radiol 1993;23(4):291–5.

65. Kumar A, Bhatnagar V. Respiratory distress in neonates. Indian J Pediatr 2005;72(5):425–8.

66. Hugosson C, Rabeeach A, Al-Rawaf A, et al. Congenital bilobar emphysema. Pediatr Radiol 1995;25:649–51.

67. Wilson RD, Hedrick HL, Liechty KW, et al. Cystic adenomatoid malformation of the lung: review of genetics, prenatal diagnosis, and in utero treatment. Am J Med Genet A 2006;140:151–5.

68. Stocker JT, Madewell JE, Drake RM. Congenital cystic adenomatoid malformation of the lung. Classification and morphologic spectrum. Hum Pathol 1977;8(2):155–71.

69. Stocker JT. Congenital pulmonary airway malformation—a new name for an expanded classification of congenital cystic adenomatoid malformation of the lung. Histopathology 2002;41(Suppl 2):424–31.

70. Cachia R, Sobonya RE. Congenital cystic adenomatoid malformation of the lung with bronchial atresia. Hum Pathol 1981;12(10):947–50.

71. Imai Y, Mark EJ. Cystic adenomatoid change is common to various forms of cystic lung diseases of children: a clinicopathologic analysis of 10 cases with emphasis on tracing the bronchial tree. Arch Pathol Lab Med 2002;126(8):934–40.

72. Gutweiler JR, Labelle J, Suh MY, et al. A familial case of pleuropulmonary blastoma. Eur J Pediatr Surg 2008;18(3):192–4.

73. Oliveira C, Himidan S, Pastor AC, et al. Discriminating preoperative features of pleuropulmonary blastoma (PPB) from congenital adenomatoid malformations (CCAM): a retrospective, age-matched study. Eur J Pediatr Surg 2011;21(1):2–7.

74. Hill DA, Jarzembowski JA, Priest JR, et al. Type 1 pleuropulmonary blastoma: pathology and biology study of 51 cases from the international pleuropulmonary blastoma registry. Am J Surg Pathol 2008; 32(2):282–95.

75. Hill DA, Ivanovich J, Priest JR, et al. DICER1 mutations in familial pleuropulmonary blastoma. Science 2009;325(5943):965.

76. Argent AC, Cremin BJ. Computed tomography in agenesis of the lung in infants. Br J Radiol 1992; 65:221–4.

77. Knowles S, Thomas RM, Lindenbaum RH, et al. Pulmonary agenesis as part of the VACTERL sequence. Arch Dis Child 1988;63:723–6.

78. Lee EY. MDCT and 3D evaluation of type 2 hypoplastic pulmonary artery sling associated with right lung agenesis, hypoplastic aortic arch, and long segment tracheal stenosis. J Thorac Imaging 2007;22(4):346–50.

79. Lee P, Westra S, Baba T, et al. Right pulmonary aplasia, aberrant left pulmonary artery, and bronchopulmonary sequestration with an esophageal bronchus. Pediatr Radiol 2006;36(5):449–52.

80. Lee EY, Boiselle PM, Shamberger RC. Multidetector computed tomography and 3-dimensional imaging: preoperative evaluation of thoracic vascular and tracheobronchial anomalies and abnormalities in pediatric patients. J Pediatr Surg 2010;45(4):811–21.

81. Lee EY, Siegel MJ. MDCT of tracheobronchial narrowing in pediatric patients. J Thorac Imaging 2007;22(3):300–9.

82. Lee EY, Siegel MJ. Pediatric airways disorders: large airways. In: Boiselle PM, Lynch DA, editors. CT of the airways. Totowa (NJ): The Humana Press; 2008. p. 351–80.

83. Currarino G, Williams B. Causes of congenital unilateral pulmonary hypoplasia: a study of 33 cases. Pediatr Radiol 1985;15:15–24.

84. Ellis K. Developmental abnormalities in the systemic blood supply to the lungs. AJR Am J Roentgenol 1991;156(4):669–79.

85. Pfefferkorn JR, Loser H, Pech G, et al. Absent pulmonary artery. Pediatr Cardiol 1982;3:283–6.

86. Lynch DA, Higgins CB. MR imaging of unilateral pulmonary artery anomalies. J Comput Assist Tomogr 1990;14:187–91.

87. Presbitero P, Bull C, Haworth SG, et al. Absent or occult pulmonary artery. Br Heart J 1984;52:178–85.

88. Debatin JR, Moon RE, Spritzer CE, et al. MRI of absent left pulmonary artery. J Comput Tomogr 1996;16:641–5.

89. Zhong YM, Jaffe RB, Zhu M, et al. CT assessment of tracheobronchial anomaly in left pulmonary artery sling. Pediatr Radiol 2010;40(11):1755–62.

90. Newman B, Meza MP, Towbin RB, et al. Left pulmonary artery sling diagnosis and delineation of associated tracheobronchial anomalies with MR. Pediatr Radiol 1996;26:661–8.

91. Berdon WE. Rings, slings, and other things: vascular compression of the infant trachea updated from the midcentury to the millennium—the legacy of Robert E. Gross, MD, and Edward B.D. Neuhauser, MD. Radiology 2000;216(3):624–32.

92. Lee EY, Litmanovich D, Boiselle PM. Multidetector CT evaluation of tracheobronchomalacia. Radiol Clin North Am 2009;47(2):261–9.

93. Lee EY, Boiselle PM. Tracheobronchomalacia in infants and children: multidetector CT evaluation. Radiology 2009;252(1):7–22.

94. Fiore AC, Brown JW, Weber TR, et al. Surgical treatment of pulmonary artery sling and tracheal stenosis. Ann Thorac Surg 2005;79(1):38–46.

95. Ho AS, Koltai PJ. Pediatric tracheal stenosis. Otolaryngol Clin North Am 2008;41(5):999–1021.

96. Drossner DM, Kim DW, Maher KO, et al. Pulmonary vein stenosis: prematurity and associated conditions. Pediatrics 2008;122(3):e656–61.

97. Remy-Jardin M, Remy J, Mayo JR, et al. Vascular anomalies of the lung. In: Remy-Jardin M, Remy J, Mayo JR, et al, editors. CT angiography of the chest. Philadelphia: Lippincott Williams & Wilkins; 2001. p. 97–114.

98. Devaney EJ, Chang AC, Ohye RG, et al. Management of congenital and acquired pulmonary vein stenosis. Ann Thorac Surg 2006;81:992–5.

99. Singh H, Singh C, Aggarwal N, et al. Angioplasty of congenital pulmonary vein stenosis. Indian Heart J 2005;57(6):709–12.

100. Spray TL, Bridges ND. Surgical management of congenital and acquired pulmonary vein stenosis. Semin Thorac Cardiovasc Surg Pediatr Card Surg Annu 1999;2:177–88.

101. Asayama J, Shiguma R, Katsume H, et al. Pulmonary varix. Angiology 1984;35:735–9.

102. Borkowski GP, O'Donovan PB, Troup BR. Pulmonary varix: CT findings. J Comput Assist Tomogr 1981;5:827–9.

103. Chaise LS, Soulen R, Teplick S, et al. Computed tomographic diagnosis of pulmonary varix. J Comput Tomogr 1983;7:281–4.

104. Vanherreweghe E, Rigaute H, Bogaerts Y, et al. Pulmonary vein varix: diagnosis with multislice helical CT. Eur Radiol 2000;10:1315–7.

105. Ferretti GR, Arbib F, Bertrand B, et al. Haemoptysis associated with pulmonary varices: demonstration using computed tomography angiography. Eur Respir J 1998;12:989–92.

106. Gossage JR, Kanj G. Pulmonary arteriovenous malformation: a state of the art review. Am J Respir Crit Care Med 1998;158:643–61.

107. Shovlin CL, Letarte M. Hereditary haemorrhagic telangiectasia and pulmonary arteriovenous malformations: issues in clinical management and

review of pathogenic mechanisms. Thorax 1999; 54:714–29.

108. Srivastava D, Preminger T, Lock JE, et al. Hepatic venous blood and the development of pulmonary arteriovenous malformations in congenital heart disease. Circulation 1995;92:1217–22.

109. Shah MJ, Rychik J, Fogel MA, et al. Pulmonary AV malformations after superior cavopulmonary connection: resolution after inclusion of hepatic veins in the pulmonary circulation. Ann Thorac Surg 1997;63: 960–3.

110. Schraufnagel DE, Kay JM. Structural and pathologic changes in the lung vasculature in chronic liver disease. Clin Chest Med 1996;17:1–15.

111. Lee KN, Lee HJ, Shin WW, et al. Hypoxemia and liver cirrhosis (hepatopulmonary syndrome) in eight patients: comparison of the central and peripheral pulmonary vasculature. Radiology 1999;211:549–53.

112. Oh YW, Kang EY, Lee NJ, et al. Thoracic manifestations associated with advanced liver disease. J Comput Assist Tomogr 2000;24:699–705.

113. McAdams HP, Erasmus J, Crockett R, et al. The hepatopulmonary syndrome: radiologic findings in 10 patients. AJR Am J Roentgenol 1996;166:1379–85.

114. Lundell C, Finck E. Arteriovenous fistulas originating from Rasmussen aneurysms. AJR Am J Roentgenol 1983;140:687–8.

115. Braun RA, Buchmiller TL, Khankhanian N. Pulmonary arteriovenous malformations complicating coccidioidal pneumonia. Ann Thorac Surg 1995; 60:454–7.

116. Stagman DJ, Presti C, Rees C, et al. Septic pulmonary arteriovenous fistula: an unusual conduit for systemic embolization in right-sided valvular endocarditis. Chest 1990;97:1484–6.

117. Remy J, Remy-Jardin M, Giraud F, et al. Angioarchitecture of pulmonary arteriovenous malformations: clinical utility of three-dimensional helical CT. Radiology 1994;191:657–64.

118. Remy-Jardin M, Remy J. Spiral CT angiography of the pulmonary circulation. Radiology 1999;212: 615–36.

119. Hofmann LV, Kuszyk BS, Mitchell SE, et al. Angioarchitecture of pulmonary arteriovenous malformations: characterization using volume-rendered 3-D CT angiography. Cardiovasc Intervent Radiol 2000;23:165–70.

120. White RI Jr, Lynch-Nyhan A, Terry P, et al. Pulmonary arteriovenous malformations: techniques and long-term outcome of embolotherapy. Radiology 1988;169:663–9.

121. Lee DW, White RI Jr, Egglin TK, et al. Embolotherapy of large pulmonary arteriovenous malformations: long-term results. Ann Thorac Surg 1997; 64:930–40.

122. Donnelly LF. Chest. In: Donnelly LF, editor. Diagnostic imaging pediatrics. Salt Lake City (UT): Amirsys; 2005. p. 118–20.

123. Clark JA, Pugash RA, Faughnan ME, et al. Multidisciplinary team interested in the treatment of pulmonary arteriovenous fistulas or malformations (PAVFs). World J Surg 2001;25:254–5.

124. Cil BE, Erdogan C, Akmangit I, et al. Use of the Tri-Span coil to facilitate the transcatheter occlusion of pulmonary arteriovenous malformation. Cardiovasc Intervent Radiol 2004;27:655–8.

125. Prasad V, Chan RP, Faughnan ME. Embolotherapy of pulmonary arteriovenous malformations: efficacy of platinum versus stainless steel coils. J Vasc Interv Radiol 2004;15:451–6.

126. Woodring JH, Howard TA, Kanga JF. Congenital pulmonary venolobar syndrome revisited. Radiographics 1994;14:349–69.

127. Huddleston CB, Exil V, Canter CE, et al. Scimitar syndrome presenting in infancy. Ann Thorac Surg 1999;67:154–9.

128. Huddleston CB, Mendeloff EN. Scimitar syndrome. Adv Card Surg 1999;11:161–78.

129. Schramel FM, Westermann CJ, Kanepen PJ, et al. The scimitar syndrome: clinical spectrum and surgical management. Eur Respir J 1995;8(2): 196–201.

130. Conran RM, Stocker JT. Extralobar sequestration with frequently associated congenital cystic adenomatoid malformation, type 2: report of 50 cases. Pediatr Dev Pathol 1999;2:454–63.

131. Lee EY, Tracy DA, Mahmood SA, et al. Preoperative MDCT evaluation of congenital lung anomalies in children: comparison of axial, multiplanar, and 3D images. AJR Am J Roentgenol 2011;196(5): 1040–6.

132. Lee KH, Sung KB, Yoon HK, et al. Transcatheter arterial embolization of pulmonary sequestration in neonates: long term follow-up results. J Vasc Interv Radiol 2003;14(3):363–7.

133. Lee BS, Kim JT, Kim EA, et al. Neonatal pulmonary sequestration: clinical experience with transumbilical arterial embolization. Pediatr Pulmonol 2008; 43(4):404–13.

Chest Trauma in Children: Current Imaging Guidelines and Techniques

Michael A. Moore, MB BCh[a], E. Christine Wallace, MB BCh[b], Sjirk J. Westra, MD[c],*

KEYWORDS

- Trauma • Chest • Pediatric • CT • Radiography
- Ultrasound • Algorithms • Techniques

Trauma to the pediatric chest, occurring in isolation or with polytrauma, may result in a variety of injuries, from minor to life-threatening. The challenge in pediatric trauma imaging is to implement a problem-oriented approach that addresses the specific mechanism of injury and clinical presentation. Taking into account that major trauma does not respect anatomic boundaries and may lead to multisystem injury, this approach should be diagnostically accurate, cost-effective, and provide for efficient treatment decisions, using the lowest possible radiation dose. The currently available imaging modalities for evaluating chest trauma include chest radiography, ultrasound, and CT scan. Chest radiography is a relatively low radiation-dose study and ultrasound does not use ionizing radiation, but they both have limitations in the setting of chest trauma in children. Multidetector CT (MDCT) scan enables rapid acquisition of data sets with accurate anatomic detail, delivering valuable multiplanar and three-dimensional information regarding the morphologic features of chest injuries. However, such rapid high-resolution imaging comes with the distinct disadvantage of delivering higher radiation doses. In this article, epidemiology and pathophysiology, imaging techniques, characteristic imaging findings, and evidence-based imaging algorithms for pediatric chest trauma are discussed.

EPIDEMIOLOGY AND PATHOPHYSIOLOGY

The most common cause of morbidity and mortality in children aged 1 to 14 years is trauma.[1] The National Pediatric Trauma Registry reported the incidence of major chest injury to be 6%.[2] It is second only to brain injury as a cause of pediatric trauma-related death, with mortality rates of 15% to 25%.[2,3] The presence of serious chest injury in a multiregional trauma patient is an indication of the overall severity of the child's injuries, increasing the mortality 20-fold compared with children without chest trauma.[3–5] The demonstration of clinically silent concomitant chest injury in patients with known head, cervical spine, abdominal, or extremity injury substantially affects the prognosis, especially in children.[6] In patients with chest injury, there is multiregional involvement (ie, polytrauma) in 50% to 81%.[7] Mortality with isolated chest injury is 5%, with one additional body part involvement 25% to 29%, and with more than two regions involved is 33% to 40%. The

The authors have nothing to disclose.
[a] Department of Radiology, Cork University Hospital, Wilton, Cork, Ireland
[b] Department of Radiology, UMass Memorial Medical Center, University of Massachusetts Medical School, 55 Lake Avenue North, Worcester, MA 01655, USA
[c] Division of Pediatric Radiology, Department of Radiology, Massachusetts General Hospital, Harvard Medical School, 55 Fruit Street, White 246, Boston, MA 02114, USA
* Corresponding author.
E-mail address: swestra@partners.org

Radiol Clin N Am 49 (2011) 949–968
doi:10.1016/j.rcl.2011.06.002

combination of major chest trauma and traumatic brain injury results in a mortality of 40% to 70%.[1,3] In polytrauma, deaths in children with chest trauma are due to nonthoracic causes in 66% to 75% of cases.[7]

An age-based classification of the causes of major chest trauma shows that infants and toddlers (0–4 years) are usually passive victims of child abuse and motor vehicle accidents. School-going children (5–9 years) sustain injuries as pedestrians. Older children (10–17 years) suffer transport-related injuries with bicycles and skateboards.[8] Older teenagers are usually injured during high-risk, high-impact sporting activities, motor vehicle accidents (including all-terrain vehicle accidents[9]), violence, and suicide.[1] Boys tend to participate in riskier activities, accounting for a male to female ratio for chest injury between 2.6 and 3.0.[8] Blunt chest trauma is about six times as common as penetrating chest injury. Penetrating injury occurs almost exclusively in teenagers, typically because of stab wounds or gun shots.[7] Of fatalities associated with blunt chest injury, only 14% are due to the chest injury; whereas the cause of death in patients with penetrating chest injury is directly attributable to this injury in 97% of cases.[2]

Rib fractures, flail chest, aortic injury, and diaphragmatic rupture are more common in adults, whereas pulmonary contusion, pneumothorax, and intrathoracic injury without bony injury predominate in children.[8] The differing pattern of injury may be explained by the anatomic and physiologic differences between children and adults. The trachea is relatively narrow, short, and more readily compressible in children, so that small changes in airway caliber from external compression or inhaled foreign body may result in respiratory compromise that is more significant. Furthermore, children have higher metabolic rates and consume more oxygen per kilogram body weight than adults consume. This results in a greater vulnerability to develop rapid hypoxia in the context of major chest trauma.[1,3] Injuries from seatbelts, ejection from a car restraining device, or airbag deployment often have unique features that can be explained by poor adjustment of these devices to variable pediatric sizes and proportions.[4,5] In general, the pediatric body is more flexible, lighter, and proportioned differently than the mature individual, leading to unique patterns of injury. In adults, whose inflexible ribcages are more likely to fracture, more energy is absorbed by the chest wall and there is relative sparing of the underlying soft-tissues. The ribs of young children are less mineralized than in adults, which, together with increased ligamentous laxity,

confer greater chest wall flexibility and pliability. This permits the transference of energy to the underlying soft-tissues. Pulmonary contusions and pneumothorax are more common in children, with comparatively fewer rib fractures.[1,3,8] Therefore, imaging protocols developed for adults do not necessarily apply to children of all age groups.

IMAGING TECHNIQUE
Radiography

Upright frontal and lateral chest radiographs are optimal to evaluate chest injury. However, in the polytrauma setting, supine radiographs are usually performed owing to the need for patient immobilization. Attention to technical factors such as proper collimation and adequate exposure factors to optimally demonstrate skeletal structures, lung parenchyma, and mediastinal contours (such as paraspinal lines) is important.

Ultrasound

Bedside ultrasonography of the lower chest may be combined with the focused assessment with sonography for trauma (FAST) examination of the abdomen.[10–12] Once pleural fluid is encountered, it is important to screen the entire pleural space, not just the lung bases. Lower frequency (3.5–7 MHz) sector transducers can be used for initial overview through intercostal and subcostal scanning, whereas higher frequency (10–12.5 MHz) linear transducers provide for more detail in the near field, before marking for needle placement. For certain indications, such as the search for an occult pneumothorax or a hemopericardium, employ an anterior approach.[13–17]

CT Scan

Once the decision to perform a CT scan has been made, it is imperative that the appropriate measures are taken to minimize radiation dose while obtaining a diagnostic study. On multidetector scanners, the authors use a kV of 80 to120 and mA adjusted to both patient weight and age.[18] More recently, we have implemented automatic longitudinal dose adjustment based on the measured attenuation on the scanogram and preset noise levels that are adapted to the patient's age, weight, and clinical indication. Radiation dose can be further lowered by novel iterative image reconstruction techniques that reduce noise.[19] All studies are preferably obtained with single-phase CT angiography technique, including (1) the use of a power injector, (2) rapid bolus injection, (3) scan acquisition initiated 20 seconds after the start of the contrast injection, and (4) the shortest available tube-rotation time and the fastest available table speed.[4,5]

SPECTRUM OF IMAGING FINDINGS
Skeletal Injury

Generally, in the setting of trauma, the rib fracture rate is as low as 1% to 2%. However, it rises substantially in the context of major pediatric chest trauma to 30% to 60%.[3,7] Seventy percent of children with two or more rib fractures had multisystem injuries, compared to12% of children with a single fractured rib.[20] The sites of rib fractures in children differ from those in adults, being more often posterior than lateral.[21] A flail chest is rare in children, with a rate of approximately 1%.[3,7] Fractures of the lower three ribs are associated with hepatic and splenic injuries. It is rarely the rib fractures, but predominantly the associated injuries, that determine the mortality of children with chest trauma.[3,20] Rib fractures in the 0 to 3 year old age group are the result of child abuse in 39% to 80% of cases.[3] Rib fractures are found in 5% to 27% of abused children, and are the only skeletal manifestation in 29%.[1,22] Multiple aligned posterior rib fractures in a child less than 3 years has a positive predictive value of 95% for child abuse, which rises to 100% in the absence of a clear history of major trauma or underlying metabolic condition predisposing to fractures.[22,23]

Acute nondisplaced rib fractures are notoriously difficult to identify on anteroposterior (AP) chest radiographs (**Fig. 1**A). With the exception of suspected child abuse, multiple radiographic projections in the search of a suspected isolated rib fracture are not routinely indicated, as accurate identification does not typically alter management. A CT scan is capable of more reliably detecting nondisplaced fractures.[4,5] Notwithstanding this increased sensitivity of a CT scan, only those rib fractures that were seen on radiography predicted the development of respiratory failure.[24] In suspected child abuse, acute nondisplaced rib fractures are best detected with skeletal scintigraphy.[25] However, owing to the delay in clinical presentation that is typical in child abuse, healing fractures with callus (see **Fig. 1**B) are more prevalent and these are usually well seen on skeletal surveys, especially when supplemented by oblique views. For these reasons, the skeletal survey in combination with scintigraphy when indicated continues to be the standard of care for the evaluation of suspected child abuse.[4,5]

Fractures of the upper three ribs signify high-energy impact and are often associated with fractures in the shoulder girdle and vascular injury.[4,5] Scapular and clavicular fractures (**Fig. 2**) and posterior sternoclavicular dislocations (**Fig. 3**), are often seen in high-impact motor vehicle accidents involving a shoulder seatbelt. They are also associated with a high incidence of vascular and cardiac injury.[4,26,27] Sternal fractures or segmental dislocations are more commonly associated with child abuse but may occur with other forms of chest trauma.[28]

Incomplete ossification of vertebrae, lax ligamentous attachments, and incompletely developed supporting musculature result in greater spinal flexibility. The thoracic spine is distinguished by the presence of the ribcage, which restricts motion and adds stiffness to the spine.

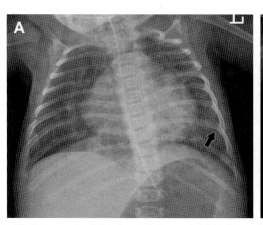
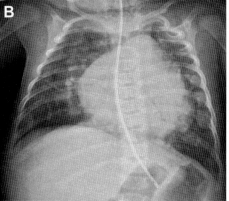

Fig. 1. Rib fractures in child abuse. A 3-month-old infant with Down syndrome and congenital heart disease, who presented to the emergency room with mild congestive heart failure. (A) Left lateral rib fracture (arrow) was not initially detected. Upon return 5 weeks later, multiple healing rib fractures were seen (B), and the child was placed into protective custody.

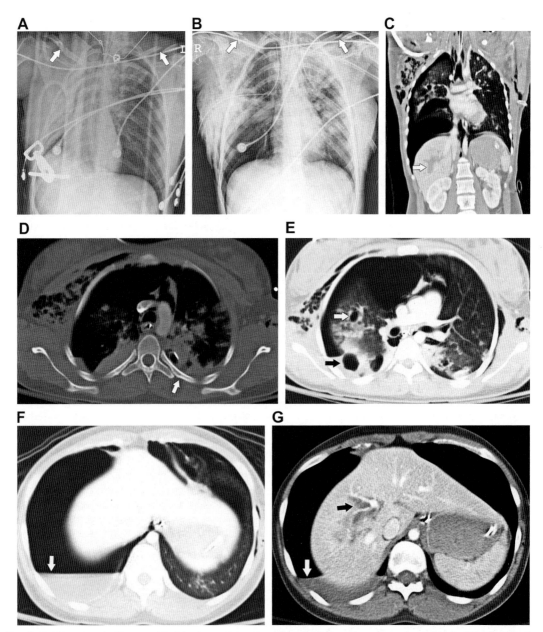

Fig. 2. Polytrauma. A 16-year-old girl who was involved in a high-speed motorcycle accident. (*A*) Chest radiograph upon admission shows large, left-sided tension pneumothorax and bilateral clavicular fractures (*arrows*). (*B*) Repeat radiograph after bilateral chest tube insertion demonstrates decompression of left tension pneumothorax, but interval development of a moderately sized, right-sided pneumothorax (note deep sulcus sign), despite presence of a chest tube. Note extensive chest wall emphysema, right greater than left, and again the bilateral clavicular fractures (*arrows*). Corresponding findings on coronal (*C*) and axial (*D–G*) CT scan images. Additional findings on CT scanning were a liver laceration (*arrow* in *C*, *black arrow* in *G*), a nondisplaced, left posterior rib fracture (*arrow* in *D*), extensive pulmonary contusion and several right-sided lung lacerations (*arrows* in *E*) and a right-sided hemopneumothorax (fluid levels in *F* [*arrow*] and *G* [*white arrow*]). The patient made a rapid and complete recovery without the need for surgery.

This provides the thoracic spine with additional strength and energy-absorbing capacity. Therefore, the presence of a displaced thoracic spine fracture signifies a high-impact injury. Owing to the relatively narrow anteroposterior diameter of the thoracic spinal canal, there is a high incidence of spinal cord injury and neurologic deficit with vertebral injury.[29]

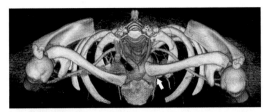

Fig. 3. Traumatic sternoclavicular dislocation. A 15-year-old boy who sustained a direct-impact football injury to his left clavicle. Superior view of three-dimensional volume rendition of CT angiogram demonstrates a left-sided posterior sternoclavicular dislocation (*arrow*). Despite this finding, there was no vascular injury demonstrated.

On chest radiography, an abrupt change in alignment in the thoracic spine indicates spinal injury. Above the T10 level, most spinal injuries produce a basic pattern of an anterior fracture-dislocation of two contiguous vertebrae, often with neurologic impairment.[30] The presence of abnormal kyphosis, pleural fluid, rib fractures, dislocations at the costovertebral joints, or widening of the interpediculate distance suggests thoracic spinal injury.[30] An important imaging finding of subtle thoracic spinal fractures is widening of paraspinal lines, indicative of a hematoma (**Fig. 4**). Upper thoracic spine injuries are often poorly demonstrated on frontal chest radiographs. Therefore, CT scan is the imaging modality of choice for both initial diagnosis and assessment of complications of surgical immobilization.[4,31] MRI is superior to CT scan in the evaluation of spinal cord injury and posttraumatic disk herniation.[30]

Pleural Injury

Pneumothorax and/or hemothorax are the second most common injuries in pediatric chest trauma, with an overall incidence of 41% to 51%. The rate of pneumothorax at 23% to 27% is higher in

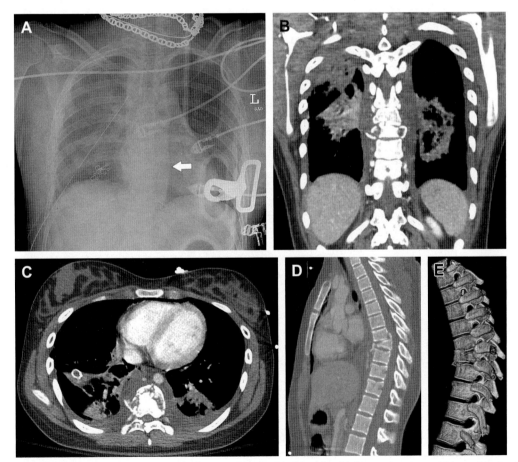

Fig. 4. Thoracic spine fracture with cord injury. A 16-year-old girl with a high speed motor vehicle accident, who presented with paralysis of the lower extremities. (*A*) Chest radiograph upon admission demonstrates paraspinal widening on the left (*arrow*). CT scan shows corresponding findings of a T6 wedge compression fracture on coronal (*B*), axial (*C*), sagittal (*D*) and three-dimensional volume rendered (*E*) images. Note the impingement of fracture fragments into the spinal canal on *D*. Also, note right lung contusion and bilateral pleural fluid.

children than in adults, whereas the rate of hemo-thorax at 7% to 29% is lower in children than in adults. Hemopneumothorax occurs in approximately 11% of children with chest trauma.[2,3,8] In children, the mortality associated with pneumothorax is 16%, and as much as 23% to 51% for hemothorax.[2,3] One-third of pneumothoraces occur in isolation, but the rest have associated other intrathoracic and/or extrathoracic injuries.[1] Causes of pneumothorax include direct penetrating injury to the chest wall, an air leak into the pleural space from a pulmonary laceration or a primary pneumomediastinum, or a traumatic tracheobronchial air leak. The increased mobility of the pediatric mediastinum relative to adults results in a greater risk for the development of significant cardiorespiratory compromise from pneumothorax or hemothorax.[3,32] In one series, the incidence of tension pneumothorax in pediatric chest trauma was 23%, almost three times the adult rate.[8]

The diagnosis of pneumothorax (see **Fig. 2**; **Fig. 5**) is usually straightforward on upright chest radiographs, with demonstration of the visceral pleural line outlined by radiolucent free pleural air and absent vascular markings in the periphery or apex of the chest. Obtaining expiration radiographs may enhance the visibility of pneumothoraces. Unfortunately, the polytrauma patient is typically radiographed in the supine position, rendering pneumothoraces more difficult to diagnose. In this situation, the correct identification of indirect imaging findings of pneumothorax is important. Such indirect imaging findings include (1) hyperlucency of the affected hemithorax (see **Fig. 5**B), (2) an unduly sharp heart or mediastinal border, (3) a deep and abnormally lucent costophrenic sulcus with sharp margins (the "deep sulcus sign," **Fig. 2**B), and (4) the "double diaphragm sign" when air adjacent to the anterior and posterior aspects of the diaphragm produces two diaphragmatic silhouettes.[26] Decubitus positioning, which would be optimal to demonstrate the visceral pleural line, is often not possible owing to the need for patient immobilization. The cross-table lateral view is relatively insensitive for demonstrating small, anteriorly located pleural air collections, and often cannot determine laterality.[4,5] A tension pneumothorax (see **Fig. 2**A) is a life-threatening emergency occurring when intrapleural air under pressure causes a mediastinal shift, reduced venous blood return to the heart, and rapid decline in cardiac output. Once identified, the presence of

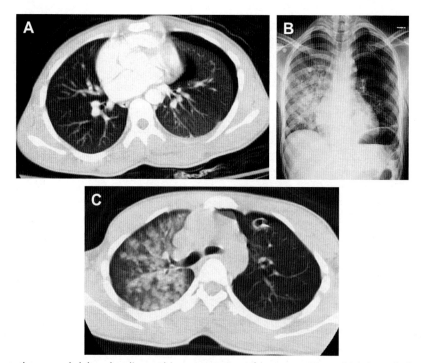

Fig. 5. Pneumothorax and delayed radiographic presentation of lung opacities, which is typical of pulmonary contusion. An 18-year-old male with blunt left chest injury was diagnosed with a left-sided pneumothorax on admission CT scan. (A) Note that the right lung was clear at that time. Following chest tube insertion, a chest radiograph (B) demonstrated development of right pulmonary parenchymal opacities. Follow up chest CT scan, 8 hours after A (C) shows the subpleural sparing, which is typical of pulmonary contusion. The patient made a rapid and complete recovery.

a tension pneumothorax should be rapidly communicated with the treatment team. Mediastinal shift to the contralateral side, depression of the ipsilateral diaphragm, and rapid expansion on serial radiographs are the typical indicators that a pneumothorax is under tension. However, a tension pneumothorax can be small and may not exhibit any mass effect, especially when occurring bilaterally in a patient on positive pressure ventilation.[4,33] As expected, a CT scan is more sensitive for small pneumothoraces than chest radiography. In one adult series, the CT scan identification of a pneumothorax not seen on chest radiography (a so-called occult pneumothorax) resulted in alteration in patient management in 43% of cases,[34] although this was not confirmed in a later pediatric series.[35] The true clinical significance and appropriate management of occult pneumothoraces is controversial.[36] Most of these occult pneumothoraces remain clinically silent. However, if positive pressure ventilation needs to be instituted for any cause, they may enlarge, causing cardiorespiratory compromise.[26] Although some advocate for the prompt drainage of all traumatic pneumothoraces,[1,34] it appears that, in children, in the absence of a need for positive pressure ventilation, thoracostomy drainage of occult pneumothoraces may not be required.[35]

Pleural fluid is readily identified on upright chest radiographs as it collects in the dependent portions of the chest, obliterating the lateral costophrenic sulcus and typically forming a meniscus. On supine chest radiography, pleural fluid manifests as "veil-like" increased density over the involved hemithorax with preserved visibility of pulmonary vascular markings. In the case of larger amounts of fluid,

thickening of the lateral pleural line may be seen.[4,26] The differential diagnostic considerations for fluid accumulating in the pleural space include infusothorax from a misplaced central venous line, reactive effusion secondary to pulmonary parenchymal injury, traumatic chylothorax, and hemothorax. Hemothorax (**Fig. 6**) may result from injury to pulmonary parenchyma or to any of the intrathoracic vessels. Rib fractures may lacerate intercostal veins or arteries and, more rarely, major mediastinal vessels, such as the aorta or vena cava, may be the source. It may be clinically silent until a large volume of blood has accumulated within each hemithorax, which has the potential to hold 40% of a child's blood volume (see **Fig. 6**).[1,37] Ultrasound is more sensitive than and just as specific as chest radiography for the detection of hemothorax, although a CT scan is more sensitive for detecting hemothoraces of smaller volumes than can be detected with ultrasound or radiography.[10] A CT scan is superior for accurate assessment of chest tube placement and related complications, such as an intraparenchymal course and associated pulmonary contusion.[4,5] Contrast enhanced MDCT also has the ability to demonstrate active contrast extravasation into the pleural space from arterial or major (pulmonary) venous injury, thereby localizing the bleeding source.[38] Once diagnosed, blood should be promptly evacuated to avoid the development of empyema and fibrothorax.[3]

Pulmonary Parenchymal Injury

Primary trauma-related pulmonary parenchymal injuries include pulmonary contusions and lacerations.

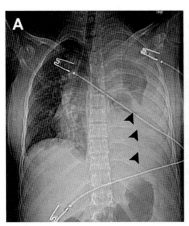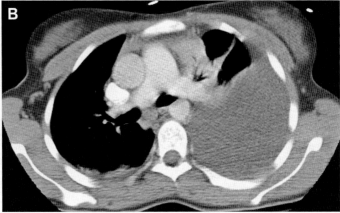

Fig. 6. Hemothorax. (*A*) CT scanogram in a 17-year-old girl with blunt chest trauma shows near-complete opacification of the left hemithorax, with shift of heart and mediastinum to the right. Note multiple left-sided rib fractures (*arrowheads*). (*B*) Axial CT scan image confirms large left-sided hemothorax, which required emergency evacuation. There was no major vascular injury demonstrated. Following a blood transfusion, the patient made a full recovery, without the need for surgery.

However, there are many other parenchymal conditions that secondarily affect pediatric trauma victims, including aspiration, fat embolism, both cardiogenic and neurogenic pulmonary edema, and intubation-related atelectasis. Additionally, as many as 20% of children with chest trauma will develop superimposed and/or hospital-acquired pneumonia. Many of these entities, if severe enough, may ultimately lead to the development of adult respiratory distress syndrome (ARDS). The reported incidence in children with chest trauma is 5% to 20%.[1,3–5] Pulmonary contusion is the most common injury in children with chest trauma, with an incidence of 43% to 53%, almost twice that observed in adults.[2,8,39] The reported mortality in children with pulmonary contusions is 10% to 20%, although this is mostly attributed to associated injuries.[3,40,41] The pliable pediatric chest wall allows for the ready transmission of energy to the underlying parenchyma, so that almost half of all children with parenchymal injury have no evidence of external chest wall injury.[3,40] Such injuries occur because of the direct impact of adjacent bony structures, such as ribs and spine, on the underlying lung parenchyma; and because of the passage of shockwaves through the lungs, causing shearing effects at tissue interfaces, resulting in alveolar hemorrhage, interstitial edema, and consolidation. The physiologic consequences include ventilation-perfusion mismatch and decreased lung compliance, resulting in hypoventilation and hypoxemia.

Contusions may occur directly at the site of impact or in the contralateral hemithorax in a contracoup fashion. Large contusions typically have a nonanatomic distribution and cross segmental boundaries because pleural fissures do not impede the passage of shock waves.[1,3,26] After an initial delay of 4 to 6 hours, chest radiographs are abnormal in the majority of cases (67%–97%) of pulmonary contusion or demonstrate ill-defined airspace opacities, frequently in a peripheral and nonanatomic distribution (see Fig. 5). However, chest radiographs may underestimate the extent of injury or not detect subtle abnormalities, and CT scanning has proven to be more sensitive for detecting pulmonary contusions.[42,43] However, the true significance of correctly detecting lung contusions is debated because many of these contusions detected by CT scan, but not by radiography, do not require additional management beyond that directed by the clinical findings.[24,41,44,45] CT scanning may have a role in predicting the need for mechanical ventilation, which was necessary with greater than 28% of lung involvement but generally not indicated if less than 18% of the lung was involved with contusions.[46] The CT scanning manifestations of pulmonary contusion include peripheral multifocal areas of airspace consolidation without air bronchograms in crescentic, amorphous, or nodular patterns. These peripheral opacities typically exhibit a thin zone of surrounding subpleural lucency that is presumed to represent a rim of relatively hypovascular lung tissue that was compressed at the moment of the injury and, therefore, relatively spared of alveolar hemorrhage and edema (see Fig. 5C). Furthermore, this subpleural sparing, which is seen 95% of cases of pulmonary contusion, is not demonstrated in cases of atelectasis, laceration, or pneumonia.[47] Most radiographic evidence of lung contusions resolves without scarring within 7 days.[4,5] It may sometimes be difficult to differentiate between aspiration and contusion. Radiographically, changes of aspiration usually evolve over 24 to 48 hours, whereas contusions are evident at about 6 hours. Aspiration is typically segmental and located in the dependent portions of the lungs, whereas contusions are nonsegmental and variably distributed.

Pulmonary lacerations are tears in the lung parenchyma leading to alveolar rupture. They are caused by penetrating injuries, such as displaced rib fractures, or by shearing blunt forces to the lung. Pulmonary lacerations are unusual in pediatric trauma; the overall incidence is just 3%. However, they are seen with higher frequency (6%) in fatal injuries because they are associated with 43% mortality.[2,48] They are typically only a few centimeters in size. If the lacerations are subpleural in location, they may be associated with a pneumothorax. When lacerations occur deeper within the lung parenchyma, the normal elastic recoil of the lung may result in cavity formation. Such a cavity may partially or completely fill with blood, which is called a pulmonary hematoma. However, the cavity may also be air-filled, either initially or with subsequent clearing of blood; it is then called a pneumatocele or pseudocyst.

On initial imaging evaluation, pulmonary lacerations (see Fig. 2E; Fig. 7C) may not be evident, particularly when they are masked by the surrounding contusions. They usually become more apparent with time as the contusions resolve relatively fast and the pneumatoceles often expand over the first 10 to 14 days, before gradually resolving.[49] In the case of large lacerations involving the pleural surface, a bronchopleural fistula (Fig. 8) may develop, and this should be suspected if there is failure of pneumothorax resolution following chest tube placement. Pulmonary hematomas have the appearance of rounded soft-tissue opacities on chest radiography, often

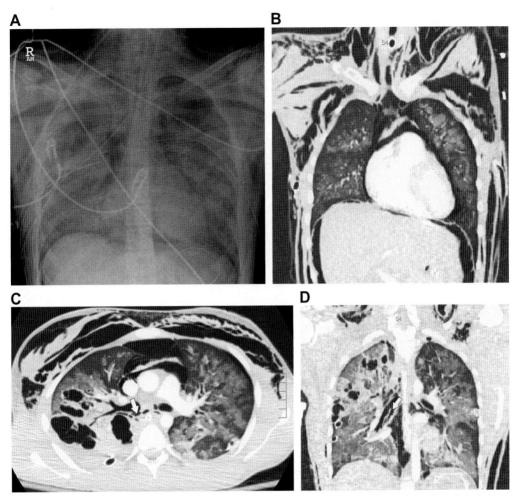

Fig. 7. Bronchial rupture. An 18-year-old male who suffered blunt trauma to the chest and face. (*A*) Chest radiograph shows extensive subcutaneous emphysema and placement of bilateral chest tubes for pneumothoraces, which evacuated air over a prolonged period. (*B–D*) Coronal (*B*), axial (*C*), and coronal (*D*) images of chest CT scan demonstrate the extensive pneumomediastinum and subcutaneous emphysema, caused by a defect in the medial and posterior wall of the right mainstem bronchus (*arrows* in *C* and *D*). Note also pneumoperitoneum in *B*. ([*A*] *From* Westra SJ, Wallace EC. Imaging evaluation of pediatric chest trauma. Radiol Clin North Am 2005;43(2):274; with permission.)

containing fluid levels. Pulmonary pseudocysts are clearly defined pockets of air within the lung parenchyma, but without a demonstrable wall and are best seen with a CT scan.[50]

Mediastinal Injury

Pneumomediastinum is reported in up to 10% of patients, of all ages, with severe blunt chest trauma.[51] It may indicate an underlying serious injury, as penetrating or blunt chest injury may result in pulmonary and pleural injuries, as well as tracheobronchial and esophageal rupture. However, air within the mediastinum in the posttraumatic setting does not always indicate chest injury as air may enter from another anatomic space. For example, pneumomediastinum may occur with penetrating head and neck trauma or with air passing through the diaphragmatic hiatus after intra-abdominal perforation of a hollow viscus.[52,53] In the absence of an obvious intrathoracic or extrathoracic source of mediastinal air, pneumomediastinum is most likely caused by the Macklin effect[51] in which an acute increase in alveolar pressure leads to alveolar rupture, followed by air dissection along bronchovascular sheaths, and eventual spreading of pulmonary interstitial emphysema into the mediastinum.

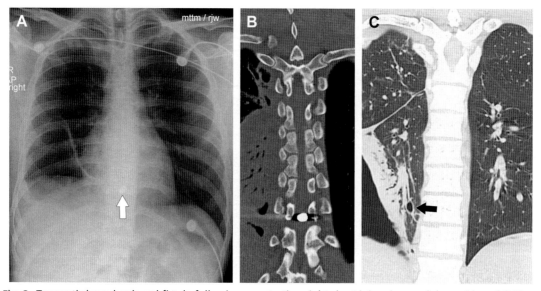

Fig. 8. Traumatic bronchopleural fistula following penetrating right chest injury in an adolescent boy. (*A*) Chest radiograph shows right loculated pneumothorax that persisted despite prolonged thoracostomy drainage. Note bullet fragment overlying the spine (*arrow*). (*B, C*) Coronal CT scan images demonstrate the bullet (*B*), which had traversed the now atelectatic right lower lobe. The bullet track (*arrow* in *C*) was found to communicate with a segmental right lower lobe bronchus and the visceral pleural surface (not shown). ([*A*] *From* Moore MA, Wallace EC, Westra SJ. The imaging of paediatric thoracic trauma. Pediatr Radiol 2009;39(5):492, Fig. 6A; with permission.)

Pneumomediastinum may be recognized on chest radiography as linear radiolucencies (see **Figs. 2**B and 7). Pneumomediastinum will frequently outline the thymus, recognized as elevation of the thymic lobes in a "spinnaker sail" or "angel wing" pattern, or the diaphragm, giving the "continuous diaphragm sign" as air outlines the superior diaphragmatic surface. An anteromedial pneumothorax may give a similar appearance to pneumomediastinum, although the two can usually be differentiated by the bilateral appearance seen with mediastinal air and the absence of demonstrable configuration change with decubitus positioning. Benign forms of pneumomediastinum generally do not require any form of follow-up with cross-sectional imaging.[4,5,51,54] Alternatively, a pneumomediastinum that ruptures through the parietal pleura to cause a pneumothorax should be further investigated with a CT scan to determine its underlying cause because this generally indicates a high-pressure air-leak. This is especially troublesome for patients requiring positive pressure ventilation and chest tube placement.

Esophageal injury resulting from chest trauma is uncommon (<1%).[2] Perforation of the esophagus may be due to penetrating injury from within, such as occurs with the ingestion of a sharp object. However, it can also result from penetrating injury from outside of the esophagus, such as gunshot wounds with a bullet trajectory traversing the posterior mediastinum. Due to the intrinsic flexibility and compliance of the esophagus and its ability to decompress into the mouth and stomach, blunt chest trauma rarely results in esophageal injury, with fewer than 10 cases reported in children.[1,3] The most common radiographic findings of esophageal perforation are unexplained pneumomediastinum and pleural fluid, usually a left-sided effusion. If the injury is suspected, an esophagram should be performed, initially with water-soluble contrast material and followed by barium.[4]

Rupture of the major airways following chest trauma is a life-threatening emergency, but fortunately is unusual in children. The reported incidence is between 0.7% and 2.9%. It is associated with a substantial mortality of 30%, of which 50% occur in the first hour after injury.[8,55] The injury may result from direct involvement by penetrating chest trauma or, in blunt trauma, either from compression of the sternum against the spine, thereby displacing the lung and disrupting the tracheobronchial tree, or from a sudden increase in intrathoracic pressure against a closed glottis. The injury typically occurs within 2.5 cm of the carina and most commonly in the proximal right mainstem bronchus.[56] When there is an associated tear in the parietal pleura, often seen with injuries that are more distal, a pneumothorax may develop. Although bilateral pneumothoraces may occur, a right-sided pneumothorax is more typical.[57] The communication between the tracheobronchial tree and the pleura often leads to a tension pneumothorax and a persistent air-leak. Segmental atelectasis may occur distal to the airway rupture.[58] Rib fractures are seen in 25% of cases of tracheobronchial rupture and, although this is nonspecific, a high proportion have involvement of the anterior ends of the first three ribs.[3,56] Unfortunately, the symptoms of tracheobronchial injury may be minimal and the radiographic findings of pneumomediastinum, pneumothorax and rib fractures are not specific for tracheobronchial injury. This may lead to a delay in diagnosis, particularly in the pediatric population.[59,60] Such an injury should be suspected when there are severe and persistent pneumothoraces and pneumomediastinum in the presence of well-functioning chest tubes.

The site of airway rupture primarily determines radiographic findings. Due to the positioning of the trachea within the mediastinum, pneumomediastinum with associated cervical emphysema is the most common radiographic finding. Not surprisingly, MDCT is more sensitive than chest radiography at diagnosing tracheobronchial injury (see **Fig. 7**) and it can accurately indentify the site of airway rupture.[61] Multiplanar reformatted images and virtual bronchoscopy are useful techniques to demonstrate the defect, and this may help in treatment planning[61–63] Fiberoptic bronchoscopy may be used for confirmation of airway rupture. Additionally, it may permit attempts at endoluminal treatment, such as occlusion of the defect or selective bronchial intubation, which are temporizing measures before final surgical repair. If there is complete transsection of the mainstem bronchus (**Fig. 9**), the collapsed lung may have an unusual lateral and inferior displacement within the hemithorax.[56,58]

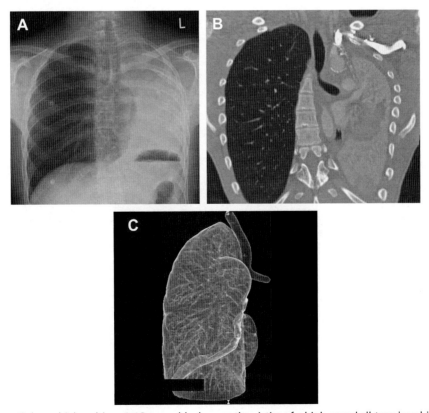

Fig. 9. Traumatic bronchial avulsion. A 16-year-old who was the victim of a high-speed all-terrain vehicle accident with chest trauma. (*A*) Chest radiograph 6 weeks after the accident demonstrate a complete collapse of the left lung. (*B*) Coronal image and (*C*) three-dimensional, volume-rendered image of the central airways and lungs demonstrate a complete occlusion of the left mainstem bronchus, which was confirmed with bronchoscopy. Surgical repair resulted in complete re-expansion with air of the left lung.

Cardiovascular Injury

Traumatic thoracic aortic injury has a high mortality, with the majority of deaths occurring at the time of injury. Only 10% to 20% of patients who suffer such injuries survive the initial injury and reach the emergency department. Of those who are alive on arrival, 30% die within 6 hours and 40% to 50% die within 24 hours if left untreated.[64] Fortunately, the overall incidence of posttraumatic aortic injuries in children is only 0.1%, which is lower than in the adult population. However, this figure rises to 1% to 7.4% in children who are admitted with blunt chest injuries, and the overall mortality is approximately 40%.[3,8,65,66] Children who sustain a traumatic thoracic aortic injury will also have important injuries to other organs, including lung contusions (100%), pelvic or long bone fractures (50%),

visceral laceration or perforation (50%), and central nervous system injury (33%). However, only half will have external evidence of chest injury.[67] Motor vehicle accidents, pedestrian accidents, and falls are the most common causes. Of traumatic aortic injuries, 77% to 90% occur at the aortic isthmus distal to the left subclavian artery and at the level of the ligamentum arteriosum. This is the site where the relatively mobile aortic arch becomes fixed as the descending aorta and, therefore, this is an area prone to injury from traumatic shearing forces. Such trauma may result in tears of the intima and media, and the adventitia is the only layer holding the aorta together, leading to the development of an unstable pseudoaneurysm, with associated high mortality.[3–5,26]

Detection of a mediastinal hematoma is important because it may be a clue to an otherwise occult traumatic aortic injury, which is often clinically

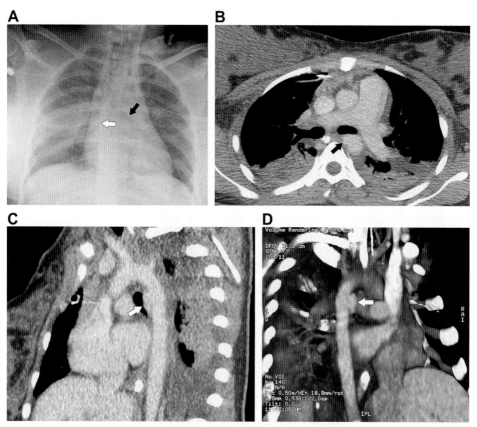

Fig. 10. Thoracic aortic injury. A 17-year-old girl who was a restrained passenger in a speed boat accident and suffered blunt chest injury. (A) Chest radiograph shows subtle findings of a mediastinal hematoma, including mediastinal widening, rightward displacement of the nasogastric tube (*white arrow*), and slight downward displacement of the left mainstem bronchus (*black arrow*). There is also a small anteromedial right pneumothorax. CT angiogram of the chest, axial image (B), coronal oblique reformat (C), and volume-rendered image (D) depict traumatic pseudoaneurysm in proximal descending aorta (*arrows*). The information provided by this study enabled the vascular surgeon to successfully place an endovascular stent for this pseudoaneurysm. ([A] *From* Moore MA, Wallace EC, Westra SJ. The imaging of paediatric thoracic trauma. Pediatr Radiol 2009;39(5):493, Fig. 7A; with permission.)

silent. Despite its limitations, a well-penetrated AP chest radiograph obtained in the trauma room is used as the initial screening for this condition. Mediastinal measurement criteria published in the adult literature have proven to lack a sufficient predictive value for traumatic thoracic aortic injury and do not necessarily apply to children.[4] The mediastinum frequently appears widened on supine chest radiographs owing to technical factors. Furthermore, the presence of the thymus in the pediatric population complicates radiographic assessment of the mediastinum.[68] Indeed, bleeding into the thymus itself has also been reported in children.[69] Other imaging findings of aortic injury on chest radiography include obliterated contour of the aortic arch, tracheal deviation to the right, displacement of the nasogastric tube to the right (**Fig. 10**A), widening of the paravertebral and paratracheal stripes, downward depression of the left mainstem bronchus, and accumulation of blood around the left apex giving the appearance of a radiodense apical "pleural cap."[70] Of note, the incidence of rib fractures is strikingly low, highlighting the issue of energy transference by the pliable chest wall to the underlying soft tissues.[67,71] Unfortunately, none of these imaging findings are sufficiently specific; therefore, the positive predictive value for detecting aortic injury with chest radiography is only 5% to 20%.[64] However, the predictive value of a normal supine chest radiograph to exclude aortic injury is significantly higher at 96%.[72] When a mediastinal hematoma is identified, the incidence of aortic injury is only 10% to 20%; the majority of mediastinal hematomas are caused by bleeding from smaller vessels for which no specific intervention is required.[4,5]

Traditionally, when one suspected traumatic thoracic aortic injury based on clinical and chest radiographic findings, conventional aortography was considered the diagnostic gold standard, especially in hemodynamically unstable patients. There is a growing body of evidence supporting the use of MDCT as the primary diagnostic tool in this clinical setting.[4,5,73–76] Because of the early mortality with the more typical aortic injuries, atypical locations may be encountered more commonly in those who survive long enough to be evaluated with a CT scan. The most common CT scan finding is a pseudoaneurysm, typically located on the anterior aspect of the proximal descending aorta, immediately distal to the aortic isthmus (see **Fig. 10**B–D). Such pseudoaneurysm should not be confused with the ductus diverticulum or "ductus bump."[26] Other signs of aortic injury demonstrated with MDCT include periaortic hematoma, intimal flaps, wall irregularities, abrupt caliber changes, occlusion of major branch vessels, luminal clots, and active contrast extravasation.[4,5,29]

Penetrating cardiac injury may result in hemopericardium or pneumopericardium, both of which may result in cardiac tamponade, a life-threatening condition requiring urgent decompression. Pneumopericardium causing tamponade has also been described with blunt chest injury, through a mechanism related to the Macklin effect causing pneumomediastinum.[77] Blunt cardiac injury represents a spectrum of injuries, including myocardial contusion or concussion, ventricular laceration or rupture, and valvular disruption. Amongst these blunt cardiac injuries, myocardial contusion is by far the most common, accounting for 95% of cases.[78] Not all blunt cardiac injuries manifest at the initial time of trauma and some of these injuries may have delayed presentations including arrhythmias and cardiac tamponade.[79,80] Most children with myocardial contusion make a full cardiac recovery, with only approximately 5% suffering any long-term sequelae such as valvular dysfunction.[78] There are no specific chest radiographic findings of cardiac injury, although associated injuries such as pulmonary contusions and rib fractures are commonly seen. Development of pulmonary edema on follow up chest radiographs is more commonly due to fluid overload from aggressive trauma resuscitation than to traumatic myocardial or valvular dysfunction.[4] CT scanning has been successfully used to demonstrate some of the structural abnormalities resulting from blunt cardiac injury, such as ventricular pseudoaneurysm.[81] Children with penetrating cardiac injury and/or hemodynamic instability generally require immediate surgical exploration. Those with myocardial contusion are typically managed in a conservative, supportive manner.[78] Clinical signs of decompensation, such as unexplained hypotension, may be further evaluated with echocardiography. Myocardial contusions may manifest as areas of impaired wall motion or ventricular hypokinesia.[3,78]

Diaphragmatic Rupture

Diaphragmatic rupture is present in 1% to 6% of all major chest injuries.[82] The incidence of diaphragmatic rupture is much higher, as much as 15%, for those with penetrating injury to the upper abdomen and lower chest than those with blunt chest trauma.[2,4,5] However, traumatic diaphragmatic rupture most commonly occurs after blunt thoracoabdominal trauma, with motor vehicle accidents accounting for 90% of cases.[82–84] Traumatic rupture is more common on the left side than the right, with reported rates of 70% to 80% on the left side, 15% to 24% on the right side and 5% to 8% bilaterally. Traditionally, the explanation for this side discrepancy was believed to be to the protective effect of the liver. More recently, this long-held belief has been questioned with evidence that right-sided diaphragmatic rupture may be more often missed clinically. Therefore, its true incidence may be underestimated.[83,84] Regardless of the side of rupture, the most common location of diaphragmatic rupture is posterolateral.[85] Given that the majority of traumatic diaphragmatic injuries occur because of major blunt trauma, it is not surprising that there are additional injuries in 75% to 100% of cases.[84,85]

When diaphragmatic rupture occurs (**Fig. 11**), the most clinically significant complication is visceral herniation with risk of strangulation and lung compression.[1] When diaphragmatic rupture occurs on the left side, the most commonly herniated organs are bowel (stomach, small bowel, and colon) and spleen. With right-sided diaphragmatic rupture, the liver is most commonly involved. With the increasing use of nonsurgical, conservative management of even severe solid abdominal injuries, there is more reliance on imaging diagnosis, and it has become even more imperative not to overlook this important lesion. Unfortunately, the most commonly performed diagnostic test, the supine chest radiograph, is not very sensitive for diagnosing diaphragmatic rupture. There is a high incidence of associated injuries, and the presence of pulmonary contusions, atelectasis, and pleural effusions can obscure the diaphragmatic rupture. Furthermore, herniation of abdominal viscera may not occur until the patient is taken off positive pressure ventilation. Although 77% of diaphragmatic rupture cases have an abnormal chest radiograph, the diagnosis is only suspected in 30% to 40%.[26] In addition, right-sided injuries are more difficult to diagnose than those on the left, with initial radiographs allowing diagnosis of 27% to 60% of left-sided injuries but only 17% of right-sided injuries.[86] The liver serves to prevent herniation of abdominal contents into the lower right side of the chest and herniation of the liver itself may be subtle and frequently overlooked. The differentiation of a herniated liver through a diaphragmatic tear from other causes of pseudoelevation of the hemidiaphragm, such as atelectasis, pleural effusion, pulmonary contusion, or laceration, is often difficult.[86] An anomalous position of a nasogastric tube tip above the left hemidiaphragm indicates herniation of the stomach, which may be confirmed with water-soluble contrast administration.[4,5] There is substantial evidence supporting the use of MDCT with multiplanar reconstructions for the diagnosis of diaphragmatic rupture. Sensitivity and specificity rates are 71% to 87% and 72% to 100%, respectively, with one study reporting 100% sensitivity.[86–89] Left-sided injuries are more readily diagnosed than right-sided injuries, with accuracy rates of 88% and 70%, respectively.[86–88] The challenges associated with accurately diagnosing diaphragmatic rupture with MDCT include the complex shape of the thin diaphragmatic muscle, the horizontal in-plane orientation of the diaphragmatic dome, and the frequency of associated traumatic abnormalities in the lung bases. Direct discontinuity of a hemidiaphragm (see **Fig. 11**), which may allow herniation of intra-abdominal mesenteric fat, parenchymal organs, or viscera, is the most sensitive imaging finding of

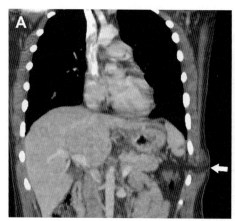
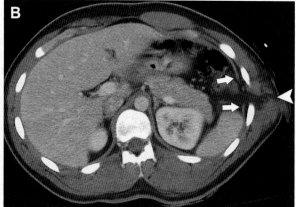

Fig. 11. Penetrating diaphragmatic tear. An 18-year-old male who sustained a stab wound to his left lower chest. Chest CT scan, coronal (*A*) and axial images (*B*) depict the trajectory of the stab wound through the chest wall (*large arrows*). Note the interruption of the left hemidiaphragm (between *small arrows* in *B*), a subtle finding that necessitated a surgical repair, to prevent future visceral herniation.

diaphragmatic rupture.[86] The "hourglass" or "collar" sign refers to the waist-like constriction of partially herniated viscera by the edges of a small diaphragmatic defect. On the right side, the same mechanism can appear as a focal indentation of the liver, termed the "rim" sign, which may be subtle and easily overlooked on axial images. Detection of this sign requires careful analysis of axial images as well as the sagittal and coronal multiplanar reformatted images. The "dependent viscera" sign describes the close contact of the herniated stomach or liver with the posterior chest wall, with no diaphragmatic leaflet holding it up against gravity, and lack of normal interposition of aerated lung tissue posteriorly.[4,5,86] Given the difficulty of reaching an accurate diagnosis, many patients are not diagnosed in the acute setting, possibly as many as 40% to 50%. A delayed diagnosis is often made days, weeks, or even years later, frequently with a complication of visceral herniation.[1,85,90]

IMAGING ALGORITHMS

When one endeavors to devise an appropriate imaging algorithm for the investigation of the child who has suffered chest trauma, three key factors have to be considered. First, the imaging modalities used should be as quick and as accurate as possible. Second, the result of these tests should positively direct patient management and help dictate treatment. Finally, the nature of the investigative tools should not have any negative effect on the child's health or, at least, that effect should be minimized. Whereas the natural inclination would be to immediately use the most accurate and sensitive test, thereby satisfying the first criterion, one has to carefully consider whether such a choice affects the other criteria positively or negatively.

MDCT is more sensitive than chest radiography for a multitude of chest injuries. Rib fracture, pneumothorax, hemothorax, pulmonary contusion and laceration, diaphragmatic rupture, and vascular injuries are all more accurately diagnosed with MDCT.[91,92] Furthermore, MDCT is quick and readily available in most trauma units. The arrival of an injured child in the trauma room is an upsetting event for all involved. Therefore, it is understandable that caregivers might choose a CT scan as their first choice investigation so as to diagnose all injuries within the shortest possible time frame. The potential advantages seem clear; not only is MDCT accurate, but a complete contiguous head-through-pelvis scan may be performed in less than a minute, without the need for repositioning of the critically injured patient. The dose from a single continuous total-body scan is less than the individual components performed separately,[93] although this in itself should not be used as a reason to include all body segments in the CT scan. The volumetric data set acquired with MDCT allows for multiplanar reconstructions, better demonstrating both soft tissue and skeletal injuries, and potentially foregoing the need for other radiographs, which might require multiple projections.[94,95] Such total body scanning is advocated by many investigators for the adult population,[96,97] but one needs to be more cautious before employing a similar policy for children, taking into consideration the second and third criteria outlined above.

With respect to the second criterion, one needs to consider whether the supplemental information provided by a CT scan, over and above the findings on chest radiography, substantially alter patient management. In a study on chest trauma in an adult population by Trupka and colleagues,[98] the routine addition of a CT scan to chest radiography did not alter patient management in 59% of cases, despite detecting significantly more injuries. A more recent adult study reported that the routine use of a CT scan in chest trauma resulted in a greater number of additional diagnoses in 43%, but resulted in a change in patient management in just 17%.[99] Moreover, in a recent pediatric study, most intrathoracic findings requiring surgical management could be identified on images of the lower chest that are part of routine abdominopelvic CT scan examinations,[100] and chest CT scan findings added relatively little to those of radiography. Therefore, rather then "routinely" scanning all potential chest trauma patients, a more selective approach guided by the nature and severity of the trauma, clinical parameters,[101] and chest radiographic findings is more prudent. This selective approach has been shown to increase the incidence of clinically significant findings demonstrated by a CT scan that actually alter patient management.[99] Given the relative infrequency of serious cardiovascular and diaphragmatic injuries in children, most abnormalities detected with a CT scan that may affect patient management relate to pneumothoraces and complications of chest tube placement.[98] Although most radiographically occult pneumothoraces that are detected with a CT scan do not require chest tube placement,[35] if left untreated, they might expand and/or develop into a tension pneumothorax following the institution of positive pressure ventilation. For this reason, a chest CT scan is nearly always indicated in children whose chest injury is severe enough to require mechanical ventilation.[4,5,102]

In our era of escalating medical costs, one also has to take into account the cost-effectiveness of expensive imaging resource use. Renton and colleagues[103] reported that if CT scans were to replace the chest radiograph as the primary tool for investigating pediatric chest trauma, 200 studies would need to be performed to detect one clinically significant finding, incurring a hospital cost of $39,600 and a patient cost of $180,000. The current medico-legal climate, which encourages defensive medicine, likely results in the over-use of CT scans, ignoring the fact that many of the injuries demonstrated do not affect patient management or treatment.[4,5,104] Another potential problem with performing CT scans is the risk of detecting "pseudodisease" and clinically unimportant findings as a result of over-interpretation of the CT scan images. This may influence clinicians to perform costly and sometimes invasive additional imaging tests and treatments that are unnecessary, which can lead to iatrogenic complications as well as added expense. In the era before the implementation of CT scans, this pseudodisease would have simply remained unnoticed, without adverse effect on patient outcome.[4]

Finally, one must consider the third criterion, which is that of radiation carcinogenesis and teratogenesis resulting from the indiscriminate use of CT scans. For a discussion of these risks and their significance, see the article by Donald Frush elsewhere in this issue. The challenge in imaging pediatric chest trauma is to incorporate all of these complex issues in an attempt to derive an appropriate imaging algorithm.[105]

The authors believe that the initial imaging evaluation of pediatric trauma should consist of the conventional trauma series (lateral cervical spine in collar, AP pelvis, and chest radiographs). The sensitivity of the conventional radiographic series may be increased by implementing a novel full-body digital radiograph system.[106] The initial radiographic findings should be interpreted in conjunction with a careful and rapid triage by an experienced clinician, taking the mechanism and force of injury into account.[4,5] This will determine the need for additional imaging. If cross-sectional imaging is required, a CT scan is not the only option. Ultrasound has been used to demonstrate pleural effusions, hemothorax, pneumothorax, pulmonary contusions, pericardial tamponade, and even sternal fractures.[10,13–17] Although ultrasound is frequently more time consuming than CT scanning, the clinical situation may allow for it and spare the patient unnecessary radiation. However, the exact place of FAST ultrasound[11,12] in the diagnostic algorithm of trauma, in particular

with regard to the qualifications of its practitioners and the optimal technique, remains somewhat controversial at this time.[107]

All patients with penetrating injury should eventually undergo a CT scan focused on the area of impact, because the risk of occult internal injury is high in these patients. Unconscious patients and those with suspicion for unstable cervical spine fractures will generally undergo a CT scan of the head and cervical spine. Factors that influence the decision to perform more extensive CT scanning include the severity of the injuries demonstrated on the initial radiographic trauma series, the degree of respiratory compromise, and the presence of hemodynamic instability. If a thoracic spine fracture is clinically suspected or demonstrated on the initial radiographic survey, a CT scan should be performed, with coronal and sagittal reformatted images. Fractures of the upper ribs, shoulder girdle, and sternum will often necessitate a contrast-enhanced CT scan to look for vascular injury. If there is persistent hemorrhagic output from chest tubes or there is radiographic evidence for progressive pneumomediastinum, a CT scan is indicated to look for bronchial and/or vascular injury. Although traumatic aortic injury in children remains rare, the associated high mortality dictates that a high index of suspicion should be maintained for this condition: unexplained hemodynamic compromise or an abnormal mediastinum on chest radiography would indicate the need for an emergent CT angiogram.

SUMMARY

Given the heterogeneous nature of pediatric chest trauma, the optimal imaging approach is one tailored to the specific patient. Chest radiography remains the most important imaging modality for initial triage. Although the role of ultrasound in the setting of trauma is currently somewhat controversial, it may suffice in specific circumstances. The decision to perform a chest CT scan should be dictated by the nature of the trauma, the clinical condition of the child, and the initial radiographic findings, taking the age-related, pretest probabilities of serious injury into account. In the conscious pediatric polytrauma patient who has a normal neurologic function, is not in respiratory failure, has no signs of hemodynamic instability, and who has a normal appearance of the mediastinum on the initial radiograph, there is sufficient evidence to support that a chest CT scan be withheld initially. If an abdominal CT scan is done for initial evaluation, proper attention should be paid to injuries that are visible in the lower thorax (including the diaphragm). Chest CT scanning is particularly important in children with chest trauma when hemodynamic instability or respiratory failure requiring intubation develops, or when there is persistent drainage of blood or air from chest tubes, suspicion for chest tube malfunction, or a progressive pneumomediastinum. In the unconscious polytrauma patient, the performance of a contiguous, head-through-pelvis MDCT may be considered. Whenever a CT scan is performed, the principles of as low as reasonably achievable (ALARA) and "Image Gently"[108] should be adhered to. Radiologists should be actively involved in trauma care. Continued education and close communication between radiologists and the clinical care team are essential to optimize patient care.

REFERENCES

1. Bliss D, Silen M. Pediatric thoracic trauma. Crit Care Med 2002;30(Suppl 11):S409–15.
2. Cooper A, Barlow B, DiScala C, et al. Mortality and truncal injury: the pediatric perspective. J Pediatr Surg 1994;29(1):33–8.
3. Sartorelli KH, Vane DW. The diagnosis and management of children with blunt injury of the chest. Semin Pediatr Surg 2004;13(2):98–105.
4. Westra SJ, Wallace EC. Imaging evaluation of pediatric chest trauma. Radiol Clin North Am 2005; 43(2):267–81.
5. Moore MA, Wallace EC, Westra SJ. The imaging of paediatric thoracic trauma. Pediatr Radiol 2009; 39(5):485–96.
6. Furnival R. Controversies in pediatric thoracic and abdominal trauma. Clin Pediatr Emerg Med 2001; 2(1):48–62.
7. Tovar JA. The lung and pediatric trauma. Semin Pediatr Surg 2008;17(1):53–9.
8. Nakayama DK, Ramenofsky ML, Rowe MI. Chest injuries in childhood. Ann Surg 1989;210(6):770–5.
9. Shah CC, Ramakrishnaiah RH, Bhutta ST, et al. Imaging findings in 512 children following all-terrain vehicle injuries. Pediatr Radiol 2009;39(7): 677–84.
10. McEwan K, Thompson P. Ultrasound to detect haemothorax after chest injury. Emerg Med J 2007; 24(8):581–2.
11. Patel NY, Riherd JM. Focused assessment with sonography for trauma: methods, accuracy, and indications. Surg Clin North Am 2011;91(1):195–207.
12. Korner M, Krotz MM, Degenhart C, et al. Current role of emergency US in patients with major trauma. Radiographics 2008;28(1):225–42.
13. Jin W, Yang DM, Kim HC, et al. Diagnostic values of sonography for assessment of sternal fractures compared with conventional radiography and bone scans. J Ultrasound Med 2006;25(10):1263–8 [quiz: 1269–70].
14. Lichtenstein DA, Meziere G, Lascols N, et al. Ultrasound diagnosis of occult pneumothorax. Crit Care Med 2005;33(6):1231–8.
15. Rocco M, Carbone I, Morelli A, et al. Diagnostic accuracy of bedside ultrasonography in the ICU: feasibility of detecting pulmonary effusion and lung contusion in patients on respiratory support after severe blunt thoracic trauma. Acta Anaesthesiol Scand 2008;52(6):776–84.
16. Soldati G, Testa A, Sher S, et al. Occult traumatic pneumothorax: diagnostic accuracy of lung ultrasonography in the emergency department. Chest 2008;133(1):204–11.
17. Testerman GM. Surgeon-performed ultrasound in the diagnosis and management of pericardial tamponade in a 20-month-old blunt injured toddler. Tenn Med 2006;99(6):37–8.
18. Singh S, Kalra MK, Moore MA, et al. Dose reduction and compliance with pediatric CT protocols adapted to patient size, clinical indication, and number of prior studies. Radiology 2009;252(1): 200–8.
19. Silva AC, Lawder HJ, Hara A, et al. Innovations in CT dose reduction strategy: application of the adaptive statistical iterative reconstruction algorithm. AJR Am J Roentgenol 2010;194(1):191–9.
20. Garcia VF, Gotschall CS, Eichelberger MR, et al. Rib fractures in children: a marker of severe trauma. J Trauma 1990;30(6):695–700.
21. Donnelly LF, Frush DP. Abnormalities of the chest wall in pediatric patients. AJR Am J Roentgenol 1999;173(6):1595–601.
22. Barsness KA, Cha ES, Bensard DD, et al. The positive predictive value of rib fractures as an indicator of nonaccidental trauma in children. J Trauma 2003;54(6):1107–10.
23. Kleinman PK, Schlesinger AE. Mechanical factors associated with posterior rib fractures: laboratory and case studies. Pediatr Radiol 1997;27(1): 87–91.
24. Livingston DH, Shogan B, John P, et al. CT diagnosis of rib fractures and the prediction of acute respiratory failure. J Trauma 2008;64(4):905–11.
25. Cadzow SP, Armstrong KL. Rib fractures in infants: red alert! The clinical features, investigations and child protection outcomes. J Paediatr Child Health 2000;36(4):322–6.
26. Hall A, Johnson K. The imaging of paediatric thoracic trauma. Paediatr Respir Rev 2002;3(3): 241–7.
27. Rozycki GS, Tremblay L, Feliciano DV, et al. A prospective study for the detection of vascular injury in adult and pediatric patients with cervicothoracic seat belt signs. J Trauma 2002;52(4): 618–23 [discussion: 623–4].

28. Pawar RV, Blacksin MF. Traumatic sternal segment dislocation in a 19-month-old. Emerg Radiol 2007; 14(6):435–7.

29. Lomoschitz FM, Eisenhuber E, Linnau KF, et al. Imaging of chest trauma: radiological patterns of injury and diagnostic algorithms. Eur J Radiol 2003;48(1):61–70.

30. el-Khoury GY, Whitten CG. Trauma to the upper thoracic spine: anatomy, biomechanics, and unique imaging features. AJR Am J Roentgenol 1993;160(1):95–102.

31. van Beek EJ, Been HD, Ponsen KK, et al. Upper thoracic spinal fractures in trauma patients - a diagnostic pitfall. Injury 2000;31(4):219–23.

32. Slimane MA, Becmeur F, Aubert D, et al. Tracheobronchial ruptures from blunt thoracic trauma in children. J Pediatr Surg 1999;34(12):1847–50.

33. Chan O, Hiorns M. Chest trauma. Eur J Radiol 1996;23(1):23–34.

34. Bridges KG, Welch G, Silver M, et al. CT detection of occult pneumothorax in multiple trauma patients. J Emerg Med 1993;11(2):179–86.

35. Holmes JF, Brant WE, Bogren HG, et al. Prevalence and importance of pneumothoraces visualized on abdominal computed tomographic scan in children with blunt trauma. J Trauma 2001; 50(3):516–20.

36. Ouellet JF, Trottier V, Kmet L, et al. The OPTICC trial: a multi-institutional study of occult pneumothoraces in critical care. Am J Surg 2009;197(5): 581–6.

37. Grisoni ER, Volsko TA. Thoracic injuries in children. Respir Care Clin N Am 2001;7(1):25–38.

38. Taylor GA, Kaufman RA, Sivit CJ. Active hemorrhage in children after thoracoabdominal trauma: clinical and CT features. AJR Am J Roentgenol 1994;162(2):401–4.

39. Balci AE, Kazez A, Eren S, et al. Blunt thoracic trauma in children: review of 137 cases. Eur J Cardiothorac Surg 2004;26(2):387–92.

40. Allen GS, Cox CS Jr, Moore FA, et al. Pulmonary contusion: are children different? J Am Coll Surg 1997;185(3):229–33.

41. Allen GS, Cox CS Jr. Pulmonary contusion in children: diagnosis and management. South Med J 1998;91(12):1099–106.

42. Elmali M, Baydin A, Nural MS, et al. Lung parenchymal injury and its frequency in blunt thoracic trauma: the diagnostic value of chest radiography and thoracic CT. Diagn Interv Radiol 2007;13(4): 179–82.

43. Schild HH, Strunk H, Weber W, et al. Pulmonary contusion: CT vs plain radiograms. J Comput Assist Tomogr 1989;13(3):417–20.

44. Kwon A, Sorrells DL Jr, Kurkchubasche AG, et al. Isolated computed tomography diagnosis of pulmonary contusion does not correlate with increased morbidity. J Pediatr Surg 2006;41(1): 78–82 [discussion: 78–82].

45. Deunk J, Poels TC, Brink M, et al. The clinical outcome of occult pulmonary contusion on multidetector-row computed tomography in blunt trauma patients. J Trauma 2010;68(2):387–94.

46. Wagner RB, Jamieson PM. Pulmonary contusion. Evaluation and classification by computed tomography. Surg Clin North Am 1989;69(1):31–40.

47. Donnelly LF, Klosterman LA. Subpleural sparing: a CT finding of lung contusion in children. Radiology 1997;204(2):385–7.

48. Peclet MH, Newman KD, Eichelberger MR, et al. Thoracic trauma in children: an indicator of increased mortality. J Pediatr Surg 1990;25(9): 961–5 [discussion: 965–6].

49. Stathopoulos G, Chrysikopoulou E, Kalogeromitros A, et al. Bilateral traumatic pulmonary pseudocysts: case report and literature review. J Trauma 2002; 53(5):993–6.

50. Tsitouridis I, Tsinoglou K, Tsandiridis C, et al. Traumatic pulmonary pseudocysts: CT findings. J Thorac Imaging 2007;22(3):247–51.

51. Wintermark M, Schnyder P. The Macklin effect: a frequent etiology for pneumomediastinum in severe blunt chest trauma. Chest 2001;120(2): 543–7.

52. Bars N, Atlay Y, Tulay E, et al. Extensive subcutaneous emphysema and pneumomediastinum associated with blowout fracture of the medial orbital wall. J Trauma 2008;64(5):1366–9.

53. Marwan K, Farmer KC, Varley C, et al. Pneumothorax, pneumomediastinum, pneumoperitoneum, pneumoretroperitoneum and subcutaneous emphysema following diagnostic colonoscopy. Ann R Coll Surg Engl 2007;89(5):W20–1.

54. Chapdelaine J, Beaunoyer M, Daigneault P, et al. Spontaneous pneumomediastinum: are we overinvestigating? J Pediatr Surg 2004;39(5):681–4.

55. Jackimczyk K. Blunt chest trauma. Emerg Med Clin North Am 1993;11(1):81–96.

56. Harvey-Smith W, Bush W, Northrop C. Traumatic bronchial rupture. AJR Am J Roentgenol 1980; 134(6):1189–93.

57. Ein SH, Friedberg J, Shandling B, et al. Traumatic bronchial injuries in children. Pediatr Pulmonol 1986;2(1):60–4.

58. Mahboubi S, O'Hara AE. Bronchial rupture in children following blunt chest trauma. Report of five cases with emphasis on radiologic findings. Pediatr Radiol 1981;10(3):133–8.

59. Hrkac Pustahija A, Vukelic Markovic M, Ivanac G, et al. An unusual case of bronchial rupture—pneumomediastinum appearing 7 days after blunt chest trauma. Emerg Radiol 2009;16(2):163–5.

60. Ozdulger A, Cetin G, Erkmen Gulhan S, et al. A review of 24 patients with bronchial ruptures: is

delay in diagnosis more common in children? Eur J Cardiothorac Surg 2003;23(3):379–83.

61. Scaglione M, Romano S, Pinto A, et al. Acute tracheobronchial injuries: impact of imaging on diagnosis and management implications. Eur J Radiol 2006;59(3):336–43.

62. Le Guen M, Beigelman C, Bouhemad B, et al. Chest computed tomography with multiplanar reformatted images for diagnosing traumatic bronchial rupture: a case report. Crit Care 2007;11(5):R94.

63. Wan YL, Tsai KT, Yeow KM, et al. CT findings of bronchial transection. Am J Emerg Med 1997; 15(2):176–7.

64. Sinclair DS. Traumatic aortic injury: an imaging review. Emerg Radiol 2002;9(1):13–20.

65. Heckman SR, Trooskin SZ, Burd RS. Risk factors for blunt thoracic aortic injury in children. J Pediatr Surg 2005;40(1):98–102.

66. Spouge AR, Burrows PE, Armstrong D, et al. Traumatic aortic rupture in the pediatric population. Role of plain film, CT and angiography in the diagnosis. Pediatr Radiol 1991;21(5):324–8.

67. Trachiotis GD, Sell JE, Pearson GD, et al. Traumatic thoracic aortic rupture in the pediatric patient. Ann Thorac Surg 1996;62(3):724–31 [discussion: 731–2].

68. Buffo-Sequeira I, Fraser DD. Widened mediastinum in a child with severe trauma. CMAJ 2007;177(10): 1181–2.

69. Gschwentner M, Gruber G, Oberladstatter J, et al. Mediastinal widening after blunt chest trauma in a child: a very rare case of thymic bleeding in a child and possible differential diagnosis. J Trauma Inj Infect Crit Care 2007;63(2):E51–4.

70. Lowe LH, Bulas DI, Eichelberger MD, et al. Traumatic aortic injuries in children: radiologic evaluation. AJR Am J Roentgenol 1998;170(1):39–42.

71. Bertrand S, Cuny S, Petit P, et al. Traumatic rupture of thoracic aorta in real-world motor vehicle crashes. Traffic Inj Prev 2008;9(2):153–61.

72. Mirvis SE, Bidwell JK, Buddemeyer EU, et al. Value of chest radiography in excluding traumatic aortic rupture. Radiology 1987;163(2):487–93.

73. Anderson SA, Day M, Chen MK, et al. Traumatic aortic injuries in the pediatric population. J Pediatr Surg 2008;43(6):1077–81.

74. Ng CJ, Chen JC, Wang LJ, et al. Diagnostic value of the helical CT scan for traumatic aortic injury: correlation with mortality and early rupture. J Emerg Med 2006;30(3):277–82.

75. Sammer M, Wang E, Blackmore CC, et al. Indeterminate CT angiography in blunt thoracic trauma: is CT angiography enough? AJR Am J Roentgenol 2007;189(3):603–8.

76. Pabon-Ramos WM, Williams DM, Strouse PJ. Radiologic evaluation of blunt thoracic aortic injury in pediatric patients. AJR Am J Roentgenol 2010; 194(5):1197–203.

77. Markarian MK, MacIntyre DA, Cousins BJ, et al. Adolescent pneumopericardium and pneumomediastinum after motor vehicle crash and ejection. Am J Emerg Med 2008;26(4):515.e511–2.

78. Dowd MD, Krug S. Pediatric blunt cardiac injury: epidemiology, clinical features, and diagnosis. Pediatric Emergency Medicine Collaborative Research Committee: Working Group on Blunt Cardiac Injury. J Trauma Inj Infect Crit Care 1996; 40(1):61–7.

79. Murillo CA, Owens-Stovall SK, Kim S, et al. Delayed cardiac tamponade after blunt chest trauma in a child. J Trauma Inj Infect Crit Care 2002;52(3): 573–5.

80. Sakka SG, Huettemann E, Giebe W, et al. Late cardiac arrhythmias after blunt chest trauma. Intensive Care Med 2000;26(6):792–5.

81. Palacio D, Swischuk L, Chung D, et al. Posttraumatic ventricular pseudoaneurysm in a 7-year-old child diagnosed with multidetector CT of the chest: a case report. Emerg Radiol 2007;14(6):431–3.

82. Eren S, Kantarci M, Okur A. Imaging of diaphragmatic rupture after trauma. Clin Radiol 2006; 61(6):467–77.

83. Ramos CT, Koplewitz BZ, Babyn PS, et al. What have we learned about traumatic diaphragmatic hernias in children? J Pediatr Surg 2000;35(4):601–4.

84. Sharma AK, Kothari SK, Gupta C, et al. Rupture of the right hemidiaphragm due to blunt trauma in children: a diagnostic dilemma. Pediatr Surg Int 2002;18(2–3):173–4.

85. Soundappan SV, Holland AJ, Cass DT, et al. Blunt traumatic diaphragmatic injuries in children. Injury 2005;36(1):51–4.

86. Iochum S, Ludig T, Walter F, et al. Imaging of diaphragmatic injury: a diagnostic challenge? Radiographics 2002;22(Spec No):S103–16 [discussion: S116–8].

87. Mihos P, Potaris K, Gakidis J, et al. Traumatic rupture of the diaphragm: experience with 65 patients. Injury 2003;34(3):169–72.

88. Nchimi A, Szapiro D, Ghaye B, et al. Helical CT of blunt diaphragmatic rupture. AJR Am J Roentgenol 2005;184(1):24–30.

89. Bodanapally UK, Shanmuganathan K, Mirvis SE, et al. MDCT diagnosis of penetrating diaphragm injury. Eur Radiol 2009;19(8):1875–81.

90. Alper B, Vargun R, Kologlu MB, et al. Late presentation of a traumatic rupture of the diaphragm with gastric volvulus in a child: report of a case. Surg Today 2007;37(10):874–7.

91. Shanmuganathan K, Mirvis SE. Imaging diagnosis of nonaortic thoracic injury. Radiol Clin North Am 1999;37(3):533–51.

92. Sivit CJ, Taylor GA, Eichelberger MR. Chest injury in children with blunt abdominal trauma: evaluation with CT. Radiology 1989;171(3):815–8.

93. Ptak T, Rhea JT, Novelline RA. Radiation dose is reduced with a single-pass whole-body multidetector row CT trauma protocol compared with a conventional segmented method: initial experience. Radiology 2003;229(3):902–5.

94. Griffey RT, Ledbetter S, Khorasani R. Changes in thoracolumbar computed tomography and radiography utilization among trauma patients after deployment of multidetector computed tomography in the emergency department. J Trauma Inj Infect Crit Care 2007;62(5):1153–6.

95. Kessel B, Sevi R, Jeroukhimov I, et al. Is routine portable pelvic X-ray in stable multiple trauma patients always justified in a high technology era? Injury 2007;38(5):559–63.

96. Anderson SW, Lucey BC, Varghese JC, et al. Sixty-four multi-detector row computed tomography in multitrauma patient imaging: early experience. Curr Probl Diagn Radiol 2006;35(5):188–98.

97. Self ML, Blake AM, Whitley M, et al. The benefit of routine thoracic, abdominal, and pelvic computed tomography to evaluate trauma patients with closed head injuries. Am J Surg 2003;186(6): 609–13 [discussion: 613–4].

98. Trupka A, Waydhas C, Hallfeldt KK, et al. Value of thoracic computed tomography in the first assessment of severely injured patients with blunt chest trauma: results of a prospective study. J Trauma Inj Infect Crit Care 1997;43(3):405–11 [discussion: 411–2].

99. Brink M, Deunk J, Dekker HM, et al. Added value of routine chest MDCT after blunt trauma: evaluation of additional findings and impact on patient management. AJR Am J Roentgenol 2008;190(6): 1591–8.

100. Patel RP, Hernanz-Schulman M, Hilmes MA, et al. Pediatric chest CT after trauma: impact on surgical and clinical management. Pediatr Radiol 2010;40(7):1246–53.

101. Holmes JF, Sokolove PE, Brant WE, et al. A clinical decision rule for identifying children with thoracic injuries after blunt torso trauma. Ann Emerg Med 2002;39(5):492–9.

102. Traub M, Stevenson M, McEvoy S, et al. The use of chest computed tomography versus chest X-ray in patients with major blunt trauma. Injury 2007;38(1):43–7.

103. Renton J, Kincaid S, Ehrlich PF. Should helical CT scanning of the thoracic cavity replace the conventional chest x-ray as a primary assessment tool in pediatric trauma? An efficacy and cost analysis. J Pediatr Surg 2003;38(5):793–7.

104. Jindal A, Velmahos GC, Rofougaran R. Computed tomography for evaluation of mild to moderate pediatric trauma: are we overusing it? World J Surg 2002; 26(1):13–6.

105. Markel TA, Kumar R, Koontz NA, et al. The utility of computed tomography as a screening tool for the evaluation of pediatric blunt chest trauma. J Trauma 2009;67(1):23–8.

106. Deyle S, Wagner A, Benneker LM, et al. Could full-body digital X-ray (LODOX-Statscan) screening in trauma challenge conventional radiography? J Trauma 2009;66(2):418–22.

107. Mirvis SE, Shanmuganathan K. The 2008 RadioGraphics monograph issue: emergency imaging in adults. Radiographics 2008;28(6):1539–40.

108. Strauss KJ, Goske MJ, Kaste SC, et al. Image gently: ten steps you can take to optimize image quality and lower dose for pediatric patients. AJR Am J Roentgenol 2010;194:868–73.

Congenital Thoracic Vascular Anomalies: Evaluation with State-of-the-Art MR Imaging and MDCT

Jeffrey C. Hellinger, MD[a],*, Melissa Daubert, MD[b],
Edward Y. Lee, MD, MPH[c,d], Monica Epelman, MD[e]

KEYWORDS

- Aortic arch anomalies • Pulmonary artery anomalies
- Thoracic systemic venous anomalies
- Pulmonary venous anomalies • CT angiography
- MR imaging • MR angiography

Congenital thoracic vascular anomalies occur in the thoracic aorta and branch arteries, pulmonary arteries, thoracic systemic veins, and the pulmonary veins (**Table 1**). Technological innovations in magnetic resonance (MR) imaging and multidetector-row computed tomography (MDCT) have greatly advanced the noninvasive diagnosis of these anomalies in pediatric patients in recent years. From the neonate to the adolescent, high-resolution two-dimensional (2D) and three-dimensional (3D) MR imaging (MRI), noncontrast MR angiography (MRA), 3D contrast-enhanced MRA, and 3D MDCT angiography (CTA) datasets provide comprehensive multiprojectional, anatomic displays for interactive interpretation, treatment planning, and postoperative and postendovascular evaluation.

Effective use and interpretation of MRI-MRA (**Fig. 1**) and CTA (**Fig. 2**) for the evaluation of congenital thoracic vascular anomalies in pediatric patients require fundamental understandings of imaging techniques, anatomic embryology and characteristics, and underlying clinical pathophysiology. Imagers should have knowledge of strategies to optimize protocols to deliver accurate and safe cardiovascular imaging based on the suspected lesion(s) and the clinical stability of the patient. Equally important is the ability to adeptly use advanced postprocessing visualization techniques for image display, interpretation, and clinical management. This article assists the reader in these objectives. Imaging strategies and MR imaging-MR angiography/CTA techniques are reviewed, followed by a discussion on the commonly encountered thoracic congenital vascular anomalies, with emphasis on embryology, clinical manifestations, and characteristic imaging findings.

[a] Advanced Cardiovascular Imaging, Advanced Imaging and Informatics Laboratory, Stony Brook Long Island Children's Hospital, Stony Brook University School of Medicine, Stony Brook, NY, USA
[b] Stony Brook University School of Medicine, Stony Brook, NY, USA
[c] Division of Thoracic Imaging, Department of Radiology, Children's Hospital Boston and Harvard Medical School, Boston, MA, USA
[d] Pulmonary Division, Department of Medicine, Children's Hospital Boston and Harvard Medical School, Boston, MA, USA
[e] Neonatal Imaging, The Children's Hospital of Philadelphia, University of Pennsylvania School of Medicine, Philadelphia, PA, USA
* Corresponding author.
E-mail address: jeffrey.hellinger@yahoo.com

Radiol Clin N Am 49 (2011) 969–996
doi:10.1016/j.rcl.2011.06.013

Table 1
Congenital thoracic vascular anomaly

Arterial		Venous	
Thoracic Aorta	**Pulmonary Artery**	**Systemic Veins**	**Pulmonary Veins**
Obstructive aortic arch lesions	Pulmonary sling	Persistent LSVC	PAPVR
Tubular hypoplasia	Hypoplasia	With an RSVC	TAPVR
Interruption of the aortic arch	Agenesis	Mirror image drainage	Type I
Aortic coarctation	Stenosis	Retroaortic left BCV	Type II
Aortic arch anomalies			Type III
Left aortic arch			Mixed
Aberrant RSCA			
Circumflex right DsAo			
Double aortic arch			
Right aortic arch			
Aberrant LSCA/BCA			
Mirror image branching			
Circumflex left DsAo			
Cervical aortic arch			
Innominate artery compression			

Abbreviations: BCA, brachiocephalic artery; BCV, brachiocephalic vein; DsAo, descending aorta; LSVC, left superior vena cava; PAPVR, partial anomalous pulmonary venous return; RSCA, right subclavian artery; RSVC, right superior vena cava; TAPVR, total anomalous pulmonary venous return.

IMAGING STRATEGIES

Chest radiography, echocardiography, vascular ultrasound, esophagography, MRI-MRA, CTA, catheter angiography, or a combination thereof may be performed for diagnostic evaluation of congenital thoracic vascular anomalies. In the past, catheter angiography was regarded as the standard for angiographic evaluation of these disorders but, in the past decade, MR angiography and CTA have gradually replaced catheter angiography for diagnostic purposes. Currently, catheter-based angiography is reserved for endovascular interventions and obtaining direct hemodynamic measurements.

In most pediatric patients presenting with a suspected congenital thoracic vascular anomaly, a frontal (and preferably also a lateral) chest radiograph is the initial imaging modality. The chest radiograph is a fast and inexpensive means to obtain initial direct or indirect evidence for a congenital vascular lesion. Although the chest radiograph may not always yield the specific diagnosis, it is useful to exclude other potential causes, guide initial management, and direct selection of subsequent imaging for confirmation and characterization.

If cardiovascular symptoms predominate (eg, congestive heart failure, systemic hypoperfusion,

cyanosis) transthoracic echocardiography (TTE) is usually obtained next. TTE, which requires no radiation, is readily performed and can assess morphology and function (eg, flow dynamics, pressure gradients). However, TTE is limited by the acoustic window (inversely related to patient age and size), acoustic impedance (air), operator skill, and the ability to visualize peripheral vascular segments (eg, pulmonary arteries, pulmonary veins, and supra-aortic branch arteries).

MR imaging-MR angiography or CTA are indicated based on the TTE findings and performance. State-of-the-art MRI-MRA with parallel imaging should be considered before CTA in pediatric patients, because it does not require radiation or iodinated contrast medium and can evaluate vascular hemodynamics as well as vascular morphology with high-resolution anatomic detail. MDCT angiography is indicated when MR imaging-MR angiography is not available, is contraindicated, is nondiagnostic, or has a high pretest probability for being nondiagnostic. CTA should be considered in the patient at high risk with sedation or anesthesia and when airway, lung parenchyma, and other noncardiovascular structures require more detailed imaging.

If respiratory symptoms predominate (eg, stridor, exercise intolerance, apnea, cyanosis, recurrent

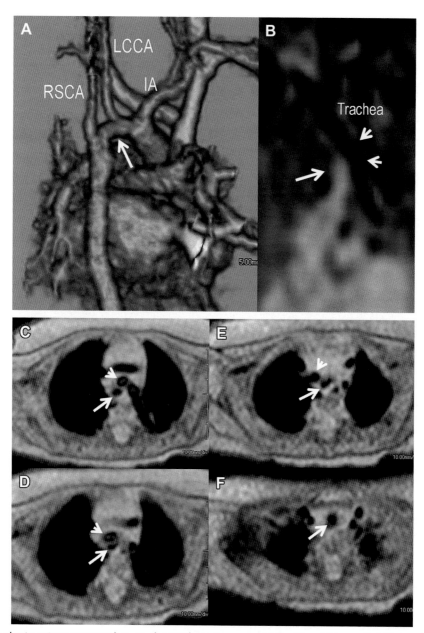

Fig. 1. Innominate artery compression on the trachea. A young child with a history of stridor underwent MR imaging-MR angiography for assessment of a possible vascular ring. (*A*) Sagittal 3D volume rendered image of the MR angiography shows a left aortic arch with normal 3 vessel branches and slightly horizontal course (*arrow*) of the innominate artery (IA). (*B*) Oblique MPR projection from a single-shot fast spin echo dark blood acquisition shows the relationship of the IA (*long arrow*) to the trachea (*short arrows*). (*C–F*) Transverse dark blood images show slightly more than 50% extrinsic compression on the trachea (*arrow*) by the IA (*arrowhead*), as the IA courses from left to right. LSCA, left subclavian artery; MPR, multiplanar reconstruction; RSCA, right subclavian artery.

upper and lower respiratory infections), MR imaging-MR angiography or CTA is performed following chest radiography per the guidelines discussed earlier. Echocardiography is indicated after a positive MR imaging-MR angiography or CTA to further evaluate cardiac morphology, assess function, and exclude other congenital cardiovascular lesions. In this clinical setting, CTA is advantageous to assess for tracheobronchomalacia, tracheal rings, and extrinsic tracheal compression. Paired inspiration-expiration MDCT angiographic techniques with controlled ventilation have proved

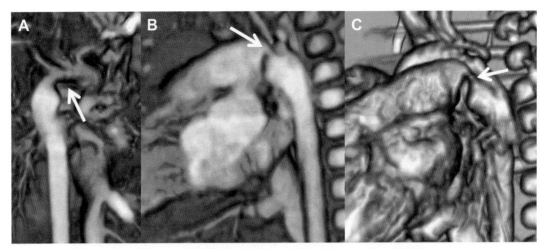

Fig. 2. Tubular hypoplasia of the aortic arch. A neonate with congenital aortic stenosis underwent MDCT angi-ography to further define aortic arch anatomy. (A–C) 3D volume rendered images show moderate to severe tubular hypoplasia of the aortic arch (A, arrow) with a small patent ductus arteriosus (B, C; arrow).

to be a reliable means to diagnose clinically signif-icant tracheomalacia and innominate artery compression on the trachea in pediatric patients.[1] If gastrointestinal symptoms predominate (eg, feeding intolerance, failure to thrive, dysphagia, aspiration), an esophagram may be obtained following chest radiography. MRI-MRA or CTA is performed if the esophagram is positive, based on the guidelines discussed earlier. If symptoms persist following a negative esophagram and there remains a high index of suspicion for a thoracic vascular anomaly, consideration should be given to either MR imaging-MR angiography or CTA. Following a positive MRI-MRA or CTA, if previ-ously obtained, TTE may be indicated to assess for congenital heart structural abnormalities.

IMAGING TECHNIQUES
MR Imaging and MDCT Protocols

MR imaging and MDCT angiographic protocols are designed to accurately evaluate cardiac and vascular morphology, and to provide detailed assessments of the central airway and its relation-ship to cardiac chambers and vascular structures. To minimize the examination duration, only essen-tial scan acquisitions should be used, because patients may become hemodynamically unstable or may develop respiratory distress. Before imaging, it is recommended to review the patient's clinical presentation, prior medical history, prior imaging studies, current management, and other relevant clinical data. Such information helps in the selection of the most appropriate imaging modality and optimal acquisition and contrast injection protocols. Clinical review also helps to determine the most appropriate location and size

for an intravenous catheter (eg, CEMRA, CTA) and whether sedation or anesthesia is required.

MR imaging-MR angiography

A standard MRI-MRA protocol for evaluation of pediatric thoracic vascular anomalies includes electrocardiogram-gated black-blood and bright-blood sequences in conjunction with an angio-graphic sequence. Black-blood and bright-blood MR imaging sequences provide comprehensive anatomic detail, in particular vessel course, caliber, and arterial branching or venous drainage pattern. Black-blood imaging is also applied to evaluate the central airway. Techniques for black-blood MR imaging typically include either single-shot fast spin echo with double inversion recovery or half-Fourier, single-shot fast spin echo with double inversion recovery. Bright-blood imaging in most current practices is achieved with 2D or 3D balanced steady-state free precession. Phase contrast (PC) MR imaging is an optional sequence that is used to evaluate flow direction and velocity, and assess vascular physiology.

Angiographic techniques include time of flight (TOF) MR angiography, PC-MR angiography, and multiphase (arterial and venous) 3D T1-weighted CEMRA. CEMRA is most frequently performed, whereas TOF-MR angiography and PC-MR angi-ography are reserved for when gadolinium is con-traindicated. To maximize 3D displays, CEMRA slice thickness should not be greater than 1.5 mm. When parallel imaging techniques are applied with CEMRA, isotropic, submillimeter datasets can be obtained, yielding the highest possible spatial resolution and robust 3D structural displays on par with those from an MDCT angiogram.

Acquisitions may be in the coronal or sagittal plane, depending on the required anatomic coverage and breath-hold duration.

MDCT angiography

Because of its inherent dependence on radiation for generating images, low-dose helical and volumetric pediatric MDCT angiography protocols strive for only 1 core series, namely a single-phase angiographic scan. This single scan is acquired with a slice thickness of 0.5 to 1.5 mm and is synchronized with the arrival of contrast to generate arterial, venous, or equilibrium phase datasets. A noncontrast acquisition is a consideration in the postsurgical or endovascular patient to assess the presence, location, and integrity of high-density material that may degrade vascular interpretation or may be obscured by the contrast (eg, metallic stents, surgical clips, embolization coils). Additional vascular phases should only be considered if image quality is suboptimal. Ultralow radiation dose volumetric, time-resolved, dynamic CTA with intermittent 2-second to 3-second data acquisitions in 10 to 15 seconds is a promising new technique that can be performed on a 320-channel MDCT scanner; similar to CEMRA, isolated arterial and venous phases can be acquired, providing temporal flow information and more direct imaging of vascular physiology with MDCT. With all pediatric CTA protocols, radiation dose reduction strategies should be used to achieve the lowest possible radiation exposure that will render an interpretable examination for the reader. These radiation dose reduction strategies include using the lowest possible voltage (eg, 80 kVp), the lowest possible amperage (eg, weight-based milliampere seconds), the minimum amount of coverage (with shielding of nontarget regions), and the shortest possible scan time (eg, fastest scan rotation, high-pitch helical, wide-collimation helical, and volumetric MDCT techniques).[2]

Interpretation and Advanced Visualization

MR imaging-MR angiography and CTA interpretation address vascular morphology and physiology, as detailed in Tables 2 and 3. Evaluation for associated cardiovascular and noncardiovascular abnormalities is imperative. Postoperative and endovascular evaluations should assess luminal patency and exclude aneurysms, pseudoaneurysms, and iatrogenic injury. For patients who have undergone stent placement, stent migration, fatigue, and disruption should be excluded.

Display and interpretation of thoracic MRA and CTA datasets are most effective when applying advanced workstation visualization techniques (Table 4). Techniques are selected in a complementary manner according to their strengths, using adjustable angiographic window and level settings, including a wide window setting to account for noise and high vascular contrast. Datasets are interrogated in real time with user-defined interaction of the techniques and related workstation tool functions. Alternatively, protocol-driven static postprocessed single and batch-serial images are generated for review along with the source images. The spatial detail of angiographic anatomy is best displayed using 3D volume rendering (VR) and 2D maximum intensity projection (MIP). Both require sliding thin slabs or prerendering editing to remove bone and other anatomic structures that may obscure vascular visualization. However, structural detail is assessed with the highest accuracy using 2D multiplanar reformations (MPR) and curved planar reformations (CPR). Although minimum intensity projection (MinIP) and ray sum (thick MPR) have limited applications in MR and CT angiography MinIP is useful with CTA datasets to show cardiac

---

Table 2
Interpretive review: congenital thoracic arterial anomalies

Aorta		Aortic Arch			Ductus		Pulmonary Arteries		Vascular
AsAo	DsAo	Transverse segment	Isthmus	Branch arteries	Arteriosus		Central	Peripheral	Physiology
Location	Location	Location	Caliber	Number	Patent		Presence	Course	Gradient
Course	Course	Number	Contour	Order	Closed		Location	Caliber	Collaterals
Caliber	Caliber	Sidedness Caliber	Coarctation Preductal Juxtaductal Postductal	Course Caliber	Diverticulum Dimple		Course Caliber		

Abbreviations: AsAo, ascending aorta; DsAo, descending aorta.

Table 3
Interpretive review: congenital thoracic venous anomalies

SVC	IVC	Innominate Vein	Coronary Sinus	Pulmonary Veins	Cardiac Chambers	Pulmonary Arteries	Airways	Lungs
Sidedness	Sidedness	Sidedness	Presence	Number	Connections	Caliber	Lobar Anatomy	Lobar Anatomy
Right	Right	Right	Caliber	Course	Size	Central	Hypoplasia	Hypoplasia
Left	Left	Left		Caliber	Atria	Peripheral	Partial agenesis	Partial agenesis
Course	Course	Course		Insertion	Ventricles	Patency		Mosaic attenuation
Caliber	Caliber	Flow direction		Patency	Septae			
Insertion	Insertion				Defects Flattening			

Abbreviations: IVC, inferior vena cava; SVC, superior vena cava.

Table 4
Cardiovascular advanced visualization techniques

	Display	Principal Use	Advantages	Disadvantages
MPR	2D	Structural detail Quantitative analysis	Slice through dataset in coronal, sagittal, and oblique projections Real-time multiplanar interrogation Simplify image interpretation	Limited spatial perception
CPR	2D	Structural detail Centerline display Simplify MPR	Single anatomic display Longitudinal cross-sectional anatomic display	Operator dependent
Ray sum	2D	Structural overview	Slice through dataset in axial, coronal, sagittal, and oblique projections Real-time multiplanar interrogation Radiograph-like display	Loss of structural detail with increased slab thickness
MIP	2D	Structural overview Angiographic display	Slice through dataset in axial, coronal, sagittal, and oblique projections Real-time multiplanar interrogation Improved depiction Small-caliber vessels Poorly enhanced vessels Communicate findings	Anatomic overlap (vessels, bone, viscera) with increased slab thickness Visualization degraded by high-density structures (ie, bone, calcium, stents, coils) Loss of structural detail with increased slab thickness Limited grading of stent lumens
MinIP	2D	Structural overview Airway Air trapping in lung Soft tissue air	Slice through dataset in axial, coronal, sagittal, and oblique projections Real-time multiplanar interrogation Depict low-density structures Communicate findings	Anatomic overlap Loss of structural detail with increased slab thickness
VR	3D	Structural overview Angiographic display	Slice through dataset in axial, coronal, sagittal, and oblique projections Real-time multiplanar interrogation Depict structural relationships Accurate spatial perception Communicate findings	Dependent upon opacity-transfer function Anatomic overlap Loss of structural detail with increased slab thickness

Abbreviations: CPR, curved planar reformation; MinIP, minimum intensity projection; MIP, maximum intensity projection; MPR, multiplanar reformation; VR, volume rendered.

From Hellinger JC, Pena A, Poon M, et al. Pediatric computed tomographic angiography: imaging the cardiovascular system gently. Radiol Clin North Am 2010;48:457; with permission.

valves (eg, bicuspid aortic valve), airways, air trapping, and abnormal nonpulmonary air collections. Ray sum may be applied with MR angiography and CTA datasets to generate radiograph-like images for structural overview.

SPECTRUM OF THORACIC CONGENITAL VASCULAR ANOMALIES
Arterial Systems

The primitive circulatory system is initially functional by the end of the third week of fetal development; blood passes from the primitive heart to paired dorsal aorta. Subsequent development of the thoracic aorta, aortic arch branch arteries, pulmonary arteries, and ductus arteriosus occurs during the fourth to eighth weeks of life, beginning with the growth of 6 paired pharyngeal aortic arches (PAA), which bridge the aortic sac to the dorsal aortae through the pharyngeal pouches. Normal development leads to a left-sided aortic arch (LAA) and descending aorta; aortic arch branching (in order) consists of the brachiocephalic artery, the left common carotid artery (LCCA), and the left subclavian artery (LSCA) (see **Fig. 1**). The ductus arteriosus is left sided, extending from the proximal left pulmonary artery (LPA) to the aortic isthmus, the segment that is between the LSCA and the proximal descending aorta. To achieve this morphology, the aortic arches along with the dorsal aortae and the seventh intersegmental arteries, undergo selective involution and differential growth of persisting structures, as detailed in **Table 5**.[3]

THORACIC AORTA
Obstructive Aortic Arch Lesions

Tubular hypoplasia
Tubular hypoplasia of the aortic arch (THAA) is a congenital anomaly in which the transverse aorta is reduced in caliber in a short segment such that antegrade flow is reduced. Borders of the aorta in THAA are smooth, without focal narrowing (see **Fig. 2**). Obstructive physiology may be present in

affected patients depending on the length of hypoplasia and the pressure gradient (**Fig. 3**). It can occur in isolation or be associated with other left-sided obstructive lesions (LSOLs), including congenital mitral stenosis (MS), mitral atresia (MA), hypoplastic left heart syndrome (HLHS), aortic stenosis (AS), aortic atresia (AA), interrupted aortic arch (IAA), and coarctation of the aorta (COA).

The hemodynamic theory can explain the pathogenesis of aortic arch hypoplasia and its association with concomitant congenital heart defect (CHD) lesions. Normal development and size of the aortic arch is dependent on flow dynamics. In normal fetal circulation, half of the combined ventricular blood volume flows from the right ventricle to the main pulmonary artery, whereas the other half flows from the left ventricle to the ascending aorta. Most the pulmonary blood volume flows across the ductus arteriosus to the descending aorta. The majority of the ascending aortic blood volume flows to the coronary circulation and the supra-aortic arteries, resulting in approximately 15% of blood volume flowing across the isthmus and a fetal isthmus that measures up to 70% to 75% the size of the ascending aorta caliber.[4–6] Any event or lesion that results in decreased antegrade blood flow will lead to less vascular stimulation for growth of the fourth aortic arches and smaller than expected size of the aortic arch and isthmus.

MR imaging-MR angiography and CTA findings of THAA include diffuse smooth narrowing of the

Table 5
Embryologic origins and development of the left aortic arch

Structure		Outcome	Vascular Derivatives
Pharyngeal aortic arches	First	Near complete involution	Ipsilateral ECA
	Second	Near complete involution	Ipsilateral ECA
	Third	Bilateral persistence	Ipsilateral CCA and ICA
	Fourth	Left: dominant persistence	Left: midaortic arch
		Right: partial persistence	Right: BCA, RSCA
	Fifth	Never forms or involutes	None
	Sixth	Left: dominant persistence	Left
			Ventral: ipsilateral central PA
			Dorsal: ductus arteriosus
		Right: partial persistence	Right
			Ventral: Ipsilateral central PA
			Dorsal: ductal involution
Seventh segmental artery		Bilateral persistence	Left: LSCA
			Right: LSCA
Dorsal aortae		Left: dominant persistence	Left: distal aortic arch
		Right: involutes	Right: none

Abbreviations: BCA, brachiocephalic artery; CCA, common carotid artery; ECA, external carotid artery; ICA, internal carotid artery; PA, pulmonary artery.

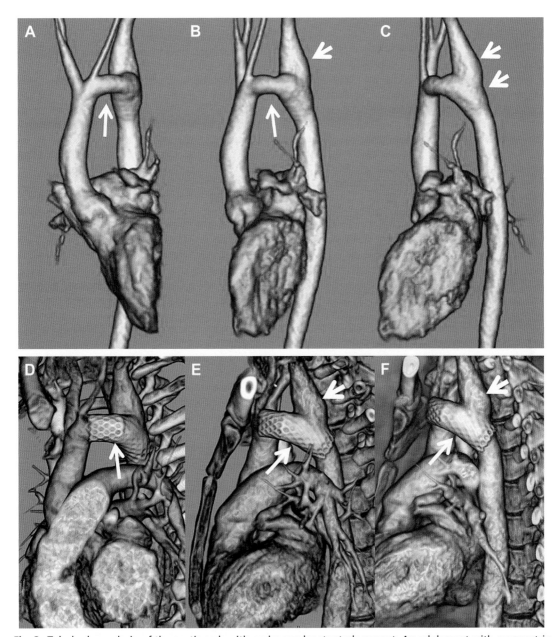

Fig. 3. Tubular hypoplasia of the aortic arch with endovascular stent placement. An adolescent with asymmetric upper extremity hypertension underwent MDCT angiography. (*A–C*) Initial diagnostic 3D volume rendered images show mild tubular hypoplasia of a mildly elongated transverse aortic arch (*A, B; long arrow*) with compensatory LSCA enlargement (*B, C short arrows*) for collateral flow. Catheter angiography confirmed a significant pressure gradient that subsequently led to endovascular stent placement. (*D–F*) 3D volume rendered CTA images after stent placement show overlapping uncovered stent placement (*long arrow*) extending from the LCCA to just past the LSCA. Note the persistent residual LSCA enlargement (*short arrow*). LCCA, left common carotid artery.

transverse aorta. Narrowing may involve the entire aortic arch or only a portion (typically midaortic arch to distal aortic arch). Search should be made for associated left-sided obstructive lesions. If MR imaging-MR angiography is performed, phase contrast imaging is essential to document the presence of a gradient. Treatment is only indicated when there is a hemodynamically significant gradient (eg, >15–20 mm Hg). If diagnosis is made by CTA, echocardiography can subsequently be performed to determine the gradient.

Interruption of the aortic arch

Interruption of the aortic arch is a rare, hemodynamically critical left-sided obstructive conotruncal anomaly in which there is discontinuity of the aortic arch, resulting in systemic perfusion that is dependent on the ductal and/or aortic branch artery. IAA accounts for 0.4% to 1.3% of CHD lesions[7,8] and 7% of CHD lesions presenting with significant physiologic compromise.[9] Arch interruption may occur at 1 of 3 levels with variable frequency: (1) type A, distal to the LSCA origin (26%); (2) type B, between the origins of the LCCA and LSCA (72%); and (3) type C, proximal to the LCCA, between the origins of the innominate and left common carotid arteries (2%).[7,10–16] Associated CHD lesions include patent ductus arteriosus (PDA), ventricular septal defect (VSD; isolated and multiple), atrial septal defect (ASD), left ventricular outflow tract obstruction (LVOTO, such as hypoplasia and subaortic, valvular, and supravalvular aortic stenosis), aortopulmonary window, truncus arteriosus, transposition of the great arteries (TGA), double outlet right ventricle, and aortic arch anomalies.[7,10–17] Evidence indicates that type A IAA occurs secondary to decreased antegrade hemodynamics from an underlying CHD lesion (eg, LVOTO lesions, left to right shunts), with presumed left fourth aortic arch involution.[17,18] By distinction, type B IAA results from genetically altered neural crest embryogenesis. In patients affected with type B IAA, approximately 50% to 82%[18–23] have a 22q11.2 deletion (most commonly Tbx1 haploinsufficiency) in which abnormal neural crest development and migration lead to an impaired epithelial remodeling of the fourth pharyngeal arch and derivatives of the third and fourth pharyngeal pouches. This condition accounts for the variably associated concomitant cardiovascular (eg, other conotruncal CHD lesions) and noncardiovascular phenotype expression (eg, DiGeorge syndrome, Velo-Cardio-Facial syndrome, conotruncal anomaly face syndrome).[24,25] IAA is also associated with CHARGE syndrome, in which CHD7 gene mutation (8q12.1 chromosome) contributes to abnormal neural crest and fourth PAA epithelial morphogenesis.[24,25]

Affected patients usually present clinically within the first few days of life and typically not more than 2 weeks of age. As with other critical LSOLs, the neonate with IAA may appear normal at birth and with no clinical cyanosis. However, as the ductus closes, systemic blood flow decreases and pulmonary venous pressure rises; congestive heart failure, respiratory distress, systemic hypoperfusion, pallor, and decreased organ function may ensue. Prompt hemodynamic stabilization, diagnosis, and surgical revision are mandatory for survival. Radiographically, IAA (and other LSOLs) shows pulmonary venous congestion, with the heart size ranging from normal to markedly increased. If a septal defect is present with left to right shunting, there may be a component of increased pulmonary vascularity. A narrow mediastinum in these patients indicates thymic aplasia (eg, DiGeorge syndrome). Echocardiography can usually define IAA with reliable accuracy. MR imaging-MR angiography or CTA may be indicated to further define the level of interruption, aortic branch arteries, and/or associated anomalies, which is key information for preoperative planning.

Coarctation of the aorta

Coarctation of the thoracic aorta is defined as a focal, eccentric, obstructive narrowing involving the aortic isthmus (**Fig. 4**). It accounts for 1.8% to 9.8% of CHD, with most studies showing an incidence of 5% to 6%.[8,26–29] COA has a slight male predominance (1.2–2.3:1).[30–37] Most cases occur sporadically, but both environmental factors and genetic causes may contribute. COA is characterized as preductal, juxtaductal, or postductal, based on its anatomic relationship to the ductus arteriosus. Preductal COA predominates in children less than 1 year of age, whereas the postductal type is more common in children greater than 1 year and in adults.

The narrowing in COA results from abnormal fibromuscular ductal tissue encircling the aorta. The ductal theory hypothesizes that, as the LSCA migrates cephalad through differential growth of the dorsal aorta, the ductal ostium from the sixth arch is pulled into the aorta, forming the circumferential sling. Obstruction at the isthmus develops when there is postnatal constriction of the ductus arteriosus. The hemodynamic theory facilitates a greater understanding of the pathogenesis and lends an explanation to the occurrence of COA with associated cardiovascular lesions. Congenital lesions with decreased antegrade flow in the ascending aorta (eg, LSOLs, left to right shunts), result in reversal of blood flow across the fetal isthmus, altering the branch point angulation, and accentuating LSCA cephalad migration, increasing the possibility for developing COA. In contrast, right-sided obstructive cardiac lesions (eg, right ventricular outflow tract obstruction, pulmonary stenosis, and pulmonary atresia) protect against coarctation, because there is dominant antegrade isthmus flow.[4–6,38–40]

The primary physiologic sequelae of coarctation is increased left ventricular afterload and decreased systemic perfusion with activation of the

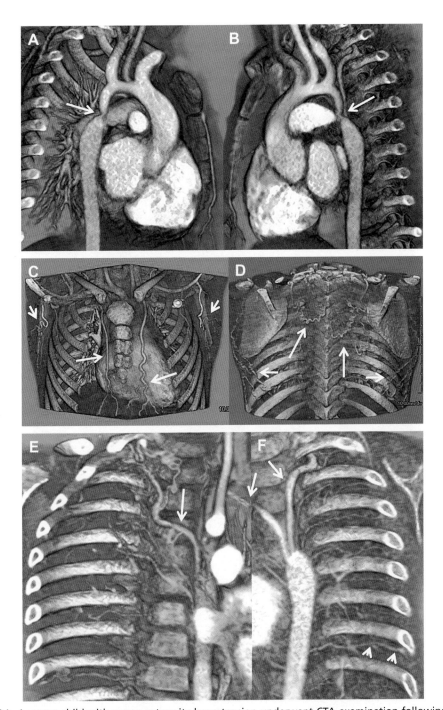

Fig. 4. COA. A young child with upper extremity hypertension underwent CTA examination following echocardiographic diagnosis of COA. (*A, B*) 3D volume rendered images show severe narrowing involving the isthmic portion of the aorta (*arrow*). (*C, D*) 3D volume rendered images show well-developed collateral pathways, including internal mammary (*C, long arrows*), thoracodorsal (*C, short arrows*), superficial paraspinal (*D, long arrows*), and parascapular (*D, short arrows*) pathways. (*E, F*) 3D volume rendered images show intercostal (*arrowhead*) and mediastinal paraspinal (*arrows*) collateral arteries.

sympathetic and renin-angiotensin systems, resulting in increased blood pressure. In neonates and infants with COA (similar to IAA), systemic perfusion is dependent on maintaining patency of

the ductus arteriosus. Prostaglandins are initiated early in the clinical course to maintain this patency. Once the ductus closes, the inability to rapidly develop collateral blood flow and counter the rising afterload may lead to left heart dysfunction with chamber enlargement and congestive heart failure. Pulmonary hypertension (with right heart dysfunction), renal insufficiency, and systemic shock may also develop. With isolated COA, when sufficient compensatory collateral flow develops to supply blood distal to the obstruction, clinical presentation is delayed until later in life. Primary collateral pathways include the subclavian, internal mammary, intercostal, cervical, scapular, and thoracodorsal arteries (see **Fig. 4**). The presence of collateral arteries and a pressure gradient are the distinguishing features between coarctation and pseudocoarctation (**Fig. 5**). In cases of pseudocoarctation, there is absence of a pressure gradient and collateral arteries.

Associated congenital cardiovascular abnormalities may occur in 44% to 84% of patients with COA; most of these patients present by 2 years of age.[30,32,41] Commonly associated abnormalities include PDA, bicuspid aortic valve, left to right shunts (eg, ASD, VSD), LSOLs, and TGA. Syndromes and genetic disorders associated with COA include Shone complex, PHACE syndrome, Williams syndrome, Noonan syndrome, Turner syndrome (45 XO karyotype), trisomy 13, and trisomy 18.

Early diagnosis and intervention are essential to minimizing morbidity and mortality in pediatric patients with COA. Untreated COA in neonates and infants has a poor prognosis (50% mortality) without urgent surgical intervention.[42] Milder forms of COA may take years or decades to become symptomatic. However, the long-term effects of systemic hypertension from aortic coarctation may lead to late cardiovascular complications, reducing life expectancy compared with the general population. Chronically increased blood

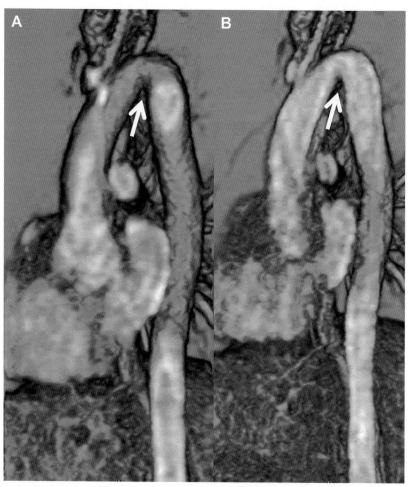

Fig. 5. Pseudocoarctation. A neonate underwent contrast-enhanced MR angiography for evaluation of underlying complex congenital heart disease. (*A, B*) 3D volume rendered images show pseudocoarctation (*arrow*) of the aortic arch, with uplifting of the aortic arch and kinking at the isthmus. Note the absence of collateral arteries.

pressure results in left ventricular hypertrophy with congestive heart failure in early to midadulthood. The increased blood pressure can lead to an increased incidence of premature coronary artery disease, ischemic heart disease, cerebral vascular accidents (eg, ischemia, hemorrhage), aortic valvular disease (eg, stenosis or insufficiency related to a bicuspid aortic valve), aortic root dilatation, aortic aneurysms (eg, proximal to a coarctation), acute aortic disease (eg, dissection, rupture), and bacterial endocarditis.

Definitive management of COA requires surgical (eg, resection with interposition graft) or endovascular (eg, angioplasty with stent placement) repair. Age at the time of coarctation repair has a predictive value for operative mortality (2%–41%, highest in infants <1 year old),[30,32,41–46] recoarctation (4%–26%, highest in infants <1 year old),[30,32,41,44–47] and residual hypertension (12.5%–21%, lowest when operated between 1 and 5 years old).[32,33,44,47] To optimize surgical outcome and minimize potential future cardiovascular risk, elective repair is recommended in early childhood (1–5 years of age) and should not be delayed past 10 years of age. Hypertension at the first postoperative evaluation and the development of postoperative paradoxic hypertension are risk factors for chronic hypertension (residual or recurrent) and acquired cardiovascular disease. Patients should be followed closely after repair for possible recurrent coarctation, progression of associated cardiac defects, and development of acquired cardiovascular disease.[33,48,49]

Chest radiography has a low to moderate sensitivity for detection of COA, dependent on the age of the patient, the degree of narrowing, and the presence of associated cardiac defects. In the neonate and infant, the heart is typically enlarged and pulmonary venous congestion is present. In the older child to young adult with isolated COA, typical imaging findings include a prominent aortic arch and proximal descending aorta silhouette with a figure-of-3 contour, inferior rib scalloping and/or sclerosis, and a normal or mildly enlarged heart size. Confirmatory diagnosis of COA in neonates and infants is most often made with TTE, which has a sensitivity of 94% to 98%[50,51] and a positive predictive value as high as 98% and 100% for neonates and infant, respectively.[51] In older children to young adults, CEMRA (sensitivity 98%, specificity 99%) is superior to TTE for depicting COA and the complete thoracic arterial system.[52] PC-MR imaging is applied to measure the gradient across the obstructive narrowing and quantify collateral flow. MDCT angiography is a highly sensitive imaging modality with an accuracy as high as 100%.[53] As with MRA, collateral pathways should be described in detail because their number and extent directly correlate with the severity of disease.

Aortic Arch Anomalies

Aortic arch anomalies (AAA) are congenital vascular abnormalities involving development of the primitive aortic arches and their derivatives, accounting for 0.5% to 1.6% of CHD lesions.[28,54] Men have a slightly greater prevalence than women (1.2:1).[55–63] Four percent of patients with these anomalies may have 22q11.2 deletion, whereas 35% of those with 22q11.2 deletion may have an isolated aortic arch anomaly.[63,64] Common AAA in pediatric patients include vascular rings, pulmonary artery slings (PAS), and innominate artery compression (IAC). The most common symptomatic AAA are a double aortic arch (49%, range 36%–72%) and right aortic arch with a left ligamentum/ductus arteriosum (28%, range 8%–49%), followed by IAC (10%, range 3.3%–27%), left aortic arch with an aberrant right subclavian artery (8%, range 1.7%–20%), and pulmonary sling (5%, range 1.8%–12.5%).[55–61,63,65,66] Associated CHD lesions occur in 18% (range 12%–32%) of patients with AAA,[55,57,59–62,65] including VSD, ASD, PDA, right-sided obstructive lesions, and COA.

The unifying characteristic of these disorders is secondary vascular compression on the central airway, the esophagus, or both. Depending on the type of lesion, severity of compression, and the presence of comorbid cardiovascular and noncardiovascular congenital disease, affected patients present with variable degrees of respiratory and gastrointestinal symptoms during the neonatal period, infancy, childhood, or young adulthood. Respiratory symptoms are more prevalent among infants and young children, whereas esophageal symptoms are more common among older children, adolescents, and adults. In addition to extrinsic compression of the central airway, concomitant intrinsic tracheomalacia may occur in up to 53% of pediatric patients with AAA, affecting the presentation and clinical management of respiratory symptoms.[1]

Vascular rings

A vascular ring occurs when the trachea and/or esophagus are surrounded and compressed by vessels (eg, aortic arch or arches, aortic arch branch arteries, pulmonary branch arteries) and the ductus or ligamentum arteriosum. A vascular ring may be complete or incomplete. Vascular rings result from abnormal persistence and involution of primitive brachial arch segments, most commonly the third, fourth, and sixth arches. They may occur with a normal left-sided arch, a double aortic arch (DAA), a right-sided aortic arch (RAA), and a cervical aortic arch (CAA). Classification of vascular rings is based on Edwards'[67] hypothetical embryologic double aortic arch model.

Left aortic arch The normal LAA, left-sided descending aorta, and left-sided ligamentum arteriosum are formed by regression of the right and persistence of the left fourth arches, eighth dorsal aorta segments, and sixth dorsal arches, respectively. Two main anomalous patterns may occur. The first is an aberrant right subclavian artery (Fig. 6), which results when right fourth arch regression occurs between the right common carotid and right subclavian arteries, rather than distal to the right subclavian artery. The aorta gives rise to the right common carotid, the left common carotid, the left subclavian, and the right subclavian arteries. The right subclavian artery courses retroesophageal. Two subdivisions are possible, namely a left-sided or right-sided ligamentum arteriosum. If there is a left-sided ligament, no vascular ring occurs; the aberrant right subclavian artery has smooth caliber throughout its course. However, a rare right-sided ligament completes a true vascular ring; it forms by persistence of the right dorsal sixth arch and passes from the right pulmonary artery (RPA) to the descending aorta, via the proximal right subclavian artery, potentially leading to fusiform dilatation of the retroesophageal aberrant segment (eg, diverticulum of Kommerell). Beyond the diverticulum, the subclavian artery is normal in caliber.

The second anomalous pattern with a LAA is a circumflex right descending aorta. With this entity, distal aortic arch and proximal descending aorta course posterior to the esophagus and trachea. It may occur with normal arch branching or an aberrant right subclavian artery.

The vascular ring is completed by the ligament passing between the RPA and the descending aorta after the retroesophageal segment.

Double aortic arch A double aortic arch (Fig. 7) results from persistence of both the right and left fourth arches and the dorsal aorta, forming a complete vascular ring. Right dominance occurs in 66% (range 37%–81%), left dominance in 16% (range 10%–20%), and codominance in 17% (range 3%–53%).[55,60–63,66] The left arch may be atretic with a fibrous segment distal to the take-off of 1 or both of the left arch branch arteries. Rarely, the right arch may be atretic. The right arch typically supplies the right common carotid and brachiocephalic arteries, whereas the left supplies the left common carotid and brachiocephalic arteries. The descending aorta is often on the left but the proximal descending aorta can be on the right or midline. The ligament is usually left sided. Less commonly, it can be right sided or bilateral. Pulmonary arteries are typically normal.

Right aortic arch A right aortic arch occurs from persistence of the right, and regression of the left, fourth arches and eighth dorsal aorta segments, respectively. A vascular ring may occur depending on the level of the left fourth arch resorption, the origins and course of the ligamentum arteriosum and the descending aorta, or a combination thereof. Three possible patterns of a RAA may occur. The first is an aberrant LSCA/ brachiocephalic artery. In this case, left fourth arch regression occurs between the left carotid

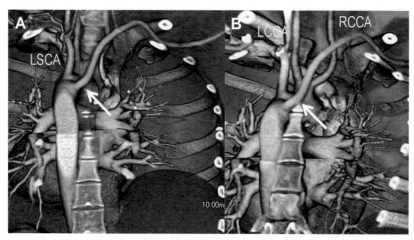

Fig. 6. Left aortic arch with an aberrant right subclavian artery. A young child underwent CTA for suspected pulmonary embolism. (A, B) 3D volume rendered images show a left aortic arch with an aberrant right subclavian artery (RSCA; arrow). The RSCA arises from the aorta as the fourth aortic branch artery, after the right common carotid artery (RCCA), LCCA, and LSCA.

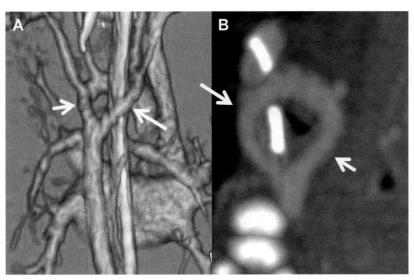

Fig. 7. Double aortic arch. A neonate with respiratory distress underwent CTA for evaluation of a vascular ring. (*A, B*) 3D volume rendered (*A*) and MIP (*B*) images show the typical vascular morphology of a double aortic arch (*arrows*) with a left descending aorta. In this instance, the right (*long arrow*) and left (*short arrow*) arches have relative codominance, forming a complete ring. (*From* Hellinger JC, Pena A, Poon M, et al. Pediatric computed tomographic angiography: imaging the cardiovascular system gently. Radiol Clin North Am 2010;48:462; with permission.)

and subclavian arteries. The aorta gives rise to the left common carotid, the right common carotid, the right subclavian, and the left subclavian arteries; the LSCA courses retroesophageal (Fig. 8). Regression before the LCCA results in an anomalous left brachiocephalic artery. The right carotid artery becomes the first branch followed by the right subclavian artery and the left brachiocephalic artery. The left brachiocephalic artery courses retroesophageal with subsequent branching into the left common carotid and subclavian arteries. In both types, when the ligament is right sided, no vascular ring is present. The left subclavian or brachiocephalic artery has a regular caliber throughout its course. When the ligament is left sided, a complete vascular ring is present; the ligament courses between the LPA and the proximal descending aorta, via the aberrant LSCA or brachiocephalic artery (Fig. 9). The retroesophageal segment of the left subclavian or brachiocephalic artery is dilated with a diverticulum of Kommerell in 15% to 21% of cases.[60,62]

The second pattern with a RAA is mirror image branching. In this condition, left fourth arch regression occurs distal to the LSCA and the aorta gives rise to the left brachiocephalic, the right common carotid, and the right subclavian arteries. In most instances, no vascular ring is present because the descending aorta and ductus/ligamentum arteriosum are ipsilateral. The right ligament passes between the right descending aorta and the RPA.

Less commonly, the ductus is contralateral. In this instance, the ligamentum usually passes between the brachiocephalic artery and the LPA without formation of a vascular ring. Rarely, however, the ligamentum arises from the proximal descending aorta and takes a retroesophageal course to the LPA, creating a vascular ring. Although the ligament may not be visualized, a small leftward-facing dimple may be present on the proximal descending aorta, at the take-off of the ligament, indicating the anomalous ligament.

The third pattern with a RAA is circumflex left descending aorta. With this entity, the descending aorta courses posterior to the esophagus and then descends on the left side, analogous to a left aortic arch with a right descending aorta. A circumflex left descending aorta can occur with an anomalous LSCA, an anomalous left brachiocephalic artery, and mirror image branching. A vascular ring is completed by a left ligamentum arteriosum coursing between the descending aorta and the LPA.

Cervical aortic arch A CAA occurs when the aortic arch is positioned above the thoracic inlet. This condition results when the third arch is the basis for aortic arch development, rather than the fourth. CAA may occur with both right and left third arches, leading to the potential formation of left-sided, right-sided, and double AAA. Most commonly, it occurs on the right side with a persistent right third aortic arch and right dorsal aorta.[68]

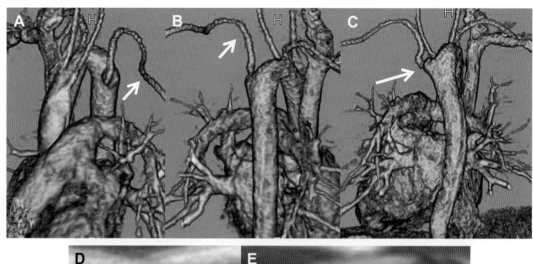

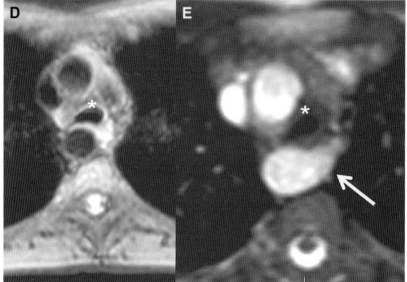

Fig. 8. Right aortic arch with an aberrant LSCA. A young child with recurrent aspiration and respiratory distress underwent MR angiography for evaluation of a vascular ring. (*A–C*) 3D volume rendered images show a right aortic arch with an aberrant LSCA (*short arrow*), a diverticulum of Kommerell (*long arrow*), and a left ligamentus arteriosum resulting in a complete vascular ring. (*D, E*) Transverse dark blood images show an approximate 50% tracheal compression (*asterisk*) by the retroesophageal LSCA (*arrow*).

Pulmonary artery sling

PAS is a condition in which the LPA typically arises from the RPA and courses between the trachea and esophagus toward the left lung (**Fig. 10**). PAS develops as a result of proximal left sixth arch involution. Although right and left ligaments are possible, only a left ligament leads to a complete vascular ring. In this instance, the left ligament connects between the main or RPA and the left descending aorta. PAS is often associated with concomitant central airway anomalies and acquired abnormalities, including tracheal rings, right upper lobe tracheal bronchus,

and tracheomalacia. Relief of symptoms requires transposing the LPA and correction of potential central airway anomalies or acquired abnormalities.

Innominate artery compression

IAC on the trachea occurs when the anterior crossing innominate artery extrinsically compresses the upper to midanterior trachea, often in an oblique manner (see **Fig. 1**). Although IAC does not constitute a traditional vascular ring, it can cause significant respiratory symptoms, particularly in infants and young children, as discussed

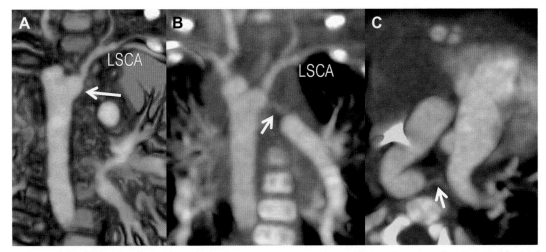

Fig. 9. Right aortic arch with an aberrant LSCA. A young child with respiratory distress underwent CTA for evaluation of a vascular ring. (A–C) 3D volume rendered (A) and MIP (B, C) images show a right aortic arch with an aberrant LSCA and a diverticulum of Kommerell (A, long arrow). A left ductus arteriosum (B, C; arrow) is patent, directly confirming the presence of a complete vascular ring.

in an article by Lee and colleagues elsewhere in this issue. IAC often results when there is accentuated horizontal angulation of the ascending aorta and compensatory angulation of the aortic arch and branch arteries. MRI-MRA or CTA can directly depict the innominate artery caliber and course as well as the degree of tracheal narrowing, which may vary from a shallow asymmetric indentation to marked anterior-posterior compression of greater than 50%. IAC has a high association with intrinsic tracheomalacia, which should be considered when choosing the imaging modality, selecting the MRI-MRA or CTA protocol, and interpreting the examination.[1]

Pulmonary Arterial Anomalies

In addition to PAS, congenital pulmonary arterial anomalies include hypoplasia, agenesis (**Fig. 11**), and stenosis. These anomalies most often occur in association with complex conotruncal congenital heart lesions, such as pulmonary valve stenosis, pulmonary valve atresia, tetralogy of Fallot, and TGA.[69] Isolated pulmonary arterial hypoplasia and agenesis, in the absence of complex CHD, are often associated with pulmonary hypoplasia and hypogenetic lung syndrome (**Fig. 12**). Isolated pulmonary arterial stenosis (PASt) is rare. Such stenoses most commonly involve the central main and branch pulmonary arteries, but

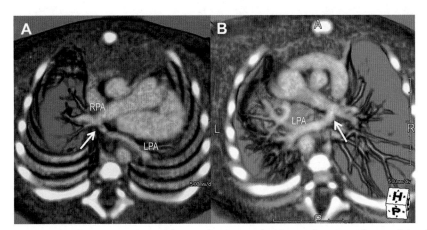

Fig. 10. Pulmonary artery sling. A neonate with complex congenital heart disease and unexplained respiratory distress who underwent CTA for evaluation of a vascular ring. (A, B) 3D volume rendered images show the LPA (arrow) arising from the RPA.

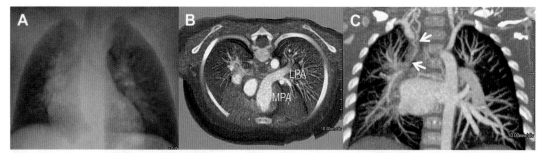

Fig. 11. Pulmonary artery agenesis. A neonate with mild respiratory distress underwent CTA following an abnormal chest radiograph. (*A*) Frontal chest radiograph shows dextroposition of the heart and mild right lung oligemia with asymmetric left greater than right pulmonary vascularity. (*B*) 3D volume rendered image shows RPA agenesis. Pulmonary blood flow (PBF) is thus from the main pulmonary artery (MPA) to the LPA. (*C*) Coronal MIP image shows right pulmonary arterial reconstitution at the lobar level from systemic to pulmonary collateral arteries (*arrows*).

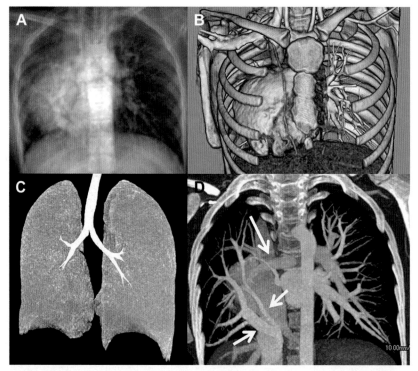

Fig. 12. Hypogenetic lung syndrome with partial pulmonary venous return to the IVC (scimitar syndrome). An adolescent with respiratory exercise intolerance underwent MDCT angiography. (*A*) Frontal chest radiograph shows increased left pulmonary vascularity and an enlarged heart with either dextrocardia or dextroposition of the heart. (*B*) 3D volume rendered image confirms dextroposition of the heart. (*C*) Coronal inverse MinIP image shows hypoplasia of the right lung with absence of the right upper lobe bronchus. (*D*) Coronal MIP image shows hypoplasia of the RPA (*long arrow*) and partial anomalous pulmonary venous return of most of the right lung into the IVC via 2 venous channels (*short arrows*). (*E*) Oblique thin-slab MIP image shows the hypoplastic RPA with compensatory LPA enlargement related to dominant PBF. (*F, G*) Cardiac 4-chamber (*F*) and short-axis (*G*) multiplanar reformations show an enlarged right atrium (RA) and right ventricle (RV) related to the right heart volume overload. LA, left atrium; LV, left ventricle. (*H, I*) 3D volume rendered images show the anomalous right lung venous drainage (*short arrows*) into the IVC. A small native right middle lobe vein (*long arrow*) drains directly into the LA.

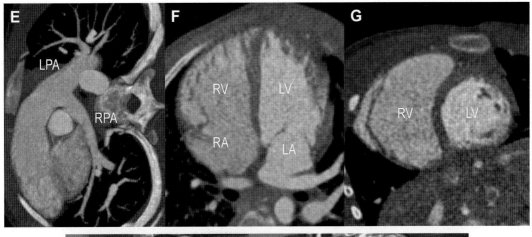

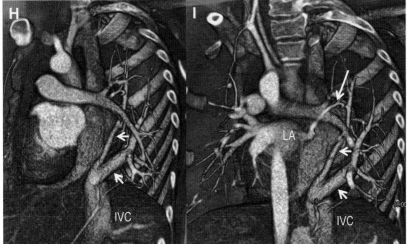

Fig. 12. (*continued*)

may occur in peripheral segments (eg, lobar and segmental divisions). Lesions may be diffuse with long segments of disease, resembling hypoplasia, or may be focal or multifocal with poststenotic dilatation. Possible underlying causes for PASt include congenital rubella, Williams syndrome, Noonan syndrome, Alagile syndrome, Ehlers-Danlos syndrome, and cutis laxa. The common pathologic finding is abnormal development of the elastic tissue of the media and increased collagen and fibrous tissue. Secondary intimal proliferation occurs with the risk of localized thrombosis. Progressive and long-standing PASt increases right ventricular afterload (pressure), leading to right ventricular hypertrophy, strain on the tricuspid valvular apparatus, and potentially tricuspid insufficiency and right heart failure.

VENOUS SYSTEMS
Systemic Venous Anomalies

Normal thoracic systemic venous anatomy consists of bilateral subclavian (SCV) and brachiocephalic (BCV) veins, draining to the right superior vena cava (RSVC) and then into the sinus venosus portion of the right atrium. Embryologically, these veins develop from the paired anterior cardinal and common cardinal veins. A communicating vein forms from the superior transverse capillary plexuses and directs blood from the left to right anterior cardinal vein. The entire right anterior cardinal vein normally persists, forming the right SCV (RSCV) and right BCV (RBCV) as well as the right internal jugular vein. The right SVC (RSVC) develops from the right anterior cardinal and common cardinal veins, which enter the sinus venosus. In distinction, the left anterior cardinal vein undergoes near complete atrophy below the level of the communicating vein, forming the ligament of the left vena cava. A residual central venous segment forms the left superior intercostal vein, which drains the second and third intercostal spaces. The remainder of left anterior cardinal vein persists to form the left SCV and internal jugular vein. The communicating vein becomes the left BCV (LBCV) and enlarges to accommodate increased left to right flow. The LBCV courses obliquely downward superior to the aortic arch and anterior to the supra-aortic branch arteries, joining with the RBCV to form the RSVC. The left common cardinal vein is incorporated into the coronary venous anatomy, becoming the oblique vein of the left atrium (vein of Marshall), draining into the coronary sinus of the right atrium.[3]

Anomalies of these systemic veins are rare. Systemic venous anomalies may occur in isolation or may be associated with cardiac disease, in particular CHD and arrhythmias. Three of the more common systemic venous anomalies are (1) a persistent left SVC (LSVC) with a native RSVC; (2) a LSVC with mirror image venous drainage (**Fig. 13**); and (3) a retroaortic left BCV (RA-LBCV, **Fig. 14**). Clear understanding of these systemic venous anomalies can facilitate planning and placement of central venous catheters, hemodynamic monitoring devices, and cardiac pacemaker and cardioverter-defibrillator leads, as well as assessment of their respective positioning on chest radiographs following placement. Recognition of a LSVC on echocardiography, MRI-MRA, or CTA is important for cardiac preoperative planning and surgical management, including cardiopulmonary bypass and procedures for CHD (eg, cavopulmonary shunts).

Persistent left superior vena cava

A persistent left superior vena cava (LSVC) has a prevalence of 0.1% to 0.5% in the general population.[70,71] It occurs more frequently in patients with CHD, with a reported prevalence of 1.3% to 5%.[72–74] Commonly associated CHD anomalies include septal defects (ventricular, atrial, and atrioventricular), tetralogy of Fallot, pulmonary atresia, bicuspid aortic valve, AS, aortic coarctation, PDA, and anomalous pulmonary venous return.[72,74] Extracardiac congenital anomalies may be found in 60% of pediatric patients with a persistent LSVC. Commonly associated disorders include VACTERL (vertebral anomalies, anal atresia, cardiovascular anomalies, tracheoesophageal fistula, esophageal atresia, renal (kidney) and/or radial anomalies, limb defects), trisomy 21, 22q11 deletion, CHARGE (coloboma of the eye, central nervous system anomalies, heart defects, atresia of the choanae, retardation of growth and/or development, genital and/or urinary defects, ear anomalies and/or deafness) syndrome, and Turner syndrome.[74] Embryologically, a persistent LSVC results from persistence of the left anterior cardinal vein. Concurrent persistence of the right anterior and common cardinal veins yields bilateral SVCs with or without a communicating brachiocephalic vein (ie, bridging vein).

Left superior vena cava with mirror image venous drainage

Involution of the right common cardinal vein and the central anterior cardinal vein, along with

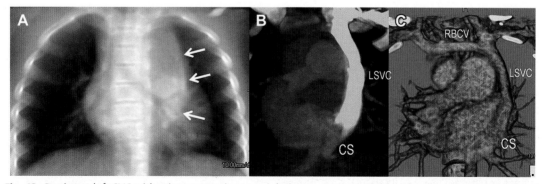

Fig. 13. Persistent left SVC with mirror systemic venous drainage. A young child with a known ASD underwent MDCT angiography after abnormal chest radiograph. (*A*) Frontal chest radiograph shows a prominent left paramediastinal shadow (*arrows*). (*B*) Coronal MIP from a direct CT venogram (CTV) shows a persistent LSVC draining into the coronary sinus (CS). (*C*) Coronal 3D volume rendered image obtained during the delayed CTV phase shows mirror image systemic venous drainage with a right brachiocephalic vein (RBCV) draining to the LSVC. The LSVC is again noted to drain to the CS.

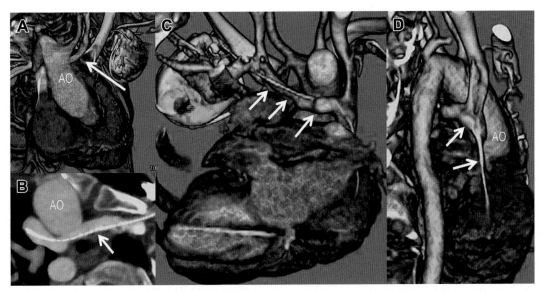

Fig. 14. Retroaortic left brachiocephalic vein. CTA was performed in a young adolescent who previously underwent tetralogy of Fallot surgical repair. (*A–D*) 3D volume rendered images (*A, C, D*) and MIP image (*B*) illustrate the course of a retroaortic left brachiocephalic vein (LBCV, *arrows*) that contains a traversing central venous catheter. The LBCV courses under the aortic arch, anterior to the central pulmonary arteries and then posterior to the ascending aorta (AO) to join the right SVC.

persistence of the communicating vein and the left anterior cardinal vein, results in mirror image thoracic systemic venous drainage (ie, right BCV and an LSVC). In most instances, the LSVC drains into the coronary sinus and the coronary sinus enlarges to accommodate flow.[74] Coronary sinus dilatation may potentially lead to left atrioventricular valve inflow obstruction, which in turn may lead to cardiac arrhythmias and/or sudden death. In addition, abnormal cardiac impulse formation and conduction may arise from abnormal morphologic development of the sinoatrial node, atrioventricular node, and bundle of His (eg, lengthening).[70] Rarely, the LSVC drains into the left atrium (ie, complete unroofing of the coronary sinus), leading to interatrial communication, right to left shunting, and cyanosis.[74]

Retroaortic left brachiocephalic vein

The retroaortic LBCV is found in 0.5% to 0.6% of patients with CHD[75,76] and in only 0.02% of patients who do not have CHD.[76] It courses posterior to the ascending aorta, underneath the aortic arch, and anterior to the central main and right pulmonary arteries, to join the RSVC at or below the ostial confluence of the azygous vein. Although it results in neither physiologic nor hemodynamic sequelae, a retroaortic left brachiocephalic vein is associated with congenital heart disease, including right side obstructive lesions (tetralogy

of Fallot, pulmonary atresia), truncus arteriosus, and AAA (eg, IAA, RAA, CAA). Embryologically, it occurs when the developing communicating vein anastomoses with the right inferior transverse capillary plexus.[75]

Pulmonary Venous Anomalies

The lung buds, developing from the foregut, initially drain via a venous plexus into the cardinal venous system.[3] A common pulmonary vein (CPV) arises from the dorsum of the left atrium and anastomoses with the venous plexus. Connections to the cardinal venous system involute with subsequent direct pulmonary venous drainage into the left atrium. CPV absorption into the wall of the left atrium results in variable pulmonary vein ostia and branching patterns, with a standard of single, bilateral superior and inferior pulmonary vein trunks.

Abnormal development of the CPV (eg, incomplete resorption) and its anastomosis with the primitive venous plexus, along with persistent connections to the systemic cardinal veins, give rise to partial anomalous pulmonary venous return (PAPVR) or total anomalous pulmonary venous return (TAPVR; 0.7%–3.2% of CHD).[8,26–28] Both PAPVR and TAPVR result in a left to right shunt with partial (PAPVR) or complete (TAPVR) admixture of deoxygenated and oxygenated blood. PAPVR and TAPVR may be associated with other congenital heart diseases, including heterotaxy; atrial, ventricular, and atrioventricular septal defects; tetralogy of Fallot; and COA.[77] Anomalous pulmonary venous return should be distinguished from pulmonary veins, which have anomalous peripheral connections and/or an aberrant course (eg, aberrant meandering vein) within the lungs, before normal drainage into the left atrium.[78] In most instances, echocardiography with gray scale and Doppler interrogation depicts the number, location, and course of pulmonary veins; detects the direction of venous blood flow; and excludes flow obstruction. MRI-MRA or CTA may be required when echocardiography cannot identify all veins or when more comprehensive evaluation is required following the diagnosis of PAPVR or TAPVR. MR imaging offers the advantage of quantifying the shunt ratio (eg, Qp/Qs) using phase contrast imaging. CTA is advantageous for its superior visualization of the central airway and lung in the evaluation of associated pulmonary developmental anomalies.

Partial anomalous pulmonary venous return

In PAPVR, 1 or more (but not all) of the pulmonary veins (segmental, lobar, or main central trunk) drain directly into systemic veins (eg, SVC, inferior vena cava [IVC], SCV, BCV, azygous vein), right atrium, or coronary sinus. Hemodynamic sequelae reflect the degree (eg, number and size of anomalous veins) and duration of shunting. When the shunt is significant, flow across the right heart and pulmonary circulation is increased (eg, increased pulmonary blood flow [PBF]). The right cardiac chambers and pulmonary vasculature (arteries and veins) are enlarged because of volume overload. Pulmonary hypertension and right heart failure may subsequently develop. Increased left atrial pressure may lead to pulmonary venous congestion; initially acyanotic, patients may become cyanotic. The right pulmonary veins are anomalous twice as often as the left. Right upper lobe venous drainage into the SVC is the most common type of PAPVR (**Fig. 15**) and may be associated with a sinus venosus defect (**Fig. 16**). The second most frequent type of PAPVR is left pulmonary venous drainage to the LBCV. The third most common form is anomalous drainage from the right lung to the IVC with an intact atrial septum. This condition may be associated with more complex pulmonary developmental anomalies in the spectrum of congenital pulmonary venolobar syndrome, including bronchopulmonary sequestration (BPS), scimitar syndrome (see **Fig. 12**), and horseshoe lung. Most associated BPS are extralobar with venous drainage into azygous or hemiazygous veins. In scimitar syndrome, also known as hypogenetic lung syndrome, an anomalous CPV (scimitar vein) drains a portion or the entire lung into the IVC either above or below the diaphragm. Alternatively, drainage may occur into hepatic veins, portal veins, azygous vein, coronary sinus, or right atrium. The right lung is almost exclusively involved and has variable hypoplasia versus partial agenesis, associated with dextroposition of the heart and ipsilateral decreased pulmonary perfusion relative to the left. Additional associated anomalies include bronchogenic cyst, BPS, horseshoe lung, accessory diaphragm, and congenital diaphragmatic hernia. Pulmonary arteries to the affected lung may have variable hypoplasia or agenesis, with or without systemic arterial supply in the absence of an associated sequestration.

Total anomalous pulmonary venous return

In TAPVR, all pulmonary veins have anomalous drainage. Affected patients typically present in the neonatal period. An obligatory ASD or patent foramen ovale is often present, leading to a right to left shunt and cyanosis. Veins may drain via a common vein into systemic veins or the right atrium (via the coronary sinus). Alternatively, veins may first drain into a venous confluence and then to a common draining vein. Depending on the level of anomalous connections, TAPVR drainage may be categorized as supracardiac (type I, **Fig. 17**), intracardiac (type II), infracardiac (type III), or mixed (**Figs. 18** and **19**). In the common form of type I TAPVR, the pulmonary veins are most commonly drained by a left ascending vertical vein to the LBCV and then the SVC, resulting in increased PBF, cardiomegaly, and a wide mediastinum radiographically. Other sites of supracardiac systemic connection are the SVC (right or left, see **Fig. 17**) and azygous vein. In type 2 TAPVR, the anomalous pulmonary veins drain into the coronary sinus (see **Fig. 18**B–D), leading to increased PBF, cardiomegaly, and a narrow mediastinum radiographically. Venous flow in types I and II TAPVR is unobstructed. Affected neonates often develop right heart volume overload, pulmonary hypertension, and right heart failure. In type 3 TAPVR (see **Fig. 19**B, C), anomalous veins drain via a descending vertical vein into the portal, hepatic, or mesenteric venous systems, with flow obstruction at or below the diaphragm, pulmonary venous congestion, a normal to small heart size, and a narrow mediastinum radiographically. This type constitutes a neonatal cardiopulmonary emergency because there is diminished cardiac output, poor systemic perfusion, and even greater cyanosis. The mixed type consists of combinations of types I to III TAPVR.

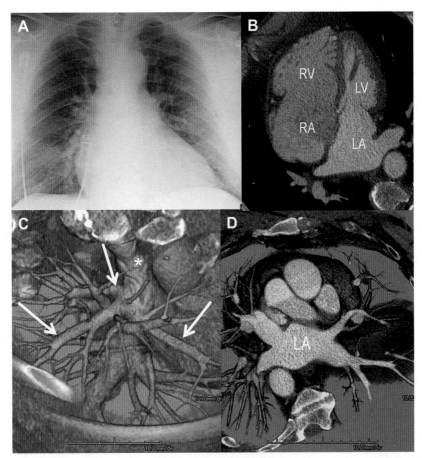

Fig. 15. Partial pulmonary venous return with intact atrial septum. An adolescent with exertional chest pressure and mild hypoxia underwent MDCT angiography. (A) Frontal chest radiograph shows moderate cardiomegaly with prominent central pulmonary vascularity. (B) Four-chamber multiplanar reformation shows an enlarged RA and RV with flattening of the interatrial and interventricular septae, related to the right heart volume overload. (C, D) 3D volume rendered images show right upper lobe segmental pulmonary veins (arrows) draining to the SVC (asterisk) with all other pulmonary veins draining into the LA.

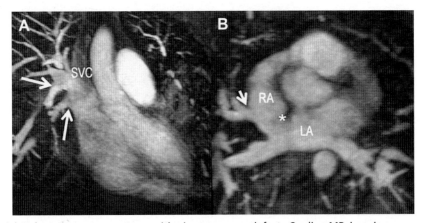

Fig. 16. Partial pulmonary venous return with sinus venosus defect. Cardiac MR imaging was performed in a young child with exertional shortness of breath and mild hypoxia. (A, B) Bright-blood MR angiography MIP images show right upper lobe anomalous pulmonary venous return into the SVC, above (arrows) or at the cavoatrial junction (arrowhead). A septal defect is present along the sinus venosus portion of the interatrial septum (asterisk), leading to communication between the RA and LA.

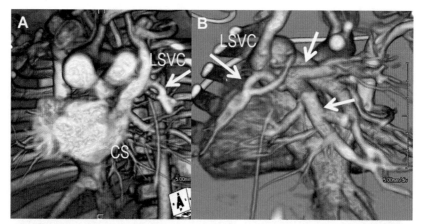

Fig. 17. TAPVR (Supracardiac Type I). A neonate with complex congenital heart disease underwent MDCT angiography. (*A, B*) 3D volume rendered images show bilateral anomalous drainage of all pulmonary veins (*arrows*) into a left SVC (LSVC). Blood then flows to the CS.

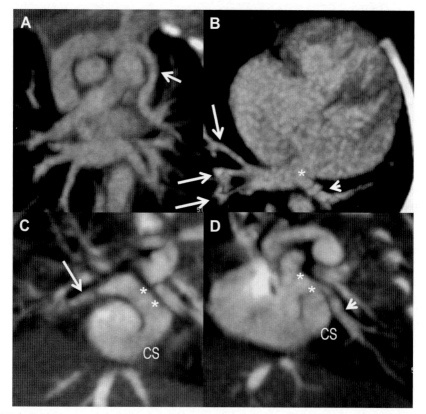

Fig. 18. TAPVR (mixed type I and II). A neonate with anomalous pulmonary veins diagnosed by echocardiography underwent low-dose MDCT angiography. (*A–D*) Variable thick, MIP images show that the left upper pulmonary veins drain into the LBCV (*A, short arrow*), whereas the left lower (*B, D; arrowheads*) and all right lung pulmonary veins (*B, C; long arrows*) drain to a retrocardiac confluence (*B, asterisk*). From the common confluence, blood drains (*C, D, asterisks*) into the CS.

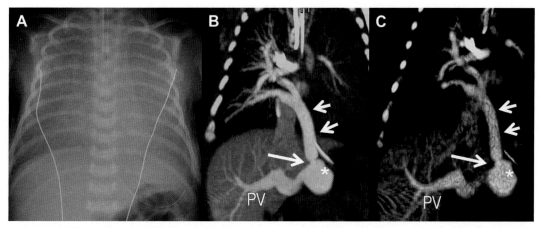

Fig. 19. TAPVR (mixed type I and III). A neonate in severe cardiopulmonary distress at 2 days of life underwent MDCT angiography. (*A*) Frontal chest radiograph shows moderate diffuse pulmonary venous congestion with a normal cardiac silhouette. (*B, C*) Coronal MIP (*B*) and 3D volume rendered (*C*) images show right pulmonary venous drainage via a common draining vein (*short arrows*). The common vein courses below the diaphragm and feeds into the confluence of the mesenteric and splenic veins (*asterisk*). Blood then drains into the portal venous (PV) system. Note the moderate obstructive stenosis (*long arrow*) in the common draining vein just above its distal outflow. Left pulmonary venous drainage was into the LBCV (not shown).

SUMMARY

Diagnostic imaging is crucial in the evaluation of thoracic congenital arterial and venous anomalies in pediatric patients. Although clinical assessment may provide insight into the possible diagnosis, imaging is usually necessary to confirm the diagnosis. Initial imaging algorithms using noninvasive modalities often begin with chest radiography followed by echocardiography. State-of-the-art MRI-MRA and MDCT angiography with advanced 3D visualization are essential in these algorithms not only for diagnosis but also treatment planning and postoperative and postendovascular evaluation. Selection between MRI-MRA and CTA should be based on their respective advantages, balanced by the suspected or known congenital vascular anomaly and patient's clinical presentation and hemodynamic stability. Understanding the embryologic basis and anatomic characteristics of thoracic congenital vascular anomalies assists in their recognition with MRI-MRA and MDCT angiography in pediatric patients.

REFERENCES

1. Lee EY, Zurakowski D, Waltz DA, et al. MDCT evaluation of the prevalence of tracheomalacia in children with mediastinal aortic vascular anomalies. J Thorac Imaging 2008;23:258–65.
2. Hellinger JC, Pena A, Poon M, et al. Pediatric computed tomographic angiography: imaging the cardiovascular system gently. Radiol Clin North Am 2010;48:439–67, x.
3. Moore KL. The cardiovascular system. In: The developing human: clinically oriented embryology. 8th edition. Philadelphia: WB Saunders; 2008. p. 286–337.
4. Rudolph AM, Heymann MA, Spitznas U. Hemodynamic considerations in the development of narrowing of the aorta. Am J Cardiol 1972;30:514–25.
5. Shinebourne EA, Elseed AM. Relation between fetal flow patterns, coarctation of the aorta, and pulmonary blood flow. Br Heart J 1974;36:492–8.
6. Rosenberg HS. Coarctation as a deformation. Pediatr Pathol 1990;10:103–15.
7. Collins-Nakai RL, Dick M, Parisi-Buckley L, et al. Interrupted aortic arch in infancy. J Pediatr 1976;88:959–62.
8. Samanek M, Voriskova M. Congenital heart disease among 815,569 children born between 1980 and 1990 and their 15-year survival: a prospective Bohemia survival study. Pediatr Cardiol 1999;20:411–7.
9. Schultz AH, Localio AR, Clark BJ, et al. Epidemiologic features of the presentation of critical congenital heart disease: implications for screening. Pediatrics 2008;121:751–7.
10. Norwood WI, Lang P, Castaneda AR, et al. Reparative operations for interrupted aortic arch with ventricular septal defect. J Thorac Cardiovasc Surg 1983;86:832–7.
11. Vouhe PR, Mace L, Vernant F, et al. Primary definitive repair of interrupted aortic arch with ventricular septal defect. Eur J Cardiothorac Surg 1990;4:365–70.

12. Jonas RA, Quaegebeur JM, Kirklin JW, et al. Outcomes in patients with interrupted aortic arch and ventricular septal defect. A multiinstitutional study. Congenital Heart Surgeons Society. J Thorac Cardiovasc Surg 1994;107:1099–109 [discussion: 1109–13].

13. Serraf A, Lacour-Gayet F, Robotin M, et al. Repair of interrupted aortic arch: a ten-year experience. J Thorac Cardiovasc Surg 1996;112:1150–60.

14. Tlaskal T, Hucin B, Hruda J, et al. Results of primary and two-stage repair of interrupted aortic arch. Eur J Cardiothorac Surg 1998;14:235–42.

15. Brown JW, Ruzmetov M, Okada Y, et al. Outcomes in patients with interrupted aortic arch and associated anomalies: a 20-year experience. Eur J Cardiothorac Surg 2006;29:666–73 [discussion: 673–4].

16. Flint JD, Gentles TL, MacCormick J, et al. Outcomes using predominantly single-stage approach to interrupted aortic arch and associated defects. Ann Thorac Surg 2010;89:564–9.

17. Van Mierop LH, Kutsche LM. Interruption of the aortic arch and coarctation of the aorta: pathogenetic relations. Am J Cardiol 1984;54:829–34.

18. Marino B, Digilio MC, Persiani M, et al. Deletion 22q11 in patients with interrupted aortic arch. Am J Cardiol 1999;84:360–1, A369.

19. Van Mierop LH, Kutsche LM. Cardiovascular anomalies in DiGeorge syndrome and importance of neural crest as a possible pathogenetic factor. Am J Cardiol 1986;58:133–7.

20. Lewin MB, Lindsay EA, Jurecic V, et al. A genetic etiology for interruption of the aortic arch type B. Am J Cardiol 1997;80:493–7.

21. Goldmuntz E, Clark BJ, Mitchell LE, et al. Frequency of 22q11 deletions in patients with conotruncal defects. J Am Coll Cardiol 1998;32:492–8.

22. Rauch A, Hofbeck M, Leipold G, et al. Incidence and significance of 22q11.2 hemizygosity in patients with interrupted aortic arch. Am J Med Genet 1998; 78:322–31.

23. Momma K, Ando M, Matsuoka R, et al. Interruption of the aortic arch associated with deletion of chromosome 22q11 is associated with a subarterial and doubly committed ventricular septal defect in Japanese patients. Cardiol Young 1999;9:463–7.

24. Randall V, McCue K, Roberts C, et al. Great vessel development requires biallelic expression of Chd7 and Tbx1 in pharyngeal ectoderm in mice. J Clin Invest 2009;119:3301–10.

25. Jyonouchi S, McDonald-McGinn DM, Bale S, et al. CHARGE (coloboma, heart defect, atresia choanae, retarded growth and development, genital hypoplasia, ear anomalies/deafness) syndrome and chromosome 22q11.2 deletion syndrome: a comparison of immunologic and nonimmunologic phenotypic features. Pediatrics 2009;123:e871–7.

26. Report of the New England Regional Infant Cardiac Program. Pediatrics 1980;65:375–461.

27. Goetzova J, Benesova D. Congenital heart diseases at autopsy of still-born and deceased children in the central Bohemian region. Cor Vasa 1981;23:8–13.

28. Samanek M, Slavik Z, Zborilova B, et al. Prevalence, treatment, and outcome of heart disease in live-born children: a prospective analysis of 91,823 live-born children. Pediatr Cardiol 1989;10:205–11.

29. Bolisetty S, Daftary A, Ewald D, et al. Congenital heart defects in central Australia. Med J Aust 2004;180: 614–7.

30. Tawes RL Jr, Aberdeen E, Waterston DJ, et al. Coarctation of the aorta in infants and children. A review of 333 operative cases, including 179 infants. Circulation 1969;39:I173–84.

31. Miettinen OS, Reiner ML, Nadas AS. Seasonal incidence of coarctation of the aorta. Br Heart J 1970; 32:103–7.

32. Cheatham JE Jr, Williams GR, Thompson WM, et al. Coarctation: a review of 80 children and adolescents. Am J Surg 1979;138:889–93.

33. Liberthson RR, Pennington DG, Jacobs ML, et al. Coarctation of the aorta: review of 234 patients and clarification of management problems. Am J Cardiol 1979;43:835–40.

34. Kish GF, Tenekjian VK, Tarnay TJ, et al. Coarctation of the thoracic aorta: an 18-year experience. Am Surg 1981;47:26–30.

35. Bobby JJ, Emami JM, Farmer RD, et al. Operative survival and 40 year follow up of surgical repair of aortic coarctation. Br Heart J 1991;65:271–6.

36. Ou P, Celermajer DS, Mousseaux E, et al. Vascular remodeling after "successful" repair of coarctation: impact of aortic arch geometry. J Am Coll Cardiol 2007;49:883–90.

37. Koller M, Rothlin M, Senning A. Coarctation of the aorta: review of 362 operated patients. Long-term follow-up and assessment of prognostic variables. Eur Heart J 1987;8:670–9.

38. Krediet P. An hypothesis of the development of coarctation in man. Acta Morphol Neerl Scand 1965; 6:207–12.

39. Hutchins GM. Coarctation of the aorta explained as a branch-point of the ductus arteriosus. Am J Pathol 1971;63:203–14.

40. Momma K, Takao A, Ando M. Angiocardiographic study of coarctation of the aorta–morphology and morphogenesis. Jpn Circ J 1982;46:174–83.

41. Kappetein AP, Zwinderman AH, Bogers AJ, et al. More than thirty-five years of coarctation repair. An unexpected high relapse rate. J Thorac Cardiovasc Surg 1994;107:87–95.

42. Glass IH, Mustard WT, Keith JD. Coarctation of the aorta in infants. A review of twelve years' experience. Pediatrics 1960;26:109–21.

43. Williams WG, Shindo G, Trusler GA, et al. Results of repair of coarctation of the aorta during infancy. J Thorac Cardiovasc Surg 1980;79:603–8.

44. Sorland SJ, Rostad H, Forfang K, et al. Coarctation of the aorta. A follow-up study after surgical treatment in infancy and childhood. Acta Paediatr Scand 1980;69:113–8.

45. Rostad H, Abdelnoor M, Sorland S, et al. Coarctation of the aorta, early and late results of various surgical techniques. J Cardiovasc Surg (Torino) 1989;30:885–90.

46. Van Son JA, Falk V, Schneider P, et al. Repair of coarctation of the aorta in neonates and young infants. J Card Surg 1997;12:139–46.

47. Nanton MA, Olley PM. Residual hypertension after coarctectomy in children. Am J Cardiol 1976;37:769–72.

48. Cohen M, Fuster V, Steele PM, et al. Coarctation of the aorta. Long-term follow-up and prediction of outcome after surgical correction. Circulation 1989;80:840–5.

49. Toro-Salazar OH, Steinberger J, Thomas W, et al. Long-term follow-up of patients after coarctation of the aorta repair. Am J Cardiol 2002;89:541–7.

50. Smallhorn JF, Huhta JC, Adams PA, et al. Cross-sectional echocardiographic assessment of coarctation in the sick neonate and infant. Br Heart J 1983;50:349–61.

51. Dodge-Khatami A, Ott S, Di Bernardo S, et al. Carotid-subclavian artery index: new echocardiographic index to detect coarctation in neonates and infants. Ann Thorac Surg 2005;80:1652–7.

52. Ming Z, Yumin Z, Yuhua L, et al. Diagnosis of congenital obstructive aortic arch anomalies in Chinese children by contrast-enhanced magnetic resonance angiography. J Cardiovasc Magn Reson 2006;8:747–53.

53. Hu XH, Huang GY, Pa M, et al. Multidetector CT angiography and 3D reconstruction in young children with coarctation of the aorta. Pediatr Cardiol 2008;29:726–31.

54. Dorfman AT, Marino BS, Wernovsky G, et al. Critical heart disease in the neonate: presentation and outcome at a tertiary care center. Pediatr Crit Care Med 2008;9:193–202.

55. Bertolini A, Pelizza A, Panizzon G, et al. Vascular rings and slings. Diagnosis and surgical treatment of 49 patients. J Cardiovasc Surg (Torino) 1987;28:301–12.

56. Hartyanszky IL, Lozsadi K, Marcsek P, et al. Congenital vascular rings: surgical management of 111 cases. Eur J Cardiothorac Surg 1989;3:250–4.

57. Rivilla F, Utrilla JG, Alvarez F. Surgical management and follow-up of vascular rings. Z Kinderchir 1989;44:199–202.

58. Chun K, Colombani PM, Dudgeon DL, et al. Diagnosis and management of congenital vascular rings: a 22-year experience. Ann Thorac Surg 1992;53:597–602 [discussion: 602–3].

59. van Son JA, Julsrud PR, Hagler DJ, et al. Surgical treatment of vascular rings: the Mayo Clinic experience. Mayo Clin Proc 1993;68:1056–63.

60. Kocis KC, Midgley FM, Ruckman RN. Aortic arch complex anomalies: 20-year experience with symptoms, diagnosis, associated cardiac defects, and surgical repair. Pediatr Cardiol 1997;18:127–32.

61. Woods RK, Sharp RJ, Holcomb GW 3rd, et al. Vascular anomalies and tracheoesophageal compression: a single institution's 25-year experience. Ann Thorac Surg 2001;72:434–8 [discussion: 438–9].

62. Backer CL, Mavroudis C, Rigsby CK, et al. Trends in vascular ring surgery. J Thorac Cardiovasc Surg 2005;129:1339–47.

63. Turner A, Gavel G, Coutts J. Vascular rings–presentation, investigation and outcome. Eur J Pediatr 2005;164:266–70.

64. McElhinney DB, McDonald-McGinn D, Zackai EH, et al. Cardiovascular anomalies in patients diagnosed with a chromosome 22q11 deletion beyond 6 months of age. Pediatrics 2001;108:E104.

65. Anand R, Dooley KJ, Williams WH, et al. Follow-up of surgical correction of vascular anomalies causing tracheobronchial compression. Pediatr Cardiol 1994;15:58–61.

66. McLaughlin RB Jr, Wetmore RF, Tavill MA, et al. Vascular anomalies causing symptomatic tracheobronchial compression. Laryngoscope 1999;109:312–9.

67. Edwards JE. Anomalies of the derivatives of the aortic arch system. Med Clin North Am 1948;32:925–49.

68. Davies M, Guest PJ. Developmental abnormalities of the great vessels of the thorax and their embryological basis. Br J Radiol 2003;76:491–502.

69. Ziolkowska L, Kawalec W, Turska-Kmiec A, et al. Chromosome 22q11.2 microdeletion in children with conotruncal heart defects: frequency, associated cardiovascular anomalies, and outcome following cardiac surgery. Eur J Pediatr 2008;167:1135–40.

70. Biffi M, Boriani G, Frabetti L, et al. Left superior vena cava persistence in patients undergoing pacemaker or cardioverter-defibrillator implantation: a 10-year experience. Chest 2001;120:139–44.

71. Gonzalez-Juanatey C, Testa A, Vidan J, et al. Persistent left superior vena cava draining into the coronary sinus: report of 10 cases and literature review. Clin Cardiol 2004;27:515–8.

72. Bjerregaard P, Laursen HB. Persistent left superior vena cava. Incidence, associated congenital heart defects and frontal plane P-wave axis in a paediatric population with congenital heart disease. Acta Paediatr Scand 1980;69:105–8.

73. Parikh SR, Prasad K, Iyer RN, et al. Prospective angiographic study of the abnormalities of systemic venous connections in congenital and acquired heart disease. Cathet Cardiovasc Diagn 1996;38:379–86.

74. Postema PG, Rammeloo LA, van Litsenburg R, et al. Left superior vena cava in pediatric cardiology associated with extra-cardiac anomalies. Int J Cardiol 2008;123:302–6.

75. Curtil A, Tronc F, Champsaur G, et al. The left retro-aortic brachiocephalic vein: morphologic data and diagnostic ultrasound in 27 cases. Surg Radiol Anat 1999;21:251–4.

76. Nagashima M, Shikata F, Okamura T, et al. Anomalous subaortic left brachiocephalic vein in surgical cases and literature review. Clin Anat 2010;23:950–5.

77. Seale AN, Uemura H, Webber SA, et al. Total anomalous pulmonary venous connection: morphology and outcome from an international population-based study. Circulation 2010;122:2718–26.

78. Sato M, Tanaka D, Nakajo M. Meandering pulmonary veins with a common inferior trunk: an anomalous left inferior pulmonary vein entering an anomalous right inferior pulmonary vein. Radiat Med 2007;25:426–9.

Cardiac MDCT in Children: CT Technology Overview and Interpretation

Hyun Woo Goo, MD

KEYWORDS

- Cardiac CT • Multidetector CT • Infants and children
- Congenital heart disease

The introduction of multidetector row CT (MDCT) has substantially increased its clinical use for cardiac CT scanning in children over the past decade.[1–5] Fast scan speeds and increased anatomic coverage, combined with a flexible ECG-synchronized scan and low radiation dose, are of critical importance in improving the image quality of cardiac CT scans and minimizing patient risks.[6] The CT scanning techniques that are currently available cannot only precisely assess the extracardiac great vessels, lungs, and airways, but must also accurately evaluate the coronary arteries and intracardiac structures regardless of the cooperation of children.[6–15] CT scan dose parameters individually adapted to body habitus and dose-saving strategies, such as low tube voltage and tube current modulation, can now minimize radiation dose in cardiac CT scan imaging in pediatric patients.[16–24] Additionally, optimization of intravenous injection protocols for cardiac CT scans can result in high levels of homogeneous vascular opacification even in pediatric patients with complex cardiac defects.[6,25–30]

When interpreting cardiac CT scan studies, it is important to understand typical preoperative and postoperative imaging findings, characteristic imaging findings related to specific interventional procedures, and imaging findings of common complications.[1–5,7–10,14,31–43] Furthermore, the recognition of abnormal hemodynamic findings on cardiac CT scans may improve understanding of underlying pathophysiologic phenomena of various cardiac defects, thereby enhancing our insights into these defects.[44] Radiologists involved in cardiac CT scan assessment of children should be able to optimally adjust cardiac CT scan techniques and accurately interpret cardiac CT scan findings. Therefore, the goal of this article is to review current cardiac CT scanning techniques and interpretation strategies for congenital heart diseases in pediatric patients.

OVERVIEW OF CURRENT TECHNOLOGY
CT Scanning with or without ECG-Synchronization

Compared with non–ECG-synchronized spiral CT scans, ECG-synchronized CT scans can effectively reduce cardiac motion artifacts. Non–ECG-synchronized spiral CT scans are usually sufficient for the evaluation of extracardiac great vessels, lungs, and airways (Fig. 1). In particular, merged or composite volume-rendered CT scan images may provide accurate information to assess often complex spatial relationships of vascular airway compression frequently associated with congenital heart disease (Fig. 2).[2,8,45] In contrast, ECG-synchronized CT scans, using either retrospective ECG-gating or prospective ECG-triggering, are necessary to evaluate coronary arteries and intracardiac structures (Fig. 3). Moreover, ECG-synchronized CT scans can now be used to accurately and reproducibly assess ventricular function and volumetry, previously assessed by cardiac

The author has nothing to disclose.
Department of Radiology and Research Institute of Radiology, Asan Medical Center, University of Ulsan College of Medicine, 88, Olympic-ro 43-gil, Songpa-gu, Seoul 138-736, South Korea
E-mail address: hwgoo@amc.seoul.kr

Radiol Clin N Am 49 (2011) 997–1010
doi:10.1016/j.rcl.2011.06.001
0033-8389/11/$ – see front matter © 2011 Elsevier Inc. All rights reserved.

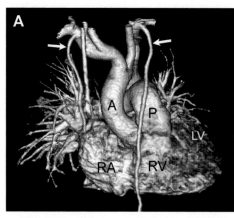
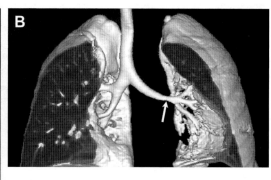

Fig. 1. Non–ECG-synchronized spiral MDCT in a 4-year-old boy following arch repair for coarctation of the aorta. (*A*) 3D volume-rendered image shows anatomic details of the extracardiac great vessels. Dilated internal mammary arteries (*arrows*) are noted. (*B*) 3D volume-rendered image demonstrates an excellent overview of the external appearance of the large airways and lungs. A mild narrowing (*arrow*) is noted at the distal left main bronchus. A, ascending aorta; LV, left ventricle; P, pulmonary trunk; RA, right atrium; RV, right ventricle.

MRI (see **Fig. 3**).[6,46,47] The advantages of cardiac CT scanning over cardiac MRI in quantifying right and left ventricular volumes include single breath-hold data acquisition, shorter scan time, higher spatial and contrast resolutions, and easier and faster segmentation. On the other hand, the temporal resolution of cardiac MRI is higher than that of cardiac CT scans. However, CT scanning volumetry has yet to be clinically validated in children with congenital heart disease. Multiphase

Fig. 2. Composite 3D volume-rendered CT image with frontal cropping in a 2-month-old boy with severe coarctation (*arrowhead*) of the aorta shows the spatial and causal relationship of vascular airway compression. A severe narrowing (*arrow*) of the left main bronchus resulting from "poststenotic dilation" of the proximal descending thoracic aorta is shown.

ECG-synchronized CT scans can be used for the four-dimensional (4D) assessment of conotruncal abnormalities throughout the cardiac cycle if clinically indicated (**Fig. 4**).[6,48] Similar to coronary CT angiography,[49] the optimal cardiac phase of ECG-synchronized cardiac CT scans in these children should be targeted, depending on heart rates and clinical indications. For anatomic evaluations, a single cardiac phase is targeted, generally either end-systolic phase in patients with high heart rates (eg, >75 beats per minute) or mid-diastolic phase in patients with low heart rates.[6] For functional evaluation, multiphase or dual-phase (ie, end-systolic and end-diastolic phases) acquisition is necessary.[6] To avoid or reduce the metallic artifacts caused by ECG leads on ECG-synchronized cardiac CT scan images, ECG leads should be placed outside the scan range.

There are currently four crucial technical considerations that can improve the image quality of cardiac CT scans in pediatric patients. First, the shortest gantry rotation time available in a CT scanning system should be selected in order to minimize motion artifacts. In this regard, dual-source CT scanning systems provide the highest temporal resolution (ie, 75–83 milliseconds), which corresponds to a quarter of the 360° rotation time.[6,50,51] The highest temporal resolution is of critical importance for obtaining diagnostic quality cardiac CT scan images in children with high heart rates. Second, axial CT scan images should be reconstructed using thinner reconstructed sections that overlap by at least 50% (eg, 0.6-mm sections and 0.3-mm reconstruction intervals), which can improve the quality of multiplanar reformatted

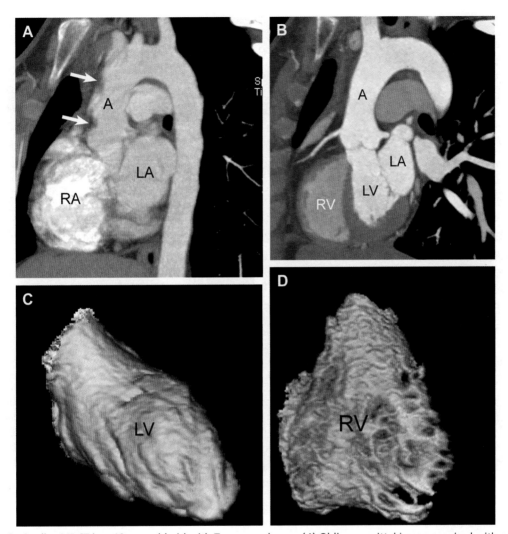

Fig. 3. Cardiac MDCT in a 19-year-old girl with Turner syndrome. (*A*) Oblique sagittal image acquired with non–ECG-synchronized spiral scanning shows cardiac pulsation artifacts (*arrows*) markedly degrading the image quality. (*B*) Oblique sagittal follow-up image acquired with retrospective ECG-gated spiral scanning shows excellent image quality without cardiac pulsation artifacts that were seen on Fig. 3A. (*C, D*) Left and right ventricular end-systolic volumes could be accurately calculated (48 mL and 59 mL, respectively). A, ascending aorta; LA, left atrium; LV, left ventricle; RA, right atrium; RV, right ventricle.

two-dimensional (2D) and three-dimensional (3D) cardiac CT scan images. Third, the z-flying focal spot technology can increase longitudinal spatial resolution by a factor of approximately 1.4 by double sampling in the z-direction, as well as reduce windmill artifacts resulting from cone beam geometry of MDCT.[52] Fourth, the image noise on cardiac CT scan can be reduced by using a 3D adaptive noise-reduction filter[53] or an iterative reconstruction kernel.[54,55]

Non–ECG-synchronized spiral CT scanning
Non–ECG-synchronized spiral CT scanning is a technique that has been widely used since the

introduction of MDCT to perform cardiac CT scanning in children with congenital heart disease. The use of newer MDCT scanners has increased longitudinal coverage and shortened gantry rotation time, resulting in a considerable decrease in cardiac and respiratory motion artifacts on non–ECG-synchronized cardiac CT scan images (**Fig. 5**). However, the greater anatomic coverage seems to almost saturate image quality with 64-detector row MDCT scanners (see **Fig. 5**). Sequential scanning with the state-of-the-art 320-MDCT scanners with a z-axis coverage of 16 cm may be used instead of spiral scanning.[56] Such z-axis detector coverage with 320-MDCT

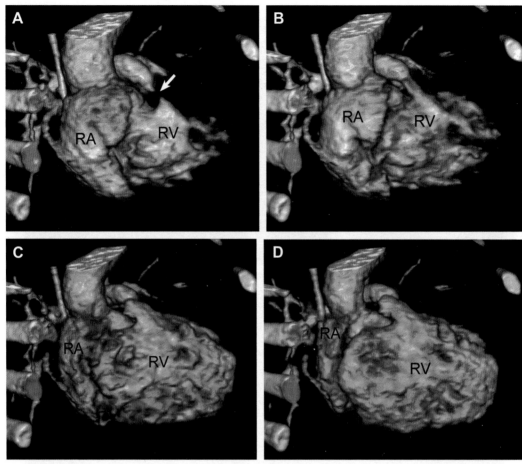

Fig. 4. Multiphase cardiac CT scan acquired with prospective ECG-triggered sequential scanning in a 1-month-old female newborn with tetralogy of Fallot. (*A–D*) Serial 3D volume-rendered images from end-systole (*A*) to end-diastole (*D*) demonstrate a severe dynamic infundibular narrowing (*arrow in A*) as well as good contractility of the right ventricle. RA, right atrium; RV, right ventricle.

scanners is sufficient to cover the entire scan range necessary for cardiac CT scans in most children in a single gantry rotation. It can eliminate stair step artifacts resulting from respiratory misregistration and differences in cardiovascular opacification between adjacent slabs not infrequently seen on typical sequential CT scan images. However, the gantry rotation time (0.35 seconds) of 320-MDCT scanners still may not be sufficient to suppress rapid cardiac motions of children. Although use of a higher pitch may reduce motion artifacts on non–ECG-synchronized spiral CT scan images, a pitch value exceeding 1.5 cannot be used in single-source spiral CT scan to obtain gapless spiral CT scan data. The recently introduced high-pitch (up to 3.0–3.4; table feed, 41.1–46.6 cm/sec) dual-source spiral CT scanner without or with ECG-triggering has been found to result in high-quality, cardiac CT scan images with minimal motion artifacts even in free-breathing children

(**Fig. 6**).[57,58] Thus, high-pitch, dual-source non–ECG-synchronized, spiral cardiac CT scan imaging is superior to conventional, single-source, non–ECG-synchronized, spiral cardiac CT scan imaging in delineating coronary arteries and intracardiac structures[11]; with the image quality of former techniques similar to that obtained with ECG-synchronized, cardiac CT scanning.[12,13,15,58] In addition, the very short scan time (approximately 0.2–0.6 seconds) of high-pitch, dual-source, non–ECG-synchronized, spiral cardiac CT scanning can make breath-hold scanning possible and reduce the need for sedation in young children aged 3 to 6 years. Unfortunately, multisection spiral scanning produces unnecessary radiation exposure outside a scan range (so-called z-overranging or z-overscanning) that is directly proportional to beam collimation, reconstructed slice thickness, and pitch.[59] Such overranging can be reduced by the adaptive collimation technology currently

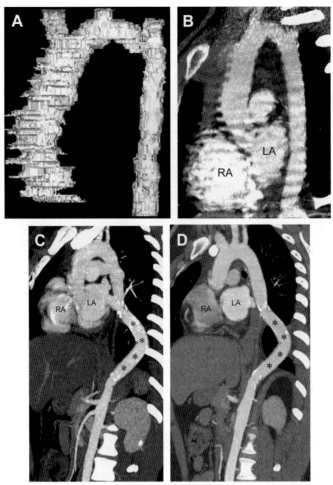

Fig. 5. Effects of technical developments in breath-hold non–ECG-synchronized multisection spiral CT scan on motion artifacts and longitudinal coverage. (*A*) 3D image of the aorta obtained with single-detector row CT scan shows severe cardiac pulsation artifacts and a short coverage that includes only the upper half of the thoracic aorta. (*B*) Oblique sagittal image obtained with 4-detector row MDCT reveals slight decrease in cardiac pulsation artifacts and a slight increase in longitudinal coverage, including the entire thoracic aorta. (*C*) Oblique sagittal image obtained with 16-detector row MDCT shows a considerable decrease in cardiac pulsation artifacts and a substantial increase in longitudinal coverage. An aortic bypass graft (*asterisks*) is noted. (*D*) Oblique sagittal image obtained with 32-detector row MDCT demonstrates that increasing the number of detector rows from 16 to 32 resulted in no further benefits in image quality or longitudinal coverage. LA, left atrium; RA, right atrium.

available from some CT scanner manufacturers.[60] However, this adaptive collimation technology cannot be currently used in high-pitch, dual-source, spiral CT scanning.

Retrospective ECG-gated spiral CT scanning

The low pitch required for obtaining gapless retrospective ECG-gated spiral CT scans is the primary reason for the high radiation dose associated with this cardiac CT scan imaging technique. Heart rate-adaptive pitch may gradually reduce radiation dose with increasing heart rate.[53] However, substantial changes in heart rate during CT scanning may degrade image quality. If heart rate changes occur during a breath-holding test, a manually selected pitch appropriate for the target heart rates may offer better image quality than the heart rate-adaptive pitch can. Although, theoretically, a multisegment reconstruction algorithm may increase temporal resolution, in reality, a single-segment reconstruction algorithm usually results in better image quality owing to a reduced scan time, thus decreasing heart rate variability. In addition, the temporal resolution of multisegment reconstruction algorithms is dependent on heart rates. The full radiation dose should target the optimal cardiac phase, whereas a reduced radiation dose, either 20% or 4% of the planned tube

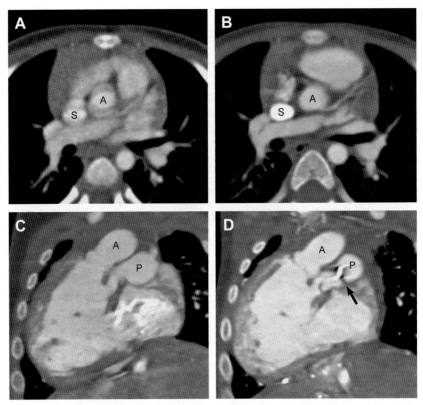

Fig. 6. High-pitch dual-source non–ECG-synchronized spiral cardiac CT scan. Axial image (*A*) obtained with single-source spiral scanning shows double lines in the superior vena cava and the ascending aorta, and image blurring due to cardiac pulsation artifacts in a free-breathing 1-year-old girl with pulmonary sequestration. In contrast, axial image (*B*) obtained with high-pitch, dual-source spiral scanning shows significant reduction of cardiac pulsation artifacts in the same patient. As a result, coronary arteries are better delineated on a high-pitch, dual-source spiral CT scan (*B*). (*C, D*) Oblique coronal image (*C*) obtained with dual-source ECG-triggered sequential scanning reveals anatomic details of intracardiac structures in a 9-month-old girl with functional single ventricle, right isomerism, pulmonary stenosis, and dextrocardia, which can be delineated on the follow-up image (*D*) obtained with high-pitch dual-source spiral scanning. The pulmonary artery banding site is noted (*arrow* in *D*). A, ascending aorta; P, pulmonary trunk; S, superior vena cava.

current, should be used for the remainder of the cardiac cycle, with the dose reduced by ECG-controlled tube current modulation. Owing to high radiation doses, up to 10 mSv, the use of the 20% of the planned tube current is strictly limited to the multiphase (10–20 phases) dynamic evaluation of myocardial wall or valve motion. In evaluating ventricular function and volumetry, two ECG-gated scans, at end-systole and end-diastole, with the 4% of the planned tube current may result in a smaller radiation dose. For the anatomic evaluation of cardiovascular structures, single-phase ECG-gated scans with 4% of the planned tube current may be performed at end-systole, mid-diastole, or end-diastole to minimize a radiation dose. The full-dose period during the cardiac cycle is freely adjustable. The entire diastole should be included in multiphase dynamic evaluation, whereas 10% of the cardiac cycle around the target cardiac phase may be an appropriate compromise between image quality and radiation dose for dual-phase and single-phase evaluations. The wider full-dose period should be used for patients with irregular heart rates. Following ECG-gated CT scanning, the optimal cardiac phase with minimal motion can be selected for image reconstruction, either manually using a preview option or automatically using a motion map.[61] Although ECG-gated spiral CT scans of free-breathing neonates have been assessed retrospectively,[12,13] breath-holding is usually recommended because image quality of the free-breathing ECG-gated spiral CT scan is reduced by respiratory motion artifacts. In fact, the overall scan time is short enough to hold his or her breath in cooperative children, usually less than 10 seconds.

Prospective ECG-triggered sequential CT scanning

In contrast to spiral CT scanning, sequential CT scanning, or "step and shoot" scanning, does not involve continuous table movement or a z-overranging effect. Compared with retrospective ECG-gated spiral scanning, prospective ECG-triggered sequential scanning delivers relatively low radiation doses, similar to those of conventional non–ECG-synchronized multisection spiral CT scans.[6,15,62] As in retrospective ECG-gated spiral scans, the optimal cardiac phase and full-dose period during the cardiac cycle of prospective ECG-triggered sequential CT scans can be adjusted to optimize image quality relative to heart rates and clinical indications, allowing either functional or anatomic evaluation. Prospective ECG-triggered sequential scanning is subject to image degradation in patients with arrhythmia, whereas ECG editing of retrospective ECG-gated spiral scans may mitigate image degradation. Stair-step artifacts resulting from respiratory misregistration between adjacent slabs may occur in free-breathing children (**Fig. 7**); however, these artifacts are fewer in free-breathing neonates and young infants, likely due to smaller tidal volumes and higher respiratory rates (see **Fig. 4**). These artifacts can be eliminated from prospective ECG-triggered sequential cardiac CT scan images by applying the respiratory triggering that has long been used in radiation oncology and nuclear medicine imaging (see **Fig. 7**). The prolonged scan time of prospective ECG-triggered sequential CT scanning may increase breath-holding difficulties, as well as differences in cardiovascular enhancement between adjacent slabs. These differences in cardiovascular enhancement may be eliminated with a multiphase intravenous injection method with decreasing injection rates, thus prolonging

peak vascular enhancement.[6,26] These disadvantages of prospective ECG-triggered sequential CT scanning have been made less problematic by increasing the longitudinal anatomic coverage, up to 16 cm, of 320-MDCT scanners.

Respiratory Dynamic CT Scans for Airways

Vascular or nonvascular airway narrowing is a common cause of respiratory difficulties or ventilator weaning failure in patients with congenital heart disease.[6,8] Tracheobronchomalacia (TBM) may be combined with a fixed airway narrowing or may be a sole source of airway narrowing. Several MDCT techniques (ie, paired end-inspiratory and end-expiratory CT scanning, paired end-inspiratory and dynamic expiratory CT scanning, and free-breathing cine-CT scanning) have been used to evaluate TBM by demonstrating excessive expiratory collapsibility of airways (**Fig. 8**).[35,63] In children, the generally accepted CT scan diagnostic criterion for the presence of TBM is greater than 50% expiratory reduction in cross-sectional area of the large airways.[64] However, CT scan findings of TBM may need to be interpreted carefully because expiratory tracheal collapsibility often exceeds the diagnostic cutoff during forced expiration, which was recently demonstrated in healthy adults.[65] Free-breathing cine-CT scans can be easily used in infants and young children because it is the CT scanning technique that does not require respiratory maneuvers for the diagnosis of TBM.[66] The 320-MDCT scanners can be used for 4D real-time dynamic evaluation of the entire large airways.[67] In addition to detecting TBM, expiratory CT scans can detect air trapping in the lungs often associated with the presence of TBM in pediatric patients.[63,68]

Dual-Energy CT Scans for Regional Lung Perfusion and Ventilation

Dual-energy CT scanning is a recently introduced CT scanning technique used to assess a specific

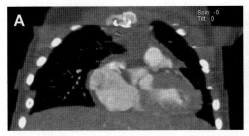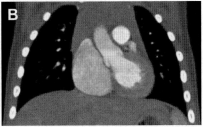

Fig. 7. Prospective ECG-triggered sequential cardiac CT scan in free-breathing young children. (*A*) Coronal image shows severe image degradation due to respiratory misregistration artifacts in a 2-year-old girl after arch repair for coarctation of the aorta. (*B*) Coronal image obtained with additional respiratory-triggering shows excellent image quality without stair-step artifacts in a 2-year-old boy with pulmonary sequestration.

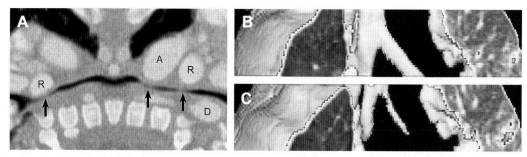

Fig. 8. Vascular bronchial compression combined with bronchomalacia in a 6-month-old girl who underwent ventricular septal defect repair, patent ductus arteriosus division, and aortopexy. (*A*) Curved multiplanar refor-matted CT scan image along the central axis of the bronchi shows three sites (*arrows*) of vascular bronchial compression by the ascending aorta and the right pulmonary artery. (*B, C*) 4D free-breathing cine-CT scan images at inspiratory (*B*) and expiratory (*C*) phases reveal excessive expiratory collapsibility of the bronchi consistent with bronchomalacia in addition to fixed bronchial narrowings. A, ascending aorta; D, descending aorta; R, right pulmonary artery.

material, such as iodine, xenon, or uric acid, by using two different kilovoltages.[69] Currently, two scan techniques are available for dual-energy CT scan data acquisition: dual-source dual-energy scanning and single-source kilovoltage switching. Dual energy CT scanning enables investigation of regional lung perfusion and ventilation,[70–72] including lung perfusion defects caused by pulmonary thromboembolism, a complication that may be associated with congenital heart disease (**Fig. 9**). Dual-energy lung ventilation CT scanning with inhaled xenon and dual-energy lung perfusion CT scanning may increase the specific diagnosis of pulmonary thromboembolism, similar to ventilation and perfusion scintigraphy.

CT Scanning Radiation Dose-Saving Strategies

To maximize the clinical usefulness of cardiac CT scanning in children, CT scan acquisition

parameters should be appropriately tailored to each patient's body and clinical indications, minimizing the radiation dose while maximizing diagnostic image quality. Establishing a body size-adapted CT scanning protocol is the first of several radiation dose-saving strategies that can be used to avoid overexposure or underexposure during cardiac CT scan imaging. Pediatric CT scan protocols that use variable tube voltages and currents are currently regarded as standard. Low tube voltage is particularly beneficial for cardiac CT scanning because it results in a higher degree of cardiovascular enhancement at a given iodine concentration.[6,19,20] Body size-adapted CT scanning protocols use several parameters, including weight, height, body mass index, cross-sectional dimensions, and attenuation.[6,17] Although body weight is the most widely used parameter for body size-adapted CT scanning protocols,[17] cross-sectional dimensions, such as

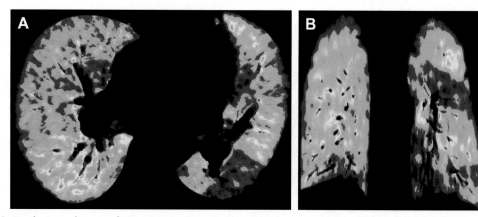

Fig. 9. Dual-energy lung perfusion CT scan in a 42-year-old man who underwent atrial septal defect repair and presented with chest pain. (*A, B*) Axial and coronal color-coded iodine maps reveal multiple, variable-sized lung perfusion defects in blue.

transverse diameter and area, are regarded as superior to body weight in adapting CT scan dose to individual patients.[18] Thus, the development of CT scanning protocols based on cross-sectional dimensions is currently an active research area in pediatric radiology. A novel and promising pediatric chest CT scan protocol was recently described that used individualized volume CT scan dose index (CTDIvol), determined by cross-sectional area and mean density of the body, at variable tube voltages and with combined tube current modulation.[73]

Tube current modulation is used to reduce CT scan dose, depending on body size, shape, and attenuation, while maintaining constant image noise. However, the references for modulation, including standard deviation, noise index, reference milliampere, and reference image, differ among manufacturers.[23] This technique may be applied along the x-y plane (angular mode), the z-axis, or a combination of both. Proper modulation of tube current requires the patient to be at the gantry isocenter. Other factors, such as tube voltage and scan direction, can affect tube current modulation.[22] The reference for modulation, however, should be selected based on the body size of each patient. Moreover, reference values are dependent on clinical indications and tube voltage. In practice, tube current modulation is used in conjunction with body size-adapted CT scanning protocols. In addition to the dose optimization achieved by body size-adapted pediatric cardiac CT scanners, radiation dose may be further reduced by 9% to 26% by combined tube current modulation.[21] Using newer MDCT scanners with fast gantry rotation and/or high-pitch dose reduction resulting from tube current modulation may, however, be limited more frequently by tube current saturation at low tube voltages (**Fig. 10**).[74] Tube current saturation can be overcome by increasing tube voltage. Ultimately, however, the benefits of tube current modulation and low kilovolt at fast gantry rotation and/or high pitch require stronger x-ray tubes.

Because an unnecessarily long scan range leads to greater radiation exposure, the scan range of cardiac CT scans should be kept to the minimum necessary for evaluation. In general, cardiac CT scanning from the aortic arch to the most caudal margin of the heart is sufficient for assessing most congenital heart diseases. A longer scan range may be necessary to assess anomalous pulmonary venous connections and major aortopulmonary collateral arteries. In contrast, a shorter scan range may be sufficient when the assessment of coronary arteries or intracardiac structures is the only indication for the cardiac

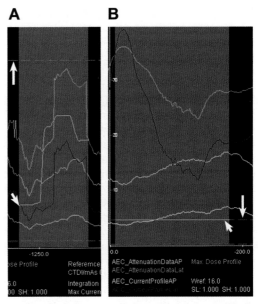

Fig. 10. Graphs showing attenuation and tube current profiles along the z-axis of a cardiac CT scan obtained at 80 kV and with combined tube current modulation. (*A*) Graph shows continuous tube current changes (*solid light brown line, short arrow*) along the z-axis below the maximal level of tube current (550 mA) (*dashed gray line, long arrow*) in a 7-day-old male newborn with coarctation of the aorta. (*B*) Graph demonstrates full saturation of tube current at 80 kV. In this situation, the fixed tube current (*solid light brown line, short arrow*) along the z-axis is identical to the maximal level of tube current (550 mA) (*dashed gray line, long arrow*) in a 4-year-old boy who underwent arch repair for coarctation of the aorta.

CT scan examination. Noise-reducing reconstruction algorithms, which may improve image quality of cardiac CT scans,[53–55] may also reduce the radiation dose of cardiac CT scans at the same image noise.[53]

Methods of Intravenous Injection of Contrast Agent

Intravenous injection of contrast agent in children with congenital heart disease should be appropriately optimized in order to achieve high and uniform enhancement of cardiovascular structures. In contrast to acquired heart disease, in which the left cardiac chambers are the primary diagnostic concern, it is usually necessary to also visualize the right cardiac chambers in patients with congenital heart disease. Thus, the injection methods used in patients with congenital heart disease differ somewhat from those used in patients with acquired heart disease. Most of these patients require 1.0 to 1.5 mL/kg iodinated contrast agent, but larger amounts, up to 2.0 mL/kg, may be necessary to avoid poor cardiovascular enhancement in patients with large intracardiac or extracardiac shunts, substantial valvular regurgitation, or severely enlarged heart. The iodine delivery rate (milligram iodine/milliliter/second), a unit including both iodine concentration and injection rate, is regarded as the best single parameter for estimating the degree of cardiovascular enhancement. In children, the injection rate should be a practical compromise between the maximally allowable and required rates. The maximally allowable rate is based on the size of the inserted angiocatheter (**Table 1**) and the estimate by a test injection of saline. The required rate is determined by a pediatric radiologist from the body weight of the patient and the time (eg, 15 seconds) required for the injection of undiluted contrast agent. The site of injection is also of critical importance in evaluating congenital heart disease and, therefore, should be chosen in advance, if possible. The leg vein is preferred for the evaluation of the aortic arch and in the presence of the bilateral superior vena cava, whereas the injection via the leg vein usually results in suboptimal pulmonary vascular enhancement in patients who have undergone bidirectional cavopulmonary connections. Of the intravenous injection methods for optimal enhancement of a Fontan pathway,[6,29,30] simultaneous injection of 50% diluted contrast agent through the arm and leg veins has been shown to be safe and effective for uniform contrast enhancement within the targeted vascular structures.

Following intravenous injection of contrast medium, a proper scan delay should be used, such that cardiac CT scanning occurs during peak vascular enhancement. A faster scan speed or a shorter scan time may require slightly longer scan delays. Three methods are currently used to determine the scan delay: empirical, test injection, and bolus tracking. The bolus tracking method is the most commonly used.[1,2,6] A long monitoring delay is used to minimize radiation dose (eg, 13 seconds for visualizing the right heart and the pulmonary circulation, and 15 seconds for visualizing the left heart and the systemic circulation). The region of interest for bolus tracking should be within the cardiac chambers or great vessels. However, the right atrium should not be used due to contrast agent-related artifacts and the nonhomogeneous mixing of opacified blood with unopacified blood, leading to faulty contrast bolus tracking.[44] The threshold CT scan attenuation in the region of interest at which the CT scan is initiated is usually set between 100 HU and 150 HU. A minimal delay between the trigger and actual scanning is generally used, in the range of 2 to 8 seconds. A longer delay is necessary for a breath-hold instruction. As a reference, peak aortic enhancement occurs approximately 5 seconds after the completion of contrast injection.[26] A test injection method may be more accurate than a bolus tracking method in acquiring CT images at peak vascular enhancement. A slightly longer delay in actual CT scanning, 3 to 5 seconds from the calculated transit time of contrast agent, may be used to adjust for the difference in the amount of contrast agent. The necessity of injecting an additional 5 to 10 mL of contrast agent, however, prevents the use of the test injection method in small children.

To obtain superb, diagnostic, quality cardiac CT scan studies, power injection is preferred to manual injection because the former provides more consistent and reproducible results. Power injection via a central venous catheter is currently controversial and a peripherally inserted central catheter should not be used for power injection. Several injection protocols have been found to result in adequate cardiovascular enhancement and to minimize perivenous artifacts in cardiac CT scan imaging.[6] A biphasic protocol involving a saline chaser reduces the amount of contrast agent and perivenous artifacts.[25] More recently, a triphasic protocol, in which undiluted contrast agent is followed by 50% to 60% diluted contrast agent and then by a saline chaser, was developed to improve opacification of the right heart and pulmonary artery, as well as to reduce perivenous artifacts.[28] In the author's practice, 5% to 10% diluted contrast agent is used instead of saline for the third phase of the triphasic protocol, and is administered at a slow injection rate. This slight modification mitigated perivenous artifacts and improved visualization of intrathoracic systemic veins on cardiac CT scan studies. Typical examples of the biphasic and triphasic intravenous injection protocols used in the author's institution are described in **Table 2**.

Table 1
Maximally allowable injection rate of contrast agent associated with the size of the inserted angiocatheter for cardiac CT scanning in children

Catheter Size (Gauge)	Maximally Allowable Injection Rate (ml/sec)
24	1.5
22	2.0
20	3.0
18	4.0

Table 2
Typical examples of intravenous injection protocols used for cardiac CT scanning in a 10 kg child

	Biphasic Protocol	Triphasic Protocol
Total amount of contrast agent	15 mL	
Scan delay with bolus tracking method	20–25 sec	
First phase	15 mL of undiluted contrast agent at 1.0 mL/sec	12 mL of undiluted contrast agent at 0.8 mL/sec
Second phase	15 mL of saline at 1.0 mL/sec	4 mL of 50% diluted contrast agent at 0.8 mL/sec
Third phase	NA	10–20 mL of 5–10% diluted contrast agent at 0.6 mL/sec

Abbreviation: NA, not applicable.

PRACTICAL CARDIAC CT SCAN INTERPRETATION

Unlike other CT scan examinations, cardiac CT scan studies performed for the assessment of congenital heart disease should be interpreted on a workstation equipped with multiplanar 2D and 3D evaluation. Such 2D-3D workstations enable the complete and systematic evaluation of thoracic structures, including the cardiovascular structures and airways, followed by the lungs.[1,2,8] The practical steps for the interpretation of cardiovascular structures on cardiac CT scan studies are similar to those for echocardiography. In contrast to typical echocardiographic evaluation, however, cardiac CT scan evaluation is performed after the patient has left the CT scanning room, uses 3D or 4D volumetric CT scan data, and is not limited by sonographic acoustic window limitations or dependent on the operator. Extracardiac great vessels should be evaluated along their long axes, using at least two perpendicular imaging planes. Intracardiac structures should be evaluated along standard imaging planes, including two-chamber, four-chamber (**Fig. 11A**), and short-axis views. The so-called en face view may be useful for characterizing septal defects (see **Fig. 11B**).[1,2] Airways are evaluated by adjusting the sagittal and oblique coronal imaging planes along the tracheal long axis, with curved multiplanar reformation along the central bronchi useful in assessing vascular airway compression (see **Fig. 8A**). In evaluating the lungs, the three orthogonal imaging planes (ie, the axial, coronal, and sagittal planes) are usually sufficient. Maximum and minimum intensity projections may be used to delineate the vascular and airway structures, respectively. The target vessels may be obscured

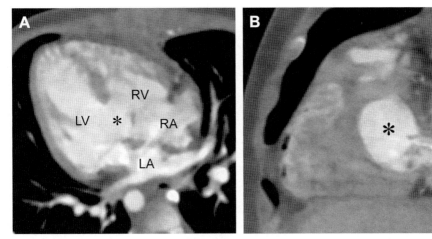

Fig. 11. A 1-year-old girl with double outlet right ventricle, a noncommitted ventricular septal defect, and dextrocardia. (*A*) Four-chamber CT scan image reveals a large ventricular septal defect (*asterisk*). (*B*) En face view of the ventricular septal defect shows its size, shape, and location (*asterisk*). LA, left atrium; LV, left ventricle; RA, right atrium; RV, right ventricle.

by adjacent cardiovascular structures on maximum intensity projection images when the slab is too thick. Volume-rendering technique can provide external overviews of cardiovascular structures and airways (see **Fig. 1**). Merged or composite volume-rendering images can demonstrate the spatial relationships between cardiovascular structures and airways in cases of vascular airway compression (see **Fig. 2**).[2,8,45] By using high-quality, 3D CT scan data and automatic software programs, it may be possible to calculate ventricular volumes and ejection fractions accurately and automatically in a very short time (see **Fig. 3**). In addition to anatomic information, a cardiac CT scan may show hemodynamic information, including extracardiac and intracardiac shunts, valvular steno-insufficiency, poor enhancement due to obstructive cardiovascular lesions, collateral vessels, preferential flow in the superior or total cavopulmonary connections, contrast regurgitation into the hepatic veins, and septal configuration, thus augmenting the role of cardiac CT scans in children with congenital heart disease.[44] Furthermore, 4D visualization on a workstation allows assessments of the dynamic obstruction of the ventricular outflow tract (see **Fig. 4**), ventricular contractility (see **Fig. 4**), and dynamic airway narrowing (see **Fig. 8**). Understanding of the wide range of cardiac CT scan findings in children with initially untreated congenital heart diseases, as well as posttreatment findings and those associated with complications of treatment, is a prerequisite for optimal interpretation of cardiac CT scan findings in children with congenital heart disease.[1–5,7–10,14,31–43]

SUMMARY

Cardiac MDCT for congenital heart disease in pediatric patients is a useful and noninvasive imaging technique that can effectively bridge the fundamental gaps among echocardiography, cardiac catheterization, and cardiac MRI. Appropriate and optimal use of this invaluable diagnostic study is based on understanding current cardiac CT scanning techniques, available postprocessing techniques, and characteristic CT scan imaging findings of congenital heart diseases in pediatric patients.

REFERENCES

1. Goo HW, Park IS, Ko JK, et al. CT of congenital heart disease: normal anatomy and typical pathologic conditions. Radiographics 2003;23(Spec No):S147–65.
2. Goo HW, Park IS, Ko JK, et al. Computed tomography for the diagnosis of congenital heart disease in pediatric and adult patients. Int J Cardiovasc Imaging 2005;21:347–65 [discussion: 367].
3. Leschka S, Oechslin E, Husmann L, et al. Pre- and postoperative evaluation of congenital heart disease in children and adults with 64-section CT. Radiographics 2007;27:829–46.
4. Sena L, Goo H. Computed tomography in congenital heart disease. In: Donogue V, editor. Radiological imaging of the neonatal chest. 2nd edition. Berlin: Springer; 2008. p. 319–46.
5. Goo HW. CT in pediatric heart disease. In: Saremi F, Achenbach S, Arbustini E, Narula J, editors. Revisiting cardiac anatomy: a computer-tomography-based atlas and reference. Oxford (UK): Wiley-Blackwell; 2010. p. 76–84.
6. Goo HW. State-of-the-art CT imaging techniques for congenital heart disease. Korean J Radiol 2010;11: 4–18.
7. Yang DH, Goo HW, Seo DM, et al. Multislice CT angiography of interrupted aortic arch. Pediatr Radiol 2008;38:89–100.
8. Goo HW. Evaluation of the airways in patients with congenital heart disease using multi-slice CT. J Korean Pediatr Cardiol Soc 2004;8:37–43.
9. Jhang WK, Park JJ, Seo DM, et al. Perioperative evaluation of airways in patients with arch obstruction and intracardiac defects. Ann Thorac Surg 2008;85:1753–8.
10. Goo HW, Jhang WK, Kim YH, et al. CT findings of plastic bronchitis in children after a Fontan operation. Pediatr Radiol 2008;38:989–93.
11. Goo HW, Park IS, Ko JK, et al. Visibility of the origin and proximal course of coronary arteries on non-ECG-gated heart CT in patients with congenital heart disease. Pediatr Radiol 2005;35:792–8.
12. Tsai IC, Lee T, Chen MC, et al. Visualization of neonatal coronary arteries on multidetector row CT: ECG-gated versus non-ECG-gated technique. Pediatr Radiol 2007;37:818–25.
13. Ben Saad M, Rohnean A, Sigal-Cinqualbre A, et al. Evaluation of image quality and radiation dose of thoracic and coronary dual-source CT in 110 infants with congenital heart disease. Pediatr Radiol 2009; 39:668–76.
14. Goo HW, Seo DM, Yun TJ, et al. Coronary artery anomalies and clinically important anatomy in patients with congenital heart disease: multislice CT findings. Pediatr Radiol 2009;39:265–73.
15. Goo HW, Yang DH. Coronary artery visibility in free-breathing young children with congenital heart disease on cardiac 64-slice CT: dual-source ECG-triggered sequential scan vs. single-source non-ECG-synchronized spiral scan. Pediatr Radiol 2010;40:1670–80.
16. Goo HW. Pediatric CT: understanding of radiation dose and optimization of imaging techniques. J Korean Radiol Soc 2005;52:1–5.

17. Yang DH, Goo HW. Pediatric 16-slice CT protocol: radiation dose and image quality. J Korean Radiol Soc 2008;59:333–47.

18. Jung YY, Goo HW. The optimal parameter for radiation dose in pediatric low dose abdominal CT: cross-sectional dimensions versus body weight. J Korean Radiol Soc 2008;58:169–75.

19. Sigal-Cinqualbre AB, Hennequin R, Abada HT, et al. Low-kilovoltage multi-detector row chest CT in adults: feasibility and effect on image quality and iodine dose. Radiology 2004;231:169–74.

20. Leschka S, Stolzmann P, Schmid FT, et al. Low kilovoltage cardiac dual-source CT: attenuation, noise, and radiation dose. Eur Radiol 2008;18:1809–17.

21. Goo HW, Suh DS. Tube current reduction in pediatric non-ECG-gated heart CT by combined tube current modulation. Pediatr Radiol 2006;36:344–51.

22. Goo HW, Suh DS. The influences of tube voltage and scan direction on combined tube current modulation: a phantom study. Pediatr Radiol 2006;36:833–40.

23. Lee CH, Goo JM, Ye HJ, et al. Radiation dose modulation techniques in the multidetector CT era: from basics to practice. Radiographics 2008;28:1451–9.

24. Herzog C, Mulvihill DM, Nguyen SA, et al. Pediatric cardiovascular CT angiography: radiation dose reduction using automatic anatomic tube current modulation. AJR Am J Roentgenol 2008;190:1232–40.

25. Hopper KD, Mosher TJ, Kasales CJ, et al. Thoracic spiral CT: delivery of contrast material pushed with injectable saline solution in a power injector. Radiology 1997;205:269–71.

26. Bae KT. Peak contrast enhancement in CT and MR angiography: when does it occur and why? Pharmacokinetic study in a porcine model. Radiology 2003;227:809–16.

27. Tsai IC, Lee T, Chen MC, et al. Homogeneous enhancement in pediatric thoracic CT aortography using a novel and reproducible method: contrast-covering time. AJR Am J Roentgenol 2007;188:1131–7.

28. Litmanovich D, Zamboni GA, Hauser TH, et al. ECG-gated chest CT angiography with 64-MDCT and triphasic IV contrast administration regimen in patients with acute non-specific chest pain. Eur Radiol 2008;18:308–17.

29. Greenberg SB, Bhutta ST. A dual contrast injection technique for multidetector computed tomography angiography of Fontan procedures. Int J Cardiovasc Imaging 2008;24:345–8.

30. Prabhu SP, Mahmood S, Sena L, et al. MDCT evaluation of pulmonary embolism in children and young adults following a lateral tunnel Fontan procedure: optimizing contrast-enhancement techniques. Pediatr Radiol 2009;39:938–44.

31. Dillman JR, Yarram SG, Hernandez RJ. Imaging of pulmonary venous developmental anomalies. AJR Am J Roentgenol 2009;192:1272–85.

32. Shih MC, Tholpady A, Kramer CM, et al. Surgical and endovascular repair of aortic coarctation: normal findings and appearance of complications on CT angiography and MR angiography. AJR Am J Roentgenol 2006;187:W302–12.

33. Katz M, Konen E, Rozenman J, et al. Spiral CT and 3D image reconstruction of vascular rings and associated tracheobronchial anomalies. J Comput Assist Tomogr 1995;19:564–8.

34. Schlesinger AE, Krishnamurthy R, Sena LM, et al. Incomplete double aortic arch with atresia of the distal left arch: distinctive imaging appearance. AJR Am J Roentgenol 2005;184:1634–9.

35. Lee EY, Zurakowski D, Waltz DA, et al. MDCT evaluation of the prevalence of tracheomalacia in children with mediastinal aortic vascular anomalies. J Thorac Imaging 2008;23:258–65.

36. Goo HW, Kim YH, Ko JK, et al. Horseshoe lung: useful angiographic and bronchographic images using multidetector-row spiral CT in two infants. Pediatr Radiol 2002;32:529–32.

37. Rajeshkannan R, Moorthy S, Sreekumar KP, et al. Role of 64-MDCT in evaluation of pulmonary atresia with ventricular septal defect. AJR Am J Roentgenol 2010;194:110–8.

38. Greil GF, Schoebinger M, Kuettner A, et al. Imaging of aortopulmonary collateral arteries with high-resolution multidetector CT. Pediatr Radiol 2006;36:502–9.

39. Ghosh S, Yarmish G, Godelman A, et al. Anomalies of visceroatrial situs. AJR Am J Roentgenol 2009;193:1107–17.

40. Gaca AM, Jaggers JJ, Dudley LT, et al. Repair of congenital heart disease: a primer—part 1. Radiology 2008;247:617–31.

41. Gaca AM, Jaggers JJ, Dudley LT, et al. Repair of congenital heart disease: a primer—Part 2. Radiology 2008;248:44–60.

42. Eichhorn JG, Jourdan C, Hill SL, et al. CT of pediatric vascular stents used to treat congenital heart disease. AJR Am J Roentgenol 2008;190:1241–6.

43. Ou P, Mousseaux E, Azarine A, et al. Detection of coronary complications after the arterial switch operation for transposition of the great arteries: first experience with multislice computed tomography in children. J Thorac Cardiovasc Surg 2006;131:639–43.

44. Goo HW. Haemodynamic findings on cardiac CT in children with congenital heart disease. Pediatr Radiol 2011;41(2):250–61.

45. Choo KS, Lee HD, Ban JE, et al. Evaluation of obstructive airway lesions in complex congenital heart disease using composite volume-rendered images from multislice CT. Pediatr Radiol 2006;36:219–23.

46. Busch S, Johnson TR, Wintersperger BJ, et al. Quantitative assessment of left ventricular function with dual-source CT in comparison to cardiac

magnetic resonance imaging: initial findings. Eur Radiol 2008;18:570–5.

47. Guo YK, Gao HL, Zhang XC, et al. Accuracy and reproducibility of assessing right ventricular function with 64-section multi-detector row CT: comparison with magnetic resonance imaging. Int J Cardiol 2010;139:254–62.

48. Schievano S, Capelli C, Young C, et al. Four-dimensional computed tomography: a method of assessing right ventricular outflow tract and pulmonary artery deformations throughout the cardiac cycle. Eur Radiol 2010;21:36–45.

49. Weustink AC, Mollet NR, Pugliese F, et al. Optimal electrocardiographic pulsing windows and heart rate: effect on image quality and radiation exposure at dual-source coronary CT angiography. Radiology 2008;248:792–8.

50. Johnson TR, Nikolaou K, Wintersperger BJ, et al. Dual-source CT cardiac imaging: initial experience. Eur Radiol 2006;16:1409–15.

51. Petersilka M, Bruder H, Krauss B, et al. Technical principles of dual source CT. Eur J Radiol 2008;68:362–8.

52. Kyriakou Y, Kachelriess M, Knaup M, et al. Impact of the z-flying focal spot on resolution and artifact behavior for a 64-slice spiral CT scanner. Eur Radiol 2006;16:1206–15.

53. McCollough CH, Primak AN, Saba O, et al. Dose performance of a 64-channel dual-source CT scanner. Radiology 2007;243:775–84.

54. Bittencourt MS, Schmidt B, Seltmann M, et al. Iterative reconstruction in image space (IRIS) in cardiac computed tomography: initial experience. Int J Cardiovasc Imaging 2010. [Epub ahead of print]. DOI: 10.1007/s10554-010-9756-3.

55. Leipsic J, Labounty TM, Heilbron B, et al. Adaptive statistical iterative reconstruction: assessment of image noise and image quality in coronary CT angiography. AJR Am J Roentgenol 2010;195:649–54.

56. Kroft LJ, Roelofs JJ, Geleijns J. Scan time and patient dose for thoracic imaging in neonates and small children using axial volumetric 320-detector row CT compared to helical 64-, 32-, and 16- detector row CT acquisitions. Pediatr Radiol 2010;40:294–300.

57. Flohr TG, Leng S, Yu L, et al. Dual-source spiral CT with pitch up to 3.2 and 75 ms temporal resolution: image reconstruction and assessment of image quality. Med Phys 2009;36:5641–53.

58. Karlo C, Leschka S, Goetti RP, et al. High-pitch dual-source CT angiography of the aortic valve-aortic root complex without ECG-synchronization. Eur Radiol 2010;21:205–12.

59. Tzedakis A, Damilakis J, Perisinakis K, et al. Influence of z overscanning on normalized effective doses calculated for pediatric patients undergoing multidetector CT examinations. Med Phys 2007;34:1163–75.

60. Deak PD, Langner O, Lell M, et al. Effects of adaptive section collimation on patient radiation dose in multisection spiral CT. Radiology 2009;252:140–7.

61. Ruzsics B, Gebregziabher M, Lee H, et al. Coronary CT angiography: automatic cardiac-phase selection for image reconstruction. Eur Radiol 2009;19:1906–13.

62. Paul JF, Rohnean A, Elfassy E, et al. Radiation dose for thoracic and coronary step-and-shoot CT using a 128-slice dual-source machine in infants and small children with congenital heart disease. Pediatr Radiol 2011;41(2):244–9.

63. Goo HW, Kim HJ. Detection of air trapping on inspiratory and expiratory phase images obtained by 0.3-second cine CT in the lungs of free-breathing young children. AJR Am J Roentgenol 2006;187:1019–23.

64. Lee EY, Boiselle PM. Tracheobronchomalacia in infants and children: multidetector CT evaluation. Radiology 2009;252:7–22.

65. Boiselle PM, O'Donnell CR, Bankier AA, et al. Tracheal collapsibility in healthy volunteers during forced expiration: assessment with multidetector CT. Radiology 2009;252:255–62.

66. Shin JH, Goo HW. Tracheomalacia in infants and children: detection by free breathing cine CT. In: Program in brief of the 96th Scientific Assembly and Annual Meeting of Radiological Society of North America. Chicago, November 30, 2010; 164.

67. Wagnetz U, Roberts HC, Chung T, et al. Dynamic airway evaluation with volume CT: initial experience. Can Assoc Radiol J 2010;61:90–7.

68. Lee EY, Tracy DA, Bastos M, et al. Expiratory volumetric MDCT evaluation of air trapping in pediatric patients with and without tracheomalacia. AJR Am J Roentgenol 2010;194:1210–5.

69. Johnson TR, Krauss B, Sedlmair M, et al. Material differentiation by dual energy CT: initial experience. Eur Radiol 2007;17:1510–7.

70. Goo HW. Initial experience of dual-energy lung perfusion CT using a dual-source CT system in children. Pediatr Radiol 2010;40:1536–44.

71. Chae EJ, Seo JB, Goo HW, et al. Xenon ventilation CT with a dual-energy technique of dual-source CT: initial experience. Radiology 2008;248:615–24.

72. Goo HW, Yang DH, Hong SJ, et al. Xenon ventilation CT using dual-source and dual-energy technique in children with bronchiolitis obliterans: correlation of xenon and CT density values with pulmonary function test results. Pediatr Radiol 2010;40:1490–7.

73. Goo HW. Individualized volume CT dose index determined by cross-sectional area and mean density of the body to achieve uniform image noise of contrast-enhanced pediatric chest CT obtained at variable kV levels and with combined tube current modulation. Pediatr Radiol 2011;41:839–47.

74. Israel GM, Herlihy S, Rubinowitz AN, et al. Does a combination of dose modulation with fast gantry rotation time limit CT image quality? AJR Am J Roentgenol 2008;191:140–4.

Preoperative and Postoperative MR Evaluation of Congenital Heart Disease in Children

L.P. Browne, MD[a],*, R. Krishnamurthy, MD[a], T. Chung, MD[b]

KEYWORDS

- Cardiovascular magnetic resonance imaging • CMR
- Congenital heart disease • Pediatric CHD

The goals of imaging in the setting of congenital heart disease (CHD) are to identify subjects with CHD, establish the need for treatment and the optimal mode of treatment, define anatomy and hemodynamics for treatment planning, monitor for complications after treatment, and determine the optimal timing of repeat intervention. Echocardiography (echo) is the primary modality used in the initial diagnosis of CHD, which can provide an excellent overview of relevant cardiovascular anatomy, flow, and function.

In the preoperative period, cardiovascular magnetic resonance imaging (CMR) can provide additional information in pediatric patients who have poor acoustic windows or when additional detail is required for surgical planning. In the postoperative period, the goals of imaging are to assess ventricular and valvular function and the status of grafts, conduits, and baffles for early detection of complications, and to determine timing of surgical intervention. Conduits are prosthetic or homograft tubes used to connect structures that are too far from each other for a direct anastomosis. Baffles are intracardiac patches that channel flow from one part to another (vein-vein, vein-chamber, chamber-artery, or artery-

artery) (**Table 1**). Complications common to conduits, baffles, and shunts include leaks, anastomotic strictures, external stenoses, and interference with adjacent native structures. Additionally, in the case of conduits, kinking or stenosis owing to the formation of a thick endothelial peal can also occur. The failure rate with echo increases in the postoperative setting and in older children with limited acoustic window. In such situations, CMR has become the gold standard noninvasive imaging modality of choice. By providing a large field of view coupled with arbitrary planes of evaluation, and 3-dimensional (3D) imaging with high spatial resolution, CMR is considered the best technique for evaluation of the right ventricle (RV) and branch pulmonary arteries, as well as conduits, baffles, and shunts created during CHD repair. CMR also provides serial accurate and reproducible measurements of ventricular function, stroke volumes, and regurgitant fractions.

In this article, current cardiac MR imaging techniques and specific questions that arise in the preoperative and postoperative evaluation of the most common CHD anomalies referred to CMR in pediatric patients are reviewed.

[a] Edward B. Singleton Department of Pediatric Radiology, Texas Children's Hospital, MC-2251, 6621 Fannin Street, Houston, TX, USA
[b] Department of Pediatric Radiology, Children's Hospital & Research Center Oakland, 747 52nd Street, Oakland, CA 94609, USA
* Corresponding author.
E-mail address: lxbrowne@texaschildrenshospital.org

Radiol Clin N Am 49 (2011) 1011–1024
doi:10.1016/j.rcl.2011.06.010

Table 1
Procedures performed on common CHD defects

Procedure	Technique	Description	CHD
Lateral tunnel Fontan procedure	Baffle	Intra-atrial tunnel between IVC and undersurface of pulmonary artery	Single ventricle anomalies (HLHS, tricuspid atresia, double inlet left ventricle)
Extracardiac Fontan procedure	Conduit	An external conduit connects the inferior vena cava to the right pulmonary artery	Single ventricle anomalies (HLHS, tricuspid atresia, double inlet left ventricle)
Rastelli procedure	Baffle and conduit	VSD closed by baffling left ventricle to aorta and a valved conduit is used to connect the RV to PA bifurcation	D-TGA and VSD or double-outlet RV and VSD
Norwood procedure	Anastomosis and conduit	Damus Kaye Stansel maneuver whereby proximal pulmonary artery is anastomosed to ascending aorta and aortic arch is augmented Atrial septectomy; Modified BT shunt or Sano modification	HLHS
Bidirectional Glenn shunt	Anastomosis	End to side anastomosis between SVC and RPA	Stage II procedure for single ventricle anomalies, TOF with pulmonary atresia
Modified Blalock-Taussig shunt	Conduit	An interposition polytetrafluoroethylene (PTFE, or Gore-Tex) graft between the subclavian artery and the pulmonary artery	Part of Stage I palliation of HLHS, TOF with pulmonary atresia
Modified Sano shunt	Conduit	A Gore-Tex graft is placed between an incision in the RVOT and bifurcation of the main pulmonary artery	Stage I palliation of HLHS, TOF with pulmonary atresia

Abbreviations: BT, Blalock Taussig; CHD, congenital heart disease; D-TGA, complete transposition of the great arteries; HLHS, hypoplastic left heart syndrome; IVC, inferior vena cava; PA, pulmonary artery; RPA, right pulmonary artery; RV, right ventricle; RVOT, right ventricular outflow tract; SVC, superior vena cava; TOF, tetralogy of Fallot; VSD, ventricular septal defect.

TECHNIQUE

The basic CMR protocol for preoperative and postoperative assessment of CHD includes evaluation of cardiovascular morphology, ventricular function, and flow.

Evaluation of Cardiovascular Morphology

Evaluation of cardiovascular anatomy, including any surgically created connections, is performed using spin-echo "black-blood" sequences or gradient-echo "bright-blood" sequences. Electrocardiogram (ECG)-triggered static black-blood techniques include fast spin-echo double-inversion recovery, or conventional spin echo with echo planar imaging (EPI) readout. Segmented cine gradient-echo imaging allows a dynamic assessment of the thoracic vasculature with multiple frames acquired throughout the cardiac cycle. Coronary artery evaluation using a free-breathing isotropic 3D steady-state free precession (SSFP) navigator respiratory gated sequence is performed in patients who are suspected to have anomalous coronary origin, and those who have undergone coronary reimplantation procedures (arterial switch and Ross procedures). Contrast-enhanced 3D magnetic resonance angiography (MRA) also provides excellent morphologic assessment of the thoracic and abdominal vasculature with time-resolved techniques enabling separation of pulmonary and systemic phases of contrast opacification.

Evaluation of Ventricular Function

Evaluation of ventricular function is performed with cine 2D steady SSFP sequences, which are optimized to provide excellent myocardial blood pool differentiation. Myocardial perfusion and viability sequences are performed in patients who have undergone coronary reimplantation procedures (Ross and arterial switch), who have segmental wall motion abnormalities, and after prolonged cardiopulmonary bypass procedure.

Evaluation of Flow

Flow evaluation is performed with cine phase-contrast sequences. It is used to assess valvular competency, measure the volume of systemic to pulmonary shunting, and estimate the pressure gradient across stenoses using the modified Bernoulli equation ($4 \times V2 = \Delta P$, where ΔP is the pressure gradient in mm Hg and V is the measured peak velocity in m/s). The Qp:Qs ratio represents the ratio of flow to the pulmonary circulation versus the systemic circulation and is usually calculated by phase-contrast imaging across the main pulmonary artery and ascending aorta. The Qp:Qs ratio is an important measurement in the presence of left-right shunts, baffle leaks, and single ventricle repair.

Suggested CMR sequences used to address specific questions in the preoperative and postoperative evaluation of common CHD anomalies are summarized in **Table 2**.

RECENT TECHNICAL ADVANCES IN CMR OF CHD

Static morphologic imaging can be efficiently performed using the whole-heart approach with 3D SSFP and respiratory navigator. A similar 3D approach can be applied to cine functional sequences. An isotropic 3D cine SSFP has been shown to be possible and newer techniques, such as real-time respiratory self-gating, to compensate for respiratory motion.[1–3] Qualitative 3D phase-contrast techniques have been used to assess the great vessels and left heart chambers in healthy volunteers with several studies validating

the results compared with conventional 2D techniques.[4,5]

Faster imaging techniques are particularly advantageous in pediatric patients with CHD, where there are specific CMR challenges including faster heart rates and inability to cooperate with breath-holding because of sedation/anesthesia. Improved temporal resolution can allow shorter breath-hold times and minimize cardiac and respiratory motion artifacts encountered during free-breathing acquisitions. Various techniques have been used to speed up acquisition, including k-space and time broad-use linear acquisition speed-up technique (k-t BLAST) and parallel imaging (SMASH, SENSE, and GRAPPA) using multiple receivers in a phased array coil. The feasibility of these techniques in enabling fast and even real-time volume SSFP acquisitions of the left ventricle (LV) and RV has been established in adults.[6]

Accelerated techniques using parallel imaging have also been applied to MRA. Time-resolved contrast-enhanced MRA consists of multiple 3D volumes (dynamics) that are acquired consecutively without interval delay. The 4D time-resolved MRA with SENSE and keyhole (4D-TRAK) implements a keyhole method of K-space filling to achieve extremely rapid volume acquisitions. Such technique has been used successfully without significant artifact in free-breathing pediatric patients with CHD.[7]

Decreased rates of cardiovascular recovery after physical or pharmacologically induced stress are associated with increased rates of mortality in patients with ischemic heart disease. CMR assessment following both supine exercise and dobutamine administration (beta 1 agonist) has been successfully used to quantify biventricular function after stress in patients with CHD who have undergone tetralogy of Fallot and transposition of great vessels repairs.[8,9] Identification of diastolic dysfunction and decreased contractility following stress, despite normal ventricular function at rest and before the onset of clinical symptoms, may improve long-term postoperative outcomes. Myocardial tagging is a method of analyzing ventricular wall motion and abnormal myocardial strain.[10] By identifying small regions of myocardial strain, myocardial tagging enables earlier detection of myocardial dysfunction. This technique has been applied to the left (non-systemic) ventricle of adult patients who have undergone transposition of the great arteries (TGA) after atrial switch procedure.[1] Such technique can demonstrate abnormal shortening patterns of the subpulmonic LV postulated to be secondary to abnormal loading arising from the anomalous ventricular geometry.[1]

Table 2
Suggested CMR sequences for evaluating common CHD anomalies

CHD	Morphology	Function	Flow Evaluation
TOF post repair	Black/bright-blood sequences to assess RVOT size and branch pulmonary artery 3D SSFP to confirm normal coronary origins	Standard planes to evaluate ventricular function with additional views of RVOT	MPA for PR fraction Branch pulmonary arteries to calculate differential pulmonary flow Aorta to evaluate Qp:Qs residual VSD
Single-ventricle anomalies	High-resolution black-blood/gradient-echo imaging to thoroughly evaluate thoracic vasculature	Standard ventricular volume assessment	Qp:Qs assessment usually requires AVV stroke volumes, stroke volume through systemic to pulmonary shunt, bilateral branch pulmonary artery and aorta volumes
D-TGA post–arterial switch procedure	Black/bright-blood sequences to assess RVOT size, branch pulmonary artery anatomy, and size of the aortic root 3D SSFP to confirm normal coronary origins	Standard planes for assessment of ventricular volumes with additional views of LVOT and RVOT	Qp:Qs with MPA and aorta. Branch pulmonary arteries to calculate differential pulmonary flow. RVOT in presence of RVOT stenosis
D-TGA post–atrial switch procedure	Black/bright-blood/ 3-d SSFP sequences to assess patency of baffles Myocardial viability assessment of the systemic RV	Standard planes for assessment of ventricular volumes	SVC, IVC, aorta, MPA and intra-atrial baffle assessment looking for evidence of baffle leak
Coarctation of aorta	Black/bright-blood sequences to assess coarctation size and transverse arch anatomy. Cine gradient echo to assess bicuspid valve, if present	Standard planes to evaluate ventricular volumes with additional views of LVOT if bicuspid aortic valve and stenosis are present	Through plane PC above coarctation and closer to diaphragm to evaluate for collateral flow in plane PC to estimate peak systolic velocity and gradient across stenotic segment

Abbreviations: AVV, arterioventricular volume; CHD, congenital heart disease; CMR, cardiovascular magnetic resonance imaging; D-TGA, complete transposition of great arteries; IVC, inferior vena cava; LVOT, left ventricular outflow tract; MPA, main pulmonary artery; PC, phase contrast; PR, pulmonary regurgitation; Qp:Qs, ratio of flow to the pulmonary circulation versus the systemic circulation; SSFP, steady-state free precession; VSD, ventricular septal defect.

CLINICAL APPLICATIONS

In this section, we address specific questions that arise in the preoperative and postoperative evaluation for the most common CHD anomalies referred to CMR in pediatric patients.

Tetralogy of Fallot

Tetralogy of Fallot (TOF) is the most common reason for referral for a CMR examination. It is actually a single pathologic defect owing to superior and anterior deviation of the conal septum, resulting in an anterior malalignment ventricular septal defect (VSD), infundibular narrowing of the right ventricular outflow tract (RVOT), right ventricular hypertrophy, and the aorta overriding the septal defect. Lillehei and colleagues[11] introduced the intracardiac repair of TOF, in which the VSD is closed and the RVOT reconstructed, usually by incorporating a transannular patch of pericardium. In severe forms of TOF, a homograft pulmonary valve, or a conduit containing a prosthetic valve, may be inserted between the RV and the pulmonary artery.

TOF may be associated with complex pulmonary artery anatomy, including pulmonary atresia, nonconfluent branch pulmonary arteries and major aorto-pulmonary collateral vessels (MAPCAs). MAPCAs most commonly arise from the descending thoracic aorta, but can arise from the subclavian arteries, coronary arteries, and abdominal aorta. In cases of pulmonary atresia with pulmonary hypoplasia or nonconfluent pulmonary arteries, these MAPCAs may be the sole source of perfusion to variable amounts of pulmonary parenchyma. Surgical corrective procedures include (1) the unifocalization procedure, whereby the MAPCAs are isolated from their systemic arterial origin and anastomosed to a central pulmonary artery; (2) early surgical relief of RVOT obstruction; and (3) VSD closure. These procedures are followed by interventional catheterization to dilate stenotic pulmonary arteries and occlude redundant MAPCAs with coils. Echo is inherently limited in its ability to visualize the distal pulmonary artery segments and MAPCAs. However, detailed depiction of the branch pulmonary artery anatomy as well as origin and course of these MAPCAs is vital for preoperative planning of possible surgical repairs.

Preoperative assessment

The intracardiac anatomy of TOF is usually well established by echo, with CMR reserved for those cases with complex pulmonary artery anatomy and MAPCAs. Traditionally, all patients with TOF underwent invasive angiography to identify the sources of pulmonary blood supply. However, time-resolved 3D MRA has been shown to be a viable alternative to catheterization, enabling a road map of pulmonary supply and major MAPCAs be created without the adverse effects of catheterization and radiation.[12] This technique can be performed from newborns to adults and may also depict any antegrade flow through the stenotic pulmonary annulus. Such technique is currently somewhat limited by (1) spatial resolution (only vessels larger than 0.5 mm will be reliably seen by MR imaging) and (2) the inability to visualize the lung parenchyma to differentiate the individual pulmonary segments.

Other anomalies encountered less frequently in the preoperative CMR evaluation of TOF include anomalous coronary arteries, anomalous pulmonary venous return, and atrial septal defects (ASDs).

Postoperative assessment

Although most patients have some degree of pulmonary regurgitation (PR), long-term results after TOF repair are currently good. The effects of chronic PR are deleterious and include arrhythmias, right ventricular volume overload, and decreased RV function. Other commonly encountered complications requiring intervention include RVOT stenosis, RVOT aneurysm, residual VSD, and branch pulmonary artery stenosis (Fig. 1). Reintervention with pulmonary valve replacement procedures using surgical or percutaneously placed conduits relieve the volume overload on the RV, resulting in remodeling and improvement in RV function. Current guidelines for valve replacement include the onset of clinical symptoms, progressive tricuspid valve regurgitation, and progressive RV dilation on imaging. CMR has been accepted as the reference standard for right ventricular evaluation, providing accurate estimation of right ventricular volumes, which is important information for the timing of pulmonary valve replacement (PVR) surgery.[13–15] Right ventricular end diastolic volume (RVEDV) thresholds used to determine PVR timing vary between centers. Normalization of RV volumes has been demonstrated with RVEDV less than 160 mL/m.^{2}[13,14] Even very large RVEDVs (190 mL/m^2) may substantially decrease after PVR.[13,14]

The aim of the postoperative TOF CMR assessment is to enable optimal timing and method of interventions by providing accurate quantification of ventricular volumes and PR fractions, in addition to depiction of the RVOT and branch pulmonary artery anatomy. Assessment for an anomalous prepulmonic course of the coronary artery anatomy may be performed before a repeat RVOT incision, although 3D SSFP image quality can be degraded by turbulent flow in the RVOT.

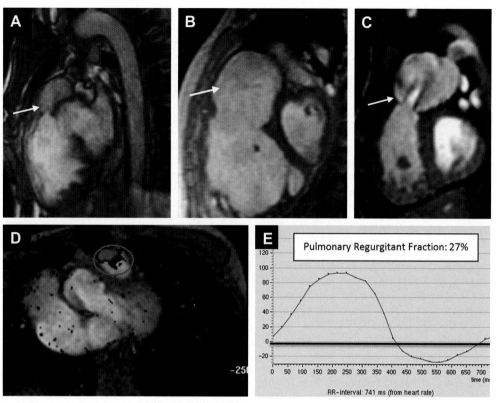

Fig. 1. Tetralogy of Fallot (TOF). (*A*) Cine SSFP image in RVOT plane showing anterior and superior deviation of the conal septum (*arrow*) in a patient with untreated TOF. (*B*) Cine SSFP image in RVOT plane in a different patient from *A* who is status post-TOF repair, showing the typical changes of RV dilatation secondary to pulmonary regurgitation, and aneurysmal changes (*arrow*) involving the outflow tract as a result of transannular RVOT patch placement. (*C*) Cine SSFP image in RVOT plane in a different patient with recurrent RVOT stenosis (*arrow*) after annulus-sparing TOF repair. (*D*) Phase-contrast sequence across the short axis of the RV outflow tract. (*E*) Flow-volume curve obtained from (*D*) demonstrating severe pulmonary regurgitation (*circle*).

MR imaging can also identify independent predictors of major adverse clinical outcomes late after TOF repair. Multivariate analysis identified severe RV dilatation and either LV or RV dysfunction as assessed by CMR as predictors of major adverse clinical events.[16]

Single-Ventricle Physiology

Hypoplastic left heart syndrome (HLHS) is the most common single-ventricle anomaly, occurring in approximately 1 in 5000 live births.[17] Other common functional single-ventricular conditions include unbalanced common atrioventricular canal, tricuspid atresia, and double-inlet left ventricle. Affected patients typically present clinically during the first few weeks of life, which coincides with the physiologic nadir in pulmonary vascular resistance. Clinical manifestations vary depending on the degree of pulmonary and systemic obstruction. Typical clinical presentations include right-ventricular failure, failure to thrive, and metabolic acidosis.[17]

For the purpose of this article, the role of CMR will be mainly focused on hypoplastic left heart physiology. HLHS has a unique first-stage surgery called the Norwood procedure, performed immediately after birth. The main pulmonary artery is tied off and resected, separating it from the right and left pulmonary arteries. The main pulmonary artery is then anastomosed to the ascending aorta (the Damus Kaye Stansel maneuver), and the narrowed aortic arch is augmented (**Fig. 2**). A modified Blalock Taussig (BT) shunt or Sano shunt (right ventricle to pulmonary artery conduit) is created to provide pulmonary arterial supply. The second stage of repair is the bidirectional superior cavopulmonary anastomosis (bidirectional Glenn shunt), performed at 6 to 9 months of life, where the superior vena cava (SVC) is anastomosed to the pulmonary artery and the BT shunt is taken down. The inferior cavopulmonary anastomosis (Fontan) operation is the final surgical stage for most patients with a functionally single ventricle. It is usually performed between 18 months and

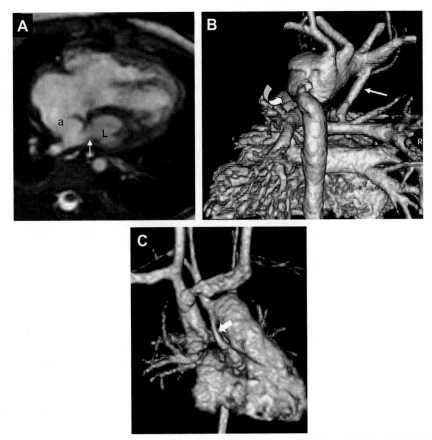

Fig. 2. Hypoplastic left heart syndrome (HLHS), status post-Norwood procedure. (*A*) Cine SSFP 4 chamber view showing severe hypoplasia of the mitral annulus (*arrow*) and left ventricle (L), and an unobstructed atrial septectomy (a) diverting pulmonary venous return to the systemic RV. (*B*) and (*C*) Posterior and anterior views of a volume-rendered 3D gadolinium-enhanced 3D MR angiogram in a different patient from (*A*) showing the expected appearance of the augmented arch and BT shunt (*straight arrow*) following a Norwood operation, but with severe recurrent coarctation (*curved arrow*) at the aortic isthmus.

4 years of age, resulting in the formation of a total cavopulmonary anastomosis. There are 2 types of Fontan currently performed: the lateral tunnel (**Fig. 3**) and the extracardiac conduit. In the lateral tunnel Fontan, an intra-atrial Gore-Tex baffle is placed in the lateral part of the right atrium connecting the inferior vena cava (IVC) with an enlarged SVC orifice, now anastomosed to the undersurface of the right pulmonary artery. A fenestration is sometimes placed through the tunnel wall into the right atrial chamber. In the extracardiac Fontan, the IVC is transected at the inferior cavoatrial junction and a Gore-Tex conduit is interposed end-to-end between the IVC and the inferior surface of the right pulmonary artery. A fenestration takes the form of a small tube graft interposed between the conduit and the right atrial appendage.

Other less widely performed HLHS procedures include the hybrid procedure (intraoperative pulmonary artery banding with percutaneous placement of ductus arteriosus stent) and orthotropic cardiac transplantation.[18] Complications of the hybrid procedure include stent migration or thrombosis, whereas transplantation is limited by organ availability, and complicated by rejection, lifelong immunosuppression, and posttransplantation lymphoproliferative conditions.

Preoperative assessment
Cardiac MR imaging has a limited role in the preoperative assessment of HLHS; however, occasionally patients with less severe forms of left-sided obstruction can benefit from a biventricular-type cardiac repair. In these instances, CMR has an advantage over echo by more accurately establishing the left ventricular end diastolic volume (LVEDV),[19] and screens for the presence of endocardial fibroelastosis, which is used as a predictor of potential outcome. Predictors of a failed biventricular repair also include a small left ventricle (LVEDVs of <15–20 mL/m^2), large

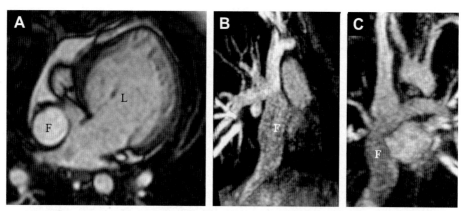

Fig. 3. Tricuspid atresia s/p lateral-tunnel Fontan procedure in a 9-year-old girl. (*A*) Cine SSFP image in a 4-chamber plane showing changes of tricuspid atresia. Functional single LV (L) and the Fontan baffle (F) lying along the right lateral wall of the atrium are seen. (*B*) and (*C*) Coronal reformatted images from a gadolinium-enhanced 3D MRA showing the superior and inferior cavopulmonary anastomoses to the right pulmonary artery, and patency of both branch pulmonary arteries and the Fontan baffle (F).

VSD with right to left systolic shunting, severe mitral annular hypoplasia, and a unicommisural aortic valve.[20,21]

Pre-Glenn assessment Routine cardiac catheterization before bidirectional Glenn operation was previously considered the standard of care in assessing anatomic and hemodynamic suitability for surgery. At this time, percutaneous interventions such as balloon dilation of aortic coarctation and coiling of systemic-pulmonary collateral vessels were also performed. However, recent studies have shown that the combination of echo and CMR can adequately evaluate Glenn suitability in selected HLHS patients without pulmonary hypertension, severe ventricular dysfunction, severe atrioventricular valvar regurgitation, known large collateral vessels, or aortic coarctation. Additionally, it is associated with lower rates of adverse events, shorter hospital stay (than patients who undergo catheterization), and no differences in immediate and short-term postoperative outcomes.[22] In these cases, a comprehensive evaluation of the thoracic vasculature and measurement of systemic and pulmonary blood flow is performed. Additional CMR applications include assessment of myocardial perfusion and viability, as the presence of extensive scarring or endocardial fibroelastosis may limit the success of the surgical repairs.[23]

Pre-Fontan assessment Patients currently undergo a cardiac catheterization as part of their pre-Fontan evaluation, necessitating jugular or subclavian catheterization to visualize the bidirectional cavopulmonary anastomosis. Retrospective studies have demonstrated that a noninvasive workup with a combination of echo and CMR can

noninvasively identify high-risk patients. Such high-risk patients are those with significant ventricular dysfunction, severe antrioventricular valvular regurgitation, aortic coarctation, major collateral vessels, or small pulmonary artery size, which are unsuitable for the Fontan procedure.[24–26] However, further validation of this practice is warranted. In select cases where pre-Fontan assessment is performed with CMR, attention is directed to evaluating the ventricular volumes, pulmonary artery size and differential pulmonary blood flow, anatomy of the systemic venous return, and the morphology of the reconstructed aortic arch.

Postoperative assessment (post-Fontan assessment)

The Fontan patient population is at risk for obstruction of the venous pathways, dilatation of the systemic venous channels with formation of collaterals, thromboembolism, dysfunction of the single systemic ventricle, compression of the pulmonary veins, and arrhythmias. The goals of a post-Fontan CMR assessment are for (1) evaluation of the systemic veins, pulmonary veins, and pulmonary arteries for evidence of obstruction or thrombosis; (2) assessment of the Fontan baffle for evidence of leaks; (3) evaluation of ventricular function and valvular regurgitation; and (4) screening for collateral vessels.

Transposition of the Great Arteries

Transposition of the great arteries (TGA) is one of the more common congenital heart diseases, accounting for 5% to 7% of all congenital cardiac lesions.[27] TGA, by definition, implies discordant ventriculoarterial connections such that the ascending aorta arises from the morphologic RV and the main pulmonary artery arises from the morphologic LV. Complete transposition of the great arteries (D-TGA) is defined by discordant ventriculoarterial connections and concordant atrioventricular connections, resulting in complete separation of systemic and pulmonary circulations. L-TGA has discordant atrioventricular and discordant ventriculoarterial connections. It is thus described as being "physiologically corrected" as pulmonary venous return reaches the systemic arteries via the right ventricle. D-TGA is encountered much more frequently than L-TGA and requires corrective surgery in the first few days of life. There are 2 major types of surgery performed for D-TGA: the atrial switch procedure (Mustard and Senning procedures) and the arterial switch procedure (Jatene). In the atrial switch procedure, intra-atrial venous baffles redirect the systemic and pulmonary venous blood returns to the appropriate atria, restoring circulating blood flow (**Fig. 4**). These baffles are created by using either in situ tissue from the right atrial wall and interatrial septum (Senning) or with autologous or synthetic material (Mustard). Ventriculoseptal defects, if present, are also closed. In the arterial switch operation (Jatene), the ascending aorta and the main pulmonary artery are transected above their valve leaflets and moved to their correct circulatory position with the pulmonary bifurcation placed anterior to the ascending aorta (Lecompte maneuver) (**Fig. 5**). The coronary arteries are then

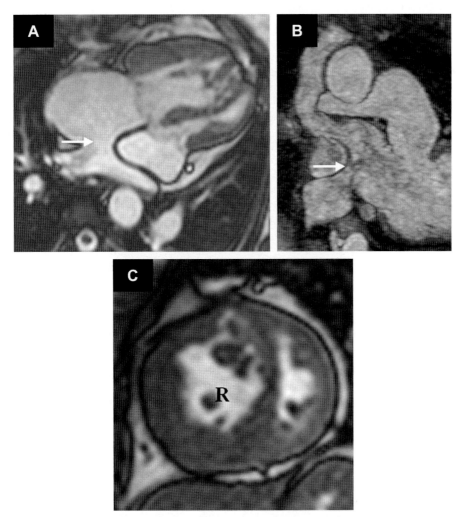

Fig. 4. D-TGA status post–atrial switch procedure in a 35-year-old woman. (*A*) Cine SSFP image in a 4-chamber plane showing pulmonary venous baffle (*arrow*). (*B*) ECG gated 3-D SSFP sequence with navigator respiratory triggering reformatted in coronal oblique plane of the systemic venous baffles demonstrating widely patent SVC baffle, but moderate stenosis of IVC baffle (*arrow*). (*C*) Cine SSFP image in short axis plane showing dilatation and hypertrophy of the systemic right ventricle (R).

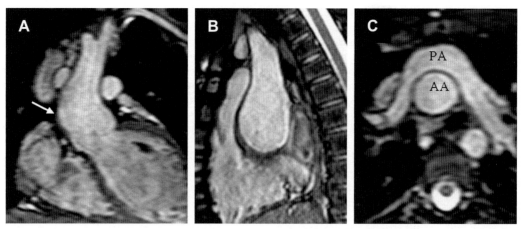

Fig. 5. D-TGA status post–arterial switch procedure evaluated with ECG-gated 3D SSFP whole heart sequence with navigator respiratory triggering in a 13-year-old boy . (*A*) Reformatted coronal plane of the LVOT showing moderate aortic root dilatation (*arrow*). (*B*) Reformatted oblique sagittal plane along the long axis of the RVOT. (*C*) Reformatted oblique axial plane of the branch pulmonary arteries (PA) straddling the ascending aorta (AA). There is no obstruction of the RVOT or the branch pulmonary arteries.

transplanted from the native aortic root to the neo-aortic root (which is the native pulmonary trunk). Septal defects, if present, are surgically closed. The arterial switch operation has superseded the Mustard and Senning procedures as the most common surgery performed in D-TGA. A less frequently performed repair is the Rastelli procedure (**Fig. 6**). This is the procedure of choice in patients with D-TGA, VSD, and pulmonary stenosis. The LV is baffled to the aorta across the VSD with a Dacron patch, and a valved conduit is placed between the right ventricle and pulmonary artery.

Many patients with L-TGA are managed medically, although most ultimately develop dysfunction of the systemic RV. In patients who have an associated anomaly such as VSD, pulmonary stenosis, or Ebstein anomaly, a surgical repair is performed using the combined atrial and arterial switch (double switch) procedure or the combined Rastelli and atrial switch procedure.[28]

Preoperative evaluation
Preoperative imaging of patients with TGA with transthoracic echo is usually adequate for surgical planning.[29] CMR is typically reserved for clarification of complex anatomy like criss-cross ventricles or coronary anatomy not adequately defined by echo.

Postoperative evaluation
Postarterial switch evaluation The main complications after the arterial switch procedure (ASO) are RVOT anastomotic narrowing and stenoses of the branch pulmonary arteries, and neo-aortic root dilatation. RVOT and pulmonary artery stenoses may lead to RV dysfunction necessitating

corrective procedures.[30] Dilatation and insufficiency of the neo-aortic root usually develops over time. Coronary abnormalities can be present in 3% to 7% of asymptomatic individuals and, although uncommon, can cause sudden death.[31] CMR using 3D SSFP navigator respiratory gated sequences can noninvasively evaluate the coronary arteries by detecting ostial stenoses or proximal kinking and screening myocardial injury using perfusion and viability sequences.[32]

Postatrial switch evaluation Patients with Mustard-type or Senning-type repair are now typically older patients. The most common complications following the atrial switch procedures are intra-atrial venous baffle stenoses and leaks. Baffle stenoses typically occur at the superior limb of the baffle where the SVC meets the right atrium. Baffle leaks are usually small but estimated to occur in approximately 25% of patients. The most important and relatively common postoperative complication after atrial switch procedure for TGA is hypertrophy and decreased function of the systemic RV. Less common complications include pulmonary arterial hypertension, residual VSD, subpulmonary stenosis, and arrhythmias.[33] CMR is considered the optimal imaging modality in determining timing and method of reintervention in patients with repaired D-TGA, providing accurate morphologic, functional, and physiologic data.[14,33]

Delayed enhancement techniques have been applied to the hypertrophied systemic RV postatrial switch in adult patients, with the presence of myocardial scarring reported to correlate with progressive ventricular dysfunction and clinical deterioration.[34]

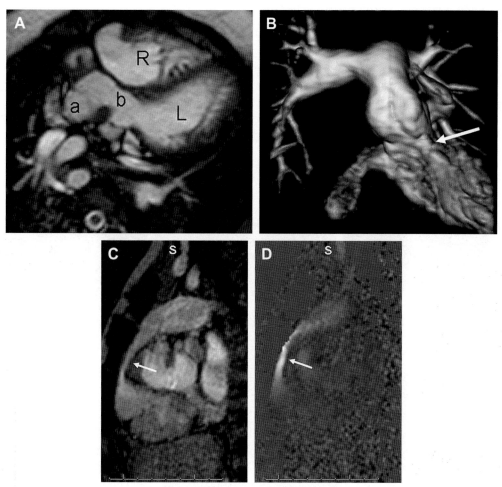

Fig. 6. D-TGA status post-Rastelli procedure with RV to PA conduit stenosis in a 7-year-old girl. (*A*) Cine SSFP image of the LVOT showing the left ventricle (L) being baffled (b) to the aorta (a). R, right ventricle. (*B*) Volume-rendered image from gadolinium-enhanced 3D MR angiogram showing stenosis of the proximal RV to PA conduit (*arrow*). (*C*) and (*D*) are magnitude and phase MR images respectively of a sagittal phase contrast sequence across the conduit, demonstrating narrowing of the proximal conduit with a high-velocity dephasing jet (*arrow*) arising from the stenosis in systole.

Coarctation of the Aorta

Coarctation of the aorta represents 5% to 10% of congenital heart disease. It can be classified into 3 types according to its location relative to the ductus arteriosus: preductal, juxtaductal, and postductal. Juxtaductal type is the most common type of the coarctation of aorta.[35] Various etiologies for the coarctation of aorta have been proposed. The ductal theory hypothesizes that coarctation results from migration of smooth muscle ductal cells that constrict and narrow the aortic lumen. The hemodynamic theory hypothesizes that coarctation results from decreased fetal arch flow secondary to left heart lesions such as bicuspid aortic valves and VSDs.[35]

A coarctation is deemed to be significant if the gradient between the upper and lower extremities exceeds 20 mm Hg.[35] Surgical procedures for significant coarctation include (1) surgical resection of the stenotic segment with end-end anastomosis, which is the preferred surgical procedure; (2) subclavian flap angioplasty using a down-turned subclavian artery to augment the stenotic segment; and (3) patch angioplasty with a prosthetic patch augmentation. Percutaneous corrective procedures include balloon angioplasty alone or balloon angioplasty combined with subsequent stent placement. In general, surgical repair is typically performed in infants with complex arch anatomy or long-segment arch hypoplasia, whereas percutaneous therapies are favored in cases of short-segment stenoses, re-coarctations, and adult patients.[36]

Preoperative assessment

Echo usually provides adequate information that can allow operative planning in most of cases of childhood coarctation. CMR provides further information in cases where the coarctation is incompletely defined because of poor acoustic windows and the coarctation is atypical/complex, such as encountered in PHACE syndrome. Phase-contrast techniques and 3D MR angiography provide most of the information required in

preoperative CMR coarctation assessment. Decisions regarding the optimal corrective procedure require information regarding the dimensions of the coarctation, involvement of the transverse arch, and the presence of a significant collateral circulation. Phase-contrast angiography along the long axis of the poststenotic jet enables quantification of peak velocity and pressure gradient (using the modified Bernoulli equation) across the narrowed region. Collateral flow via the intercostal arteries can be estimated by subtracting stroke volume proximal to the coarctation from that close to the diaphragmatic hiatus.

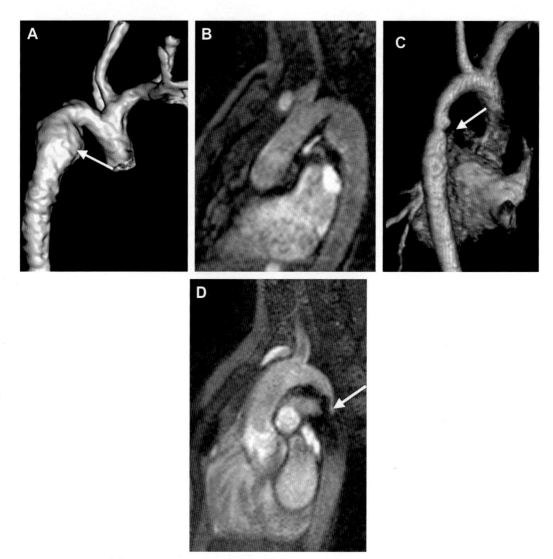

Fig. 7. Coarctation of the aorta status post–subclavian flap repair. (*A*) Volume-rendered image from gadolinium-enhanced 3D MR angiogram showing aneurysm at the site of previous repair (*arrow*). (*B*) Cine SSFP image demonstrating an aneurysm. (*C*) Volume-rendered image from gadolinium-enhanced 3D MR angiogram in different patient from *A* and *B* showing recoarctation at site of repair (*arrow*). (*D*) Sagittal oblique cine gradient-echo image demonstrating narrowing of the proximal conduit with a dephasing jet (*arrow*) arising from the stenosis.

Postoperative assessment

Complications occur after both surgical and percutaneous coarctation repairs and include re-coarctation, dissection, and aneurysm formation. Recurrent coarctation is more common with surgical repairs in infancy.[37] Aneurysm formation is most common following patch aortoplasty with a reported incidence of 27%. It is usually located at the opposite side to the patch (**Fig. 7**).[37,38] The risk of progressive aneurysmal dilatation and subsequent rupture is highest when the ratio between the caliber of the aneurysm and the caliber of the diaphragmatic aorta exceeds 1.5. It is more common in cases associated with Turner syndrome and bicuspid valves.[38] Stent migration and fracture are unique complications of percutaneous procedures for the coarctation of aorta repair. Late dissection at the repair site is a rare complication of both percutaneous and surgical procedures.

Although MR artifact from percutaneously placed stents hinders the postoperative coarctation assessment, successful evaluation for complications requiring interventions can still be performed with MR imaging. Artifact from the stent itself allows stent migration to be easily demonstrated. Aneurysms around the stent can be seen on a black-blood morphologic sequence. Restenosis is suggested by an increase in peak systolic velocity distal to the stent and persistent forward flow during diastole. Dissections outside the stent will be seen on black-blood and gradient-echo sequences.[39] However, MR imaging cannot demonstrate stent fracture or the nature of in-stent stenosis.

The incidence of complications after coarctation repair mandates continuous imaging follow-up. Clinical examination coupled with MR imaging has been shown to be a cost-effective method of screening for complications after coarctation of aorta repair.[40]

SUMMARY

CMR is a valuable and noninvasive imaging modality in the preoperative and postoperative evaluation of pediatric patients with CHD. Ongoing technical advancements have the potential to not only alleviate compromises between coverage and temporal and spatial resolution, but also provide rapid and accurate morphologic and functional assessment in free-breathing pediatric patients with CHD.

REFERENCES

1. Pettersen E, Lindberg H, Smith HJ, et al. Left ventricular function in patients with transposition of the great arteries operated with atrial switch. Pediatr Cardiol 2008;29:597–603.
2. Uribe S, Muthurangu V, Boubertakh R, et al. Whole-heart cine MRI using real-time respiratory self-gating. Magn Reson Med 2007;57:606–13.
3. Sorensen TS, Korperich H, Greil GF, et al. Operator-independent isotropic three-dimensional magnetic resonance imaging for morphology in congenital heart disease. A validation study. Circulation 2004; 110:163–9.
4. Fenchel M, Greil GF, Martirosian P, et al. Three-dimensional morphological magnetic resonance imaging in infants and children with congenital heart disease. Pediatr Radiol 2006;36:1265–72.
5. Markl M, Draney MT, Hope MD, et al. Time-resolved 3-dimensional velocity mapping in the thoracic aorta: visualization of 3-directional blood flow patterns in healthy volunteers and patients. J Comput Assist Tomogr 2004;28:459–68.
6. Davarpanah AH, Chen YP, Kino A, et al. Accelerated two- and three-dimensional cine MR imaging of the heart by using a 32-channel coil. Radiology 2010; 254(1):98–108.
7. Krishnamurthy R, Slesnick TC, Browne LP, et al. Free breathing high temporal resolution time resolved contrast enhanced MRA (4D MRA) at high rates using keyhole SENSE CENTRA in congenital heart disease. Phoenix (AZ): Society of Cardiac MRI; 2010.
8. Robbers-Visser D, Jan Ten Harkel D, Kapusta L, et al. Usefulness of cardiac magnetic resonance imaging combined with low-dose dobutamine stress to detect an abnormal ventricular stress response in children and young adults after Fontan operation at young age. Am J Cardiol 2008;101:1657–62.
9. Roest AA, Helbing WA, Kunz P, et al. Exercise MR imaging in the assessment of pulmonary regurgitation and biventricular function in patients after tetralogy of Fallot repair. Radiology 2002; 223:204–11.
10. McVeigh ER. MRI of myocardial function: motion tracking techniques. Magn Reson Imaging 1996; 14:137–50.
11. Lillehei CW, Cohen M, Warden HE, et al. Direct vision intracardiac surgical correction of the tetralogy of Fallot, pentalogy of Fallot, and pulmonary atresia defects; report of first ten cases. Ann Surg 1955; 142(3):418–42.
12. Geva T, Greil GF, Marshall AC, et al. Gadolinium-enhanced 3-dimensional magnetic resonance angiography of pulmonary blood supply in patients with complex pulmonary stenosis or atresia: comparison with x-ray angiography. Circulation 2002;106(4):473–8.
13. Oosterhof T, van Straten A, Vliegen HW, et al. Preoperative thresholds for pulmonary valve replacement in patients with corrected tetralogy of Fallot using

cardiovascular magnetic resonance. Circulation 2007;116:545–51.

14. Therrien J, Provost Y, Merchant N, et al. Optimal timing for pulmonary valve replacement in adults after tetralogy of Fallot repair. Am J Cardiol 2005; 95:779–82.

15. Greil GF, Beerbaum P, Razavi R, et al. Imaging the right ventricle. Heart 2008;94:803–8.

16. Knauth AL, Gauvreau K, Powell AJ, et al. Ventricular size and function assessed by cardiac MRI predict major adverse clinical outcomes late after Tetralogy of Fallot repair. Heart 2008;94:211–6.

17. Bardo DM, Frankel DG, Applegate KE, et al. Hypoplastic left heart syndrome. Radiographics 2001; 21:705–17.

18. Alsoufi B, Bennetts J, Verma S, et al. New developments in the treatment of hypoplastic left heart syndrome. Pediatrics 2007;119:109–17.

19. Chuang ML, Hibberd MG, Salton CJ, et al. Importance of imaging method over imaging modality in noninvasive determination of left ventricular volumes and ejection fraction: assessment by two- and three-dimensional echocardiography and magnetic resonance imaging. J Am Coll Cardiol 2000;35: 477–84.

20. Grosse-Wortmann L, Yun TJ, Al-Radi O, et al. Borderline hypoplasia of the left ventricle in neonates: insights for decision making from functional assessment with magnetic resonance imaging. J Thorac Cardiovasc Surg 2008;136:1429–36.

21. Schwartz ML, Gauvreau K, Geva T. Predictors of outcome of biventricular repair in infants with multiple left heart obstructive lesions. Circulation 2001;104:682–7.

22. Brown DW, Gauvreau K, Powell AJ, et al. Cardiac magnetic resonance versus routine cardiac catheterization before bidirectional Glenn anastomosis in infants with functional single ventricle: a prospective randomized trial. Circulation 2007;116:2718–25.

23. Lloyd TR, Evans TC, Marvin WJ Jr. Morphologic determinants of coronary blood flow in the hypoplastic left heart syndrome. Am Heart J 1986;112:666–71.

24. Ro PS, Rychik J, Cohen MS, et al. Diagnostic assessment before Fontan operation in patients with bidirectional cavopulmonary anastomosis: are noninvasive methods sufficient? J Am Coll Cardiol 2004;44:184–7.

25. Prakash A, Khan MA, Hardy R, et al. A new diagnostic algorithm for assessment of patients with single ventricle before a Fontan operation. J Thorac Cardiovasc Surg 2009;138:917–23.

26. Fogel MA, Donofrio MT, Ramaciotti C, et al. Magnetic resonance and echocardiographic imaging of pulmonary artery size throughout stages of Fontan reconstruction. Circulation 1994;90:2927–36.

27. Fyler DC. Report of the New England Regional Infant Cardiac Program. Pediatrics 1980;65(Suppl):377.

28. Graham TP Jr, Bernard YD, Mellen BG, et al. Long-term outcome in congenitally corrected transposition of the great arteries: a multi-institutional study. J Am Coll Cardiol 2000;36:255–61.

29. Wernovsky G. Transposition of the great arteries. In: Allen HD, Gutgesell HP, Clark EB, et al, editors. Moss and Adams' heart disease in infants, children, and adolescents: including the fetus and young adult. 6th edition. Philadelphia: Lippincott, Williams and Wilkins; 2000. p. 1027–84.

30. Warnes CA, Williams RG, Bashore TM, et al. ACC/ AHA 2008 Guidelines for the Management of Adults with Congenital Heart Disease: executive summary—a report of the American College of Cardiology/American Heart Association Task Force on Practice Guidelines. Circulation 2008;118: 2395–451.

31. Bonhoeffer P, Bonnet D, Piechaud JF, et al. Long-term fate of the coronary arteries after the arterial switch operation in newborns with transposition of the great arteries. Heart 1996;76:274–9.

32. Taylor AM, Dymarkowski S, Hamaekers P, et al. MR coronary angiography and late-enhancement myocardial MR in children who underwent arterial switch surgery for transposition of great arteries. Radiology 2005;234:542–7.

33. Moons P, Gewillig M, Sluysmans T, et al. Long-term outcome up to 30 years after the Mustard or Senning operation: a nationwide multicentre study in Belgium. Heart 2004;90:307–13.

34. Babu-Naravan SV, Goktekin O, Moon JC, et al. Late gadolinium enhancement cardiovascular magnetic resonance of the systemic right ventricle in adults with previous atrial redirection surgery for transposition of the great arteries. Circulation 2005;111: 2091–8.

35. Abbruzzese PA, Aidala E. Aortic coarctation: an overview. J Cardiovasc Med (Hagerstown) 2007; 8(2):123–8.

36. Zabal C, Attie F, Buendía-Hernández, et al. The adult patient with native coarctation of the aorta: balloon angioplasty or primary stenting? Heart 2003;89:77–83.

37. Konen E, Merchant N, Provost Y, et al. Coarctation of the aorta before and after correction: the role of cardiovascular MRI. AJR Am J Roentgenol 2004; 182:1333–9.

38. Mendelsohn AM, Crowley DC, Lindauer A, et al. Rapid progression of aortic aneurysms after patch aortoplasty repair of coarctation of the aorta. J Am Coll Cardiol 1992;20:381–5.

39. Rosenthal E, Bell A. Optimal imaging after coarctation. Heart 2010;96:1169–71.

40. Therrien J, Thorne SA, Wright A, et al. Repaired coarctation: a "cost-effective" approach to identify complications in adults. J Am Coll Cardiol 2000;35: 997–1002.

Nuclear Medicine and Molecular Imaging of the Pediatric Chest: Current Practical Imaging Assessment

Frederick D. Grant, MD[a,b,*], S. Ted Treves, MD[a,b]

KEYWORDS

- Pediatric chest disease • Nuclear medicine
- Pediatric oncology • Pediatric cardiopulmonary disease
- Pediatric aerodigestive disorders

All of the currently available techniques of nuclear medicine can be used in children, but as the spectrum of chest disease is different in children compared with that of adults, the indications for nuclear medicine studies are broader and more varied in children than in adults. For example, in children myocardial perfusion imaging is performed for evaluation of congenital heart disease, but is used less frequently for evaluation of coronary artery disease. ^{18}F-Fluorodeoxyglucose positron emission tomography (FDG PET) is used more commonly for evaluation of neuroblastoma than primary lung tumors. Despite these differences, pediatric nuclear medicine studies use the same radiopharmaceuticals and imaging methods that are used in adults. During the past few decades, ^{99m}Tc-labeled radiopharmaceuticals that are imaged with a gamma camera have been the mainstay of pediatric nuclear medicine. As in adult nuclear medicine, the introduction of PET, mostly using ^{18}F-FDG, has transformed pediatric nuclear medicine and, in particular, pediatric nuclear oncology. Although the radiation exposure resulting from pediatric nuclear medicine studies has always been low, concerns about radiation dose have gained prominence in the past few years.

Attempts to standardize pediatric radiopharmaceutical doses and new imaging hardware and software will allow radiation doses to be decreased even further. This article reviews imaging techniques and clinical applications of nuclear medicine studies that currently are used to evaluate chest diseases in pediatric patients.

LUNG VENTILATION/PERFUSION IMAGING

Scintigraphic methods are available for imaging and quantifying both lung ventilation (V) and perfusion (Q). The most established indication for lung ventilation/perfusion (V/Q) scans has been the diagnosis of pulmonary embolism.[1] Although less common in children than in adults, pulmonary embolism remains an indication for ventilation/perfusion scintigraphy in pediatric nuclear medicine.[2] Other important indications for lung scintigraphy in children include: (1) quantitative evaluation of differential and regional lung perfusion in children with congenital heart disease[3]; (2) evaluation of lung volumes and ventilation in patients with bronchial or parenchymal lung diseases[4]; and (3) identification of ventilation/perfusion mismatches in patients with developmental or acquired lung disease.[5,6]

[a] Division of Nuclear Medicine and Molecular Imaging, Department of Radiology, Children's Hospital Boston, Pavilion 2, 300 Longwood Avenue, Boston, MA 02115, USA
[b] Joint Program in Nuclear Medicine, Harvard Medical School, Boston, MA, USA
* Corresponding author. Division of Nuclear Medicine and Molecular Imaging, Department of Radiology, Children's Hospital Boston, Pavilion 2, 300 Longwood Avenue, Boston, MA 02115.
E-mail address: frederick.grant@childrens.harvard.edu

Radiol Clin N Am 49 (2011) 1025–1051
doi:10.1016/j.rcl.2011.06.012
0033-8389/11/$ – see front matter © 2011 Elsevier Inc. All rights reserved.

Techniques

Little patient preparation is needed before performing lung scintigraphy. Some guidelines suggest that patients should be treated to optimize control of acute or chronic airway disease before nonurgent lung scintigraphy.[7] Such prestudy preparation may decrease the likelihood that regional airway obstruction will interfere with interpretation of a study, but it is not done routinely.

99mTc-macroaggregated albumin lung perfusion

Lung perfusion scans are performed with 99mTc-labeled macroaggregated albumin (MAA). 99mTc-MAA (particle size 20–100 μm) injected into the systemic venous system circulates through the right heart into the pulmonary circulation and is trapped within the capillary beds of the lungs.[8] The distribution of 99mTc-MAA within the lungs reflects differential and regional blood flow, and region-of-interest analysis can be performed for quantitative assessment of lung perfusion. The adult dose of approximately 500,000 particles of radiolabeled MAA results in temporary occlusion of approximately 1 per 1000 capillaries. The particles have a biological half-life of a few hours[9] and have essentially no physiologic effect on normal lung function. However, a smaller number of particles is recommended for children or patients with underlying pulmonary hypertension.[10] In pediatric patients who may have a shunt from the pulmonary to systemic circulation (ie, a right-to-left shunt), a smaller number of particles should be used because of the potential for penetration of MAA particles into the systemic circulation. As few as 10,000 particles are needed for the evaluation of differential lung perfusion in infants with congenital heart disease, but at least 60,000 to 100,000 particles may be needed to ensure uniform images when higher-quality images are needed for localization of a possible pulmonary embolism.[7,11]

133Xe lung ventilation

There are several commercially available systems for inhaled administration of 133Xe gas for imaging lung ventilation. Many of these methods require some degree of cooperation from the patient, but 133Xe gas can be administered successfully to patients with limited cooperation, such as infants, and to patients intubated with an endotracheal tube. One advantage of this method is the ability to perform quantitative dynamic ventilation studies.[12] When a single breath of 133Xe gas is inhaled, its distribution in the lungs corresponds to regional ventilation. When 133Xe gas is administered with a rebreathing system, the gas can reach equilibrium within the airways of the lungs, and lung images will demonstrate the distribution of lung volume.[11] Once the patient is no longer rebreathing 133Xe, continued imaging during the washout phase is useful for identifying regional air trapping within the lungs.[13] One logistical constraint to the use of 133Xe gas for assessing lung ventilation is the requirement for trapping and exhaust of exhaled 133Xe gas.

99mTc-labeled aerosol for lung ventilation

A possible alternative to inhaled gas for lung ventilation scans is the use of radiolabeled aerosolized particles that are deposited within the airways. The most commonly used aerosol in the United States is aerosolized 99mTc-labeled diethylenetriamine penta-acetic acid (DTPA).[14] Because aerosolized DTPA persists in the lung airways, images can be acquired in multiple projections, but dynamic ventilation studies cannot be performed.[15] Persistence of tracer in the lung requires that, for a combined ventilation/perfusion scan, the second study (typically the perfusion study) be performed with a higher administered dose of radiopharmaceutical.[7] Another aerosolized ventilation agent, 99mTc-labeled carbon nanoparticles (Technigas), is not available in the United States, but has been used extensively in many centers throughout the world.[16] One potential limitation with these agents is the deposition of particles in the large airways, which can interfere with interpretation of lung images. Particles that are deposited in the throat can be swallowed, and tracer accumulation in the esophagus and stomach also can interfere with interpretation of lung images.

Pulmonary Embolism

As in adults,[17] ventilation/perfusion scans have been replaced largely by computed tomographic (CT) pulmonary angiography for the diagnosis of pulmonary embolism in most pediatric patients.[18–22] Ventilation/perfusion scans typically are performed in pediatric patients who have contraindications to CT angiography, such as an allergy to iodinated contrast, renal disease, or special concerns about radiation dose.[23] As in adults, the diagnosis of pulmonary embolism in children typically is based on the modified PIOPED (Prospective Evaluation of Pulmonary Embolism Diagnosis) II criteria.[1] However, the use of these criteria has never been fully validated in children. Recent reports of a high rate of pulmonary embolism in children receiving chronic lipid-containing hyperalimentation suggest that pulmonary embolism may be underdiagnosed in this population, but the appropriate clinical approach has not been determined.[24] Follow-up ventilation/perfusion scans can be used to confirm resolution of the embolic perfusion defects in the lungs. This approach may be most useful in patients at risk for recurrent pulmonary embolism, and in whom identification of new perfusion defects could be complicated by residual defects from prior embolic events.

Recently increased concerns about pediatric radiation exposure, particularly with CT angiography, have led to a reappraisal of the role of ventilation/perfusion scans.[23] Balancing the higher effective radiation dose of CT pulmonary angiography is the higher level of anatomic detail provided by this study. Notwithstanding concerns about the clinical meaning or significance of some small angiographic findings, this higher sensitivity of CT pulmonary angiography has been a major reason why it has replaced ventilation/perfusion scans in both pediatric and adult patients with suspected pulmonary embolism.

Another reason for the preference for CT angiography may the higher comfort level that many radiologists may have when interpreting a CT, compared with the lower level of certainty they sometimes have with ventilation/perfusion scans. However, in children, ventilation/perfusion scan may have a low rate of indeterminate studies.[2] Recent experience in adults has shown that the use of single-photon emission computed tomography (SPECT) for acquiring ventilation or perfusion images can increase both diagnostic accuracy and reader confidence in the evaluation for pulmonary embolism.[25] New diagnostic criteria, similar to PIOPED, are needed for diagnosing pulmonary embolism by lung SPECT.[26] Little experience with pulmonary SPECT has been reported in children. However, if SPECT is shown to provide similar improvements in diagnostic accuracy in children, then renewed use of ventilation/perfusion scans to diagnose pulmonary embolism could have the potential to decrease radiation exposure in children requiring evaluation for pulmonary embolism.[27]

Congenital Heart Disease

Quantitative lung perfusion scans can be used to determine differential pulmonary perfusion to each lung or to assess regional perfusion within the lungs.[11] For example, in patients with pulmonary atresia or with stenosis of a main or branch pulmonary artery, differential lung perfusion can be assessed as part of diagnosis and for routine follow-up after surgical repair.[3] With pulmonary venous occlusion or anomalous pulmonary venous return, capillary perfusion as assessed by ^{99m}Tc-MAA will reflect capillary blood flow and can provide a measure of the severity of disease. In patients undergoing balloon catheter dilation or stenting of a pulmonary vessel, postcatheterization differential lung perfusion is helpful in demonstrating improved regional blood flow and in confirming that instrumentation did not precipitate vessel occlusion (**Fig. 1**).

Pediatric patients with congenital heart disease also may have anomalous patterns of blood flow as the result of surgery. For example, in patients treated with cavopulmonary anastomosis by placement of a bidirectional Glenn shunt, venous return from the upper extremities flows to the lungs, while venous return from the inferior vena cava is returned to the systemic circulation.[28]

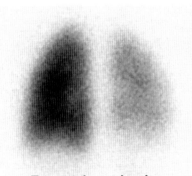 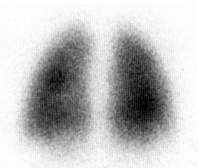

Pre-catheterization   Post-catheterization

Fig. 1. Lung perfusion scans (posterior images) in a 3-year-old girl with truncus arteriosus surgically repaired with a conduit from right atrium to pulmonary artery. Before catheterization (Pre-catheterization), a posterior image shows relative lung perfusion was left lung 77%, right lung 23%. After catheterization with balloon dilation of the conduit and left pulmonary artery (Post-catheterization), the relative lung perfusion is left lung 48% and right lung 52%. This change demonstrates that the balloon dilation procedure resulted in equalization of perfusion between the two lungs.

The pattern of perfusion seen on a perfusion lung scan will depend on the site of intravenous administration of tracer. Therefore, it is important to confirm the expected cardiopulmonary anatomy before performing a perfusion lung scan. In some cases, direct discussion with the referring physician may be necessary to determine the site of MAA administration.

Bronchial and Parenchymal Lung Disease

A lung ventilation scan can be used to quantitate differential or regional lung ventilation in patients. For example, ventilation scans can help define pulmonary function in patients with airway disease or primary lung disease, such as cystic fibrosis, bronchiectasis, or pulmonary fibrosis.[5] In patients with obstructive lung diseases, such as congenital lobar emphysema, dynamic ventilation scans can demonstrate functional airway obstruction or air trapping.[4]

In some clinical situations, a combined lung ventilation/perfusion scan is useful to compare relative ventilation and perfusion or to demonstrate a ventilation/perfusion mismatch. However, these studies must be interpreted carefully. If an airway is obstructed, the resulting hypoxia can lead to pulmonary vasoconstriction and shunting of blood flow away from the affected lung segment. Therefore, in cases of primary respiratory disease, matching ventilation and perfusion defects may reflect vasoconstriction in response to regional hypoxia.[7] However, the airways are not regulated by regional blood flow, and obstruction of a segmental pulmonary artery will not affect airflow, resulting in a ventilation/perfusion mismatch.

Ventilation/perfusion scans are used to follow pediatric patients after repair of a congenital diaphragmatic hernia (**Fig. 2**).[29] With repair of the diaphragmatic hernia, the affected lung expands and ventilation volume increases, but the response of the pulmonary blood flow may depend on the age of the patient. If a congenital diaphragmatic hernia is repaired early in life, it is possible that the affected lung might undergo some degree of further maturation. With development of additional capillary beds, pulmonary perfusion may more closely match ventilation.[30] However, the extent of this growth is unpredictable, and a ventilation/perfusion scan can help determine the degree of mismatch.[31] Combined assessment of pulmonary perfusion and ventilation also may be useful in pediatric patients with structural abnormalities of the thorax, such as pectus excavatum or severe spinal scoliosis.[32]

Pulmonary Shunting

During the performance of a lung perfusion study, a right-to-left shunt is demonstrated by systemic penetration of administered ^{99m}Tc-MAA. Shunted MAA enters the systemic circulation where it is trapped within capillary beds of other organs. MAA trapping reflects relative blood flow to an organ, so that organs receiving a greater fraction of cardiac output, such as kidneys and brain, will show accumulation of a larger amount of MAA (**Fig. 3**). Therefore in patients who may have a right-to-left shunt, the use of a smaller number of particles is advised to diminish systemic microembolization of MAA particles.[11]

Patients who have undergone a cavopulmonary anastomosis, such as a Glenn shunt, develop

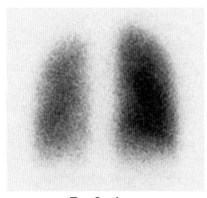
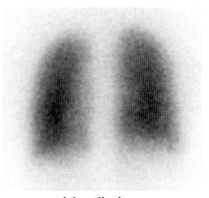

Perfusion   **Ventilation**

Fig. 2. Lung ventilation/perfusion study (posterior images) in a 9-year-old boy with history of left congenital diaphragmatic hernia repaired as an infant. Relative lung perfusion is left 30%, right 70%, but relative lung ventilation is left 49%, right 51%, demonstrating a ventilation/perfusion mismatch in the left lung. This mismatch suggests that correction of the congenital diaphragmatic hernia expanded the lung volume, but did not correct the developmental perfusion abnormality in the left lung.

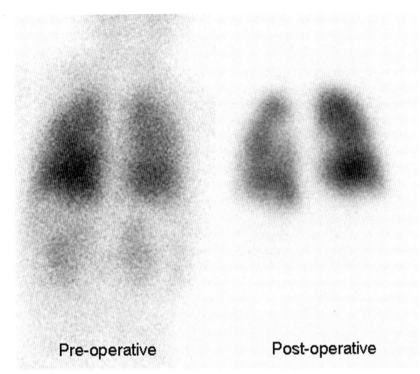

Pre-operative   Post-operative

Fig. 3. Lung perfusion scans (posterior image) in a 1-year-old girl with tetralogy of Fallot with pulmonary atresia, atrial septal defect, and ventricular septal defect. Before surgery (Pre-operative), the relative lung perfusion was left lung 53%, right lung 47%. Systemic penetration of tracer reflected a moderate right-to-left shunt. After surgery (Post-operative), the relative lung perfusion is left 37%, right 63%, and the left-to-right shunt has been corrected.

intrapulmonary arteriovenous shunting, possibly reflecting dysregulated pulmonary vasodilation.[28] In patients with a bidirectional Glenn shunt, the degree of right-to-left shunt may differ for systemic venous return into the superior and inferior venae cavae. In some circumstances, it may be appropriate to perform 2 lung perfusion scans and calculate the shunt after administration of ^{99m}Tc-MAA into either the upper or lower systemic venous circulation.[33]

Intrapulmonary arteriovenous shunting may be seen as a complication of chronic liver disease. As with cardiac shunts, an intrapulmonary shunt is characterized by systemic penetration of tracer during a perfusion lung scan.[34] A recent report showed a lung perfusion scan to be more sensitive than contrast-enhanced echocardiography in identifying physiologically significant intrapulmonary shunts in children with chronic liver disease.[35]

ESOPHAGEAL AND GASTRIC IMAGING

Nuclear medicine provides several different studies to evaluate the function of the lower pharynx and esophagus, including the gastric emptying study ("milk scan"), the salivagram, and the esophageal transit study. Some patients undergoing these studies have primarily symptoms of the upper gastrointestinal tract, such as impaired esophageal transit or vomiting. A gastric emptying study may provide a definite diagnosis in infants with suspected gastroesophageal reflux disease. However, other pediatric indications for one of these nuclear medicine studies can be upper airway disease or pulmonary disease. Symptoms such as wheezing, chronic cough, or recurrent pneumonia may reflect tracheobronchial aspiration.[36]

Gastric Emptying Study

Technique
To perform a liquid gastric emptying study,[37,38] a small dose (0.015 mCi/kg, 0.2–1.5 mCi) of ^{99m}Tc-labeled sulfur colloid is mixed with milk or formula. Ideally the gastric emptying study is performed with the child's usual formula. In some circumstances juice, or even water, can be used, but the sulfur colloid is more likely to remain suspended and widely distributed in milk or protein-based formula. For patients taking food by mouth, the radiolabeled formula is offered in a bottle or cup, as appropriate to the patient's development.

The volume of formula should either replicate the patient's typical feeding volume or approximate the volume that has been associated with symptoms. For patients receiving nutrition through a nasogastric tube or percutaneous gastrostomy, the radiolabeled formula may be administered by these routes. A nasogastric tube ideally should be removed after feeding, as it may disrupt the integrity of the gastroesophageal junction and promote gastroesophageal reflux. A false-positive study also can result from reflux of formula through the tube, which may mimic gastroesophageal reflux. In certain clinical circumstances it may be appropriate to leave a gastroesophageal tube in place. A feeding tube emptying into the duodenum or small bowel cannot be used for a gastroesophageal imaging study. The position of a feeding tube should be known before it is used for a gastric emptying study.

Due to the rapid gastric emptying of a liquid meal, dynamic images are acquired over 1 hour, while the patient is supine. It is nearly impossible for a child of any age to remain stationary in an upright position for the 1 hour of dynamic imaging.

Even small amounts of gastroesophageal reflux can be identified with the gastric emptying study. The severity of reflux can be graded by frequency of reflux and by the level that gastric contents reach within the esophagus. In addition, quantitative assessment of gastric emptying may indicate if reflux or regurgitation is exacerbated by prolonged retention of a meal.

Indication for gastric emptying study

Although the primary indication for most gastric emptying studies is assessment of gastric function, the gastric emptying study also can be used to identify and characterize gastroesophageal reflux (**Fig. 4**). In patients with poor airway protection, gastroesophageal reflux rarely may lead to tracheobronchial aspiration of gastric contents and result in either a chemical pneumonitis or infectious pneumonia. In pediatric patients with recurrent pneumonia, an abnormal milk scan provides presumptive evidence that gastroesophageal reflux is leading to aspiration pneumonia. Aspiration of radiolabeled gastric contents during the gastric emptying study is very rarely

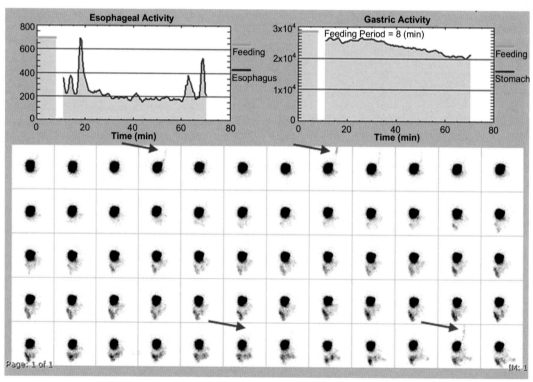

Fig. 4. Gastric emptying and gastroesophageal reflux study (milk study) in a 3-month-old girl with continued respiratory distress after repair of a tracheo-esophageal fistula. A salivagram was normal. After administration of 40mL of Tc-99m labeled formula by percutaneous gastric feeding tube, there are 4 episodes of gastroesophageal reflux (*arrows*). After 1 hour, there is limited gastric emptying (74% residual), but after 2 hours (not shown) most of the meal emptied from the stomach. A gastric emptying study performed with a liquid meal is a sensitive method for detecting gastroesophageal reflux.

demonstrated, but suggests that aspiration of gastric contents is occurring.[39] Unfortunately, these patients are at risk of pneumonia or respiratory compromise if they were to aspirate gastric contents during the study. Therefore, for the evaluation of pediatric patients in whom there is strong clinical suspicion of aspiration, it can be more appropriate to evaluate first with a radionuclide salivagram.

Radionuclide Salivagram

Technique

To perform a salivagram, a small drop of saline (approximately 100 μL) containing ^{99m}Tc-labeled sulfur colloid is placed sublingually or on the back of the tongue.[39] Sodium pertechnetate should not be used, as it is absorbed by oral and gastric mucosa. Images typically are acquired as a dynamic study over 1 hour. In a normal child, there is rapid transit of swallowed tracer though the esophagus to the stomach. Aspirated tracer can be seen accumulating at the carina and possibly spreading into the primary and secondary bronchi. In an individual with a high clinical suspicion of aspiration, delayed images can be acquired if no aspiration is seen after the first hour of imaging. If essentially all tracer is rapidly cleared from the mouth before the end of imaging, administration of a second dose can be considered, at the discretion of the interpreting physician. If tracheobronchial aspiration is identified then imaging should not be stopped, as continued imaging may demonstrate spontaneous clearance of aspirated tracer from the airways. Spontaneous clearance of tracer during the hour of imaging suggests that tracer has not penetrated the airways beyond the level of ciliated bronchial mucosa, demonstrates normal mechanisms to clear the airway, and suggests a better prognosis for the patient.[40]

Indication for radionuclide salivagram

The radionuclide salivagram is a sensitive and specific imaging method for detecting tracheobronchial aspiration of oropharyngeal contents and oral secretions.[41] The primary clinical indication is the evaluation of aspiration pneumonia, but this study also may be helpful to investigate chronic cough, atypical wheezing, or nocturnal choking episodes, particularly in pediatric and young adult patients with neurologic impairment.[42] The goal of a salivagram is to determine whether the airway is protected from spontaneous aspiration of oral secretions (**Fig. 5**).

Tracheobronchial aspiration of oropharyngeal contents usually indicates that the airway cannot be protected even from normal oral secretions. Accumulation of tracer within the airways also can occur if there is a tracheoesophageal fistula.[43] Another rare cause of a false-positive study is accumulation of tracer in an esophageal diverticulum.[44] If a salivagram does not confirm clinically suspected aspiration, some investigators have suggested repeating the test with a larger volume of liquid,[45] but this approach has not entered routine clinical use.

The radionuclide salivagram can serve as a complementary or alternative study to contrast-based swallowing studies[46] and to gastroesophageal reflux studies. These other studies use larger volumes of barium contrast or radiolabeled meal with a potentially increased risk of aspiration during the study. Of these 3 studies, the radionuclide salivagram has the highest sensitivity for detecting tracheobronchial aspiration[38] and has the lowest radiation dose. If a patient is unable to

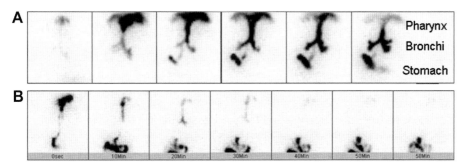

Fig. 5. Radionuclide salivagram. Radionuclide salivagrams detect tracheobronchial aspiration to determine if the airway is protected from aspiration of oropharyngeal contents. (*A*) In a 3-year-old girl with a mitochondrial disorder and frequent pneumonia, there is marked aspiration of pharyngeal contents into the trachea and branching secondary bronchi, indicating impaired protection of the airway. (*B*) In a 4-year-old boy with severe developmental delay and recurrent pneumonia, there is aspiration to the primary bronchi by 20 minutes, but by 40 minutes tracer has been cleared from the airways, indicating that the mechanisms for clearing the airway are intact and may protect the airway from aspirated material.

protect the airway from aspiration of oral secretions, identifying impaired swallowing or gastroesophageal reflux will be of secondary concern. Therefore, if the clinical concern is tracheobronchial aspiration or impaired airway protection, a radionuclide salivagram should be considered before performing other studies that require intake of larger volumes of barium contrast or radiolabeled meal.

Esophageal Transit Study

Technique

Most esophageal transit studies are performed with ^{99m}Tc-labeled sulfur colloid suspended in milk, juice, or water.[39] A solid bolus may cause greater symptoms, and may be retained in the esophagus if there is structural or functional esophageal disease. Most children are able to take up to 1 ounce (30 mL) of labeled fluid through a straw and then swallow on command.[39] Dynamic images are acquired while the patient sits upright, and region-of-interest analysis is used to map the transit of the bolus through the esophagus. Regions typically are placed over the upper, mid, and lower esophagus, and over the stomach. With normal esophageal transit, there should be anterograde transit of the radiolabeled bolus through the esophagus to the stomach. Esophageal transit of the bolus from pharynx to stomach may be as rapid as 1 second and should take no longer than 10 seconds.[47] Delayed, dyssynchronous, or retrograde transit indicates an abnormality of esophageal transit. The time-activity curves for each esophageal segment may help to localize the abnormality within the esophagus.[39] If there is normal esophageal transit of liquid bolus and the patient has no symptoms with a liquid bolus, then a repeat study may be performed with a small bolus (< one teaspoon) of soft solid food, such as scrambled egg,[48] cereal, or mashed potato.

Indication for radionuclide esophageal transit study

A radionuclide esophageal transit study can be complementary to other methods of assessing esophageal symptoms or evaluating esophageal function.[39,49] Most pediatric patients referred for nuclear medicine evaluation of esophageal transit already have undergone examination of the esophagus with direct visualization with endoscopy or indirect visualization with an upper gastrointestinal (GI) study. Endoscopy is useful in identifying an inflammatory process of the esophagus. Either endoscopy or an upper GI study may localize abnormal structural lesions of the esophagus. However, these studies cannot directly assess esophageal motility or function. Although esophageal manometry provides useful information for evaluation of primary esophageal motor disorders, a radionuclide esophageal transit study is useful in demonstrating the integrated affect of esophageal function on the transit of an ingested bolus of liquid or solid. The esophageal transit study may be particularly helpful for evaluating esophageal transit in pediatric patients with poorly defined symptoms that could be related to the esophagus. An esophageal transit study also provides a fast and noninvasive method to follow changes in esophageal function in pediatric patients with known disorders of esophageal transit. For example, an esophageal transit study can be used for follow-up in patients with a history of repaired esophageal atresia, with structural abnormalities such as achalasia or stricture, or with neuromotor diseases affecting esophageal function.[49,50]

MYOCARDIAL PERFUSION IMAGING

Myocardial perfusion imaging is among the most commonly performed nuclear medicine procedures in adults. The procedure is used less frequently in the practice of pediatric nuclear medicine, but is used to evaluate a variety of disorders of coronary artery circulation in children and young adults.

Technique

Myocardial perfusion imaging depends on the comparison of perfusion at rest and after stress. Stress protocols for myocardial perfusion testing must be clinically useful, as well as appropriate to age and postsurgical anatomy.[51] However, there are no consensus guidelines for the performance of exercise stress testing specific to children.[52] Pediatric studies have rarely used pharmacologic stress, but may use a wide variety of exercise stress protocols. Most use a treadmill, but a cycle ergometer can be more appropriate for some children.[52] Patients with surgically repaired congenital heart disease may have anatomic or physiologic limitations in exercise capacity.[53] Either ^{99m}Tc-sestamibi or ^{99m}Tc-tetrafosmin is appropriate for pediatric myocardial perfusion studies.

PET agents for myocardial imaging include the potassium analogue [82]Rb–rubidium chloride[54] and ^{13}N-ammonia.[55] Neither has been well studied in pediatric patients, in part due to the short physical half-life of each agent and the resulting need for proximity to a medical cyclotron. In addition to these logistical problems, the short physical half-life requires the use of pharmacologic stress methods that have not been well validated in children. The improved imaging characteristics of PET and the ability to quantitatively assess myocardial blood flow can make these agents alternatives for myocardial perfusion studies, especially in larger patients, and their use is likely to increase in pediatrics.

Pediatric Coronary Artery Disease

Although uncommon, coronary artery disease occurs in high-risk populations such as children with obesity or type 1 diabetes mellitus.[56] Some illnesses of childhood predispose to coronary artery disease. For example, in young children myocardial perfusion can be disrupted by Kawasaki disease, and aneurysmal dilation of coronary arteries due to Kawasaki disease is a risk factor for development of myocardial ischemia or infarction.[57,58] Because of their increased risk for myocardial ischemia, these patients may require follow-up for decades[59] even in the absence of coronary artery aneurysms.[60] Premature coronary artery disease can occur in children with systemic lupus erythematosus.[61] In a recent prospective study, myocardial perfusion imaging identified abnormal perfusion in approximately one-quarter of patients with lupus or primary antiphospholipid syndrome.[62]

Patients with anomalous coronary arteries are at risk for premature coronary ischemia and sudden death.[63] These patients come to clinical attention when they develop arrhythmias or other symptoms of myocardial ischemia. However, only one-quarter of these patients present with exertional chest pain.[64] In other patients, identification of an anomalous coronary artery is made as an incidental finding on an unrelated imaging study. In patients with the incidental finding of an anomalous coronary artery, myocardial perfusion imaging can identify exercise-induced myocardial ischemia and can help determine whether structural abnormalities in coronary arteries have functional importance.

Postsurgical Evaluation of Coronary Perfusion

Reimplantation of coronary arteries into the aorta is a necessary part of some cardiac surgical procedures, but the site of surgical reimplantation into the aorta is at risk for coronary artery stenosis. For example, the arterial switch operation procedure typically includes reimplantation of coronary arteries into the aorta. These patients are at increased risk for myocardial perfusion abnormalities with[65] or without[66] coronary artery obstruction, and they may require coronary revascularization.[67] When performing myocardial perfusion in pediatric patients with congenital heart disease, care must be taken to correctly identify the ventricles pumping the systemic and pulmonary circulation. For example, the systemic ventricle may be on the right in patients with congenitally corrected transposition.[68]

Cardiac Transplant Evaluation

Cardiac transplantation is another risk factor for premature coronary artery disease in children.[69] Up to 30% of pediatric cardiac transplant patients may develop coronary artery vasculopathy.[70] This risk likely is multifactorial, including the effects of immunosuppressive drugs[71] and older donor age.[72] These patients rarely have typical symptoms of myocardial ischemia, and require long-term follow-up, including myocardial perfusion imaging.[70]

Cardiac Function Studies

Two nuclear medicine studies for assessment of cardiac function are radionuclide ventriculography and the cardiac shunt study.

RADIONUCLIDE VENTRICULOGRAPHY
Technique

To perform a radionuclide ventriculogram, the blood pool is labeled with ^{99m}Tc-labeled red blood cells, and imaging of the heart is gated to the cardiac cycle. Images are acquired through multiple cardiac cycles, and these images are summed to produce the gated ventriculogram. The gated images show regional wall motion of the ventricles, and region-of-interest analysis is used to determine the ejection fraction of each ventricle. The radionuclide ventriculogram is an accurate and highly reproducible method of determining left ventricular ejection fraction.[73]

Indication for Radionuclide Ventriculography

Radionuclide ventriculography provides a noninvasive method to assess regional and global ventricular function. Indications for radionuclide ventriculography include congenital heart disease, myocarditis, and myocardial dysfunction. Patients receiving chemotherapy regimens that put them at risk of myocardial damage can have left ventricular function assessed as a baseline, during treatment, and as a follow-up study. In children, the current practice seems to use echocardiography to evaluate cardiac function, with nuclear ventriculography as a complementary technique.[3] Nuclear ventriculography still has the advantage of providing quantitative assessment of the physiologic consequences of cardiac disease.[74] An alternative method for evaluating myocardial function is to assess wall motion with gated myocardial perfusion imaging.[75] For example, in patients with thalassemia major, gated myocardial perfusion imaging demonstrates wall motion abnormalities in the absence of myocardial perfusion abnormalities.[76] In patients with myocarditis, gated myocardial perfusion imaging can demonstrate perfusion defects as well as ventricular dysfunction.[77]

CARDIAC SHUNT EVALUATION
Technique

To perform a cardiac shunt study, ^{99m}Tc-pertechnetate is rapidly administered in a small bolus into the systemic circulation. The tracer circulates through the pulmonary circulation to the left heart, and a left-to-right shunt is identified by detecting the rapid recirculation of tracer from the left heart back to the lungs.[73] Calculation of a left-to-right

shunt can be aided by deconvolution analysis of the time-activity curve, which is best performed with software developed specifically for this task (**Fig. 6**). A right-to-left shunt also can be detected and quantitated with this method.[3] However, a lung perfusion study using ^{99m}Tc-MAA is an easier and more routine method for assessing a right-to-left shunt.

Indication for Cardiac Shunt Study

Cardiac shunt studies are performed for the specific indication of determining the presence and magnitude of a shunt between the systemic and pulmonary circulation (left-to-right shunt). The cardiac shunt study is a quantitative, but noninvasive, method that can be useful in any patient with a suspected left-to-right shunt, for example, those at risk for developing Eisenmeger physiology. Most commonly, this is performed in a patient with a congenital heart disease (see **Fig. 6**)

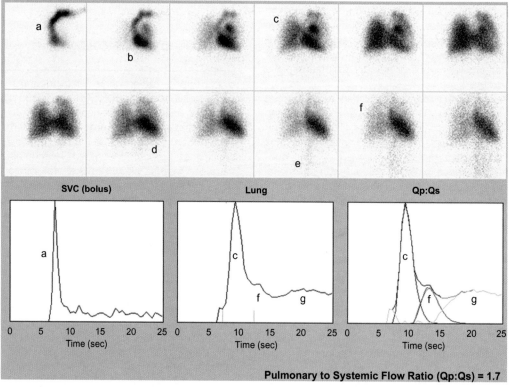

Pulmonary to Systemic Flow Ratio (Qp:Qs) = 1.7

Fig. 6. Cardiac shunt study. A cardiac shunt study quantitates a left-to-right shunt by calculating the recirculation of tracer from the left heart to the lungs. In a 7-year-old boy with a ventricular septal defect, a small bolus of tracer is injected into an indwelling catheter in the left upper arm. Tracer flows through the superior vena cava (a) to the right ventricle (b) and then to the lungs (c). On return to the left ventricle (d), most tracer enters the aorta (e) and the systemic circulation throughout the body. A fraction of tracer is shunted to the right ventricle and recirculates through the pulmonary circulation to the lungs (f). Normal recirculation of the lungs (g) occurs from bronchial arteries and venous return of tracer to the right heart. Deconvolution analysis is used to determine that the ratio of pulmonary flow (Qp) to systemic flow (Qs) is 1.7, indicating a mild left-to-right shunt.

such as a septal defect or truncus arteriosus, or in a patient with suspected aortopulmonary collaterals.[3]

LYMPHOSCINTIGRAPHY
Technique

Lymphoscintigraphy may be performed with a variety of radiolabeled nanoparticles.[78] In the United States, filtered ^{99m}Tc-labeled sulfur colloid is the most commonly used tracer. After intradermal injection of the tracer, serial images are acquired to document normal or abnormal lymphatic transit.[78] Normal lymphatic transit will carry tracer centrally to the thoracic duct and then into the systemic circulation, which is confirmed by tracer accumulation in the liver. With lymphatic obstruction, there will be an absence of tracer accumulation in lymph node stations proximal to the obstruction. In the absence of lymphangiectasia, tracer accumulation in the abdomen or thorax strongly suggests a thoracic duct leak.

Indication for Lymphoscintigraphy

Radionuclide imaging of the lymphatic system (lymphoscintigraphy) can be helpful in the evaluation of patients with suspected abnormal lymphatic drainage (Fig. 7). Abnormal lymphatic drainage may result from congenital lymphangiectasia or be due to a lymphatic duct leak. In patients with congenital lymphangiectasia, severe dilation of lymphatic channels results in poor lymphatic drainage of the affected region.[79] Congenital lymphangiectasia may be generalized or may affect only the lungs, abdomen, or extremities. Infants with involvement of the trunk present with chylous ascites or chylothorax, while involvement of the extremities presents as lymphedema. The mechanism of congenital lymphangiectasia is not known, but may occur as a primary developmental defect or secondary to lymphatic duct agenesis or obstruction. Chylothorax also may occur with a thoracic duct leak resulting from damage to the thoracic duct during cardiac or gastroesophageal surgery.[80] Obstruction of major lymphatic ducts can occur as a complication of thrombus in the left subclavian vein or right internal jugular vein.[80,81] Lymphoscintigraphy can confirm abnormal lymphatic drainage, and may help determine whether abnormal drainage represents lymphatic duct obstruction or lymphatic leak (Fig. 8).[82]

ONCOLOGY IMAGING

For many pediatric tumors, the site of primary or metastatic disease may be located in the chest. In children, the most common solid tumors that occur in the chest are lymphomas, neuroblastoma, and musculoskeletal sarcomas.[83] Evaluation of pediatric tumors frequently involves multiple imaging studies and, as in adults, the most common indication for ^{18}F-FDG PET is the evaluation of malignancy. Primary lung tumors are rare in children, but when they occur FDG PET may have a role in the management of these tumors. In children, ^{99m}Tc-labeled methyl diphosphonate (^{99m}Tc-MDP) bone scan and ^{123}I-labeled metaiodobenzylguanidine (^{123}I-mIBG) scan continue to be

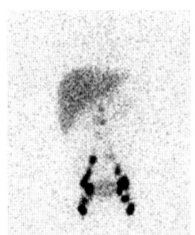
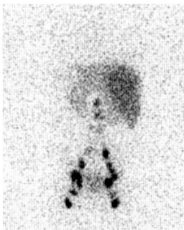

Fig. 7. Normal lymphoscintigraphy. Lymphoscintigraphy can be helpful in identifying a congenital or acquired abnormality in lymphatic drainage. In a 3-year-old boy with a protein-losing enteropathy, normal lymphatic drainage is demonstrated after intradermal administration of ^{99m}Tc–sulfur colloid in the feet. By 4 hours, appropriate tracer accumulation is seen in inguinal, pelvic, and retroperitoneal lymph nodes. Tracer accumulation in the liver confirms patency of the thoracic duct.

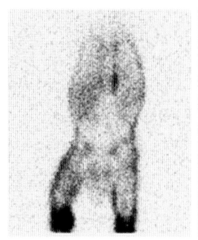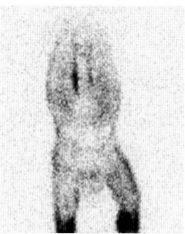

Fig. 8. Lymphoscintigraphy in a 1-year-old boy with chronic pleural effusions resulting from congenital lymphangiectasia. After intradermal administration of ^{99m}Tc–sulfur colloid in the feet, prominent cutaneous tracer accumulation in the lower legs indicates abnormal lymphatic drainage. Little tracer is seen in the lymph nodes of the trunk, but tracer accumulation is seen in prominent bilateral thoracic ducts and the chest cavity. Tracer accumulation in the liver confirms a nonobstructive disruption of lymphatic drainage.

important for evaluating specific tumors, such as neuroblastoma. At present, gallium scans are rarely indicated, and in the evaluation of Hodgkin disease, gallium scans have been replaced by FDG PET.[84]

Techniques

^{18}F-FDG PET and PET/CT

The clinical introduction of PET and PET/CT, as well as ready commercial availability of ^{18}F-FDG, has transformed the clinical practice of nuclear medicine and molecular imaging. This change has been most marked in oncology imaging, where ^{18}F-FDG has been widely used for diagnoses, staging, follow-up, and assessing the response to therapy for nearly all forms of malignancy.[85] During the past decade, the practice of PET imaging has evolved, so that most departments currently use integrated PET/CT scanners that acquire images in only 3-dimensional mode.[86]

Patient preparation is important for successful completion of a technically adequate PET.[87,88] Patients should be fasting for at least 4 hours before administration of ^{18}F-FDG and should remain fasting during the 1-hour uptake period. In selected circumstances, patient satisfaction and cooperation can be improved if the patient is allowed to eat a small snack just before the start of imaging. Similarly, if a small infant is to be imaged without sedation, then allowing the infant to breastfeed or take a bottle just before imaging may help them settle or even sleep during the study. Unless the study is to be performed under sedation or anesthesia, patients should be encouraged to continue to drink water before the study, but cautioned to avoid sweetened or caffeine-containing beverages. Before administration of FDG, a blood glucose level should be checked, preferably by using a glucometer to assay a finger-stick sample of capillary blood.

Depending on the season and the climate, brown adipose tissue uptake can be seen in up to one-third of all children undergoing FDG PET.[89] A variety of measures is used in an attempt to minimize FDG uptake in brown adipose tissue. Heating in a warm room at least half an hour before FDG administration and for the duration of the uptake period will decrease the incidence of significant brown adipose uptake from 33% to 9%.[89] Other maneuvers that have been used in an attempt to decrease FDG uptake in brown adipose tissue include oral administration of a low dose of a β-blocker such as propranolol,[90] intravenous administration of an opioid such as fentanyl,[91] or restriction to a high-fat diet for 12 hours before the study.[92]

Accurate interpretation of FDG PET of the chest requires an understanding of the normal physiologic uptake of FDG PET in children (**Fig. 9**). Physiologic uptake in skeletal muscle or brown adipose tissue can obscure sites of disease and can decrease the confidence of the interpreting physician.[87,93] Physiologic uptake of FDG in specific organs, such as the heart or thymus, can affect interpretation of FDG PET of the chest.[94] In children, cardiac FDG uptake can be variable.

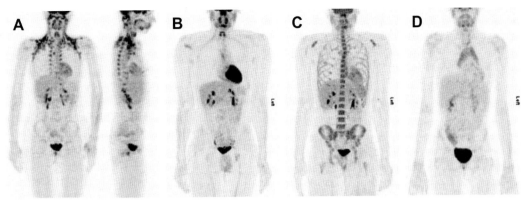

Fig. 9. Patterns of physiologic uptake of ^{18}F-FDG in children. Interpretation of FDG PET in children requires recognition of uptake patterns that may reflect physiologic uptake of ^{18}F-FDG. (*A*) FDG uptake in brown adipose tissue is seen in a typical distribution that can include brown adipose tissue in posterior cervical, supraclavicular, axillary, paravertebral, paracardiac, and suprarenal locations. Muscle uptake can reflect specific types of physical activity, such as increased FDG uptake in the thumb after use of a personal digital assistant during the uptake period. (*B*) FDG uptake in the heart is not consistent among patients, and some individuals may have intense myocardial uptake of FDG. Uptake likely reflects glucose metabolism, but cannot be predicted from the blood glucose level. (*C*) Myocardial uptake of FDG may be different on subsequent scans in the same individual. In this repeat scan, minimal FDG uptake in the heart probably reflects an alteration in glucose metabolism compared with (*B*). Widespread uptake in the expected locations of bone marrow in both the axial and appendicular skeleton may reflect physiologic activation or posttreatment stimulation. (*D*) Diffuse uptake in the thymus rarely indicates disease, and more likely reflects physiologic activation or posttreatment stimulation ("thymic rebound").

Surreptitious feeding before the study can cause insulin-mediated myocardial uptake of FDG, but intense myocardial uptake also can be seen even after well-documented fasting. Additional dietary interventions have been used in an attempt to decrease myocardial FDG uptake in adults,[95] especially those with disease located near the heart, but little experience has been reported in children. Therefore, adequate patient preparation is essential when performing FDG PET. For example, patients should be instructed to fast for at least 4 hours before imaging. In infants and small children, adequate fasting can be a challenge, and may require coordinating the imaging schedule with an infant's eating and sleeping routine.

FDG PET typically is unable to detect small tumors or metastases in the lungs, and therefore other methods such as chest CT are necessary for early identification of lung metastases. Because the CT portion of a PET/CT typically is acquired with tidal breathing to match the acquisition of the PET, a separate diagnostic CT obtained at full inspiration may be necessary to fully evaluate for pulmonary metastases.[88]

mIBG tumor imaging

Iodine-131–labeled mIBG was developed as an imaging agent for the detection and localization of pheochromocytoma,[96] but soon after its introduction it was used to image neuroblastoma.[97] In the past, mIBG labeled with iodine-123 was used by some centers,[98] but the use of ^{123}I-mIBG did not become widespread until AdreView (GE Medical) was approved for clinical use in children. Compared with ^{131}I-mIBG, ^{123}I-mIBG provides better image quality with a lower radiation dose to the patient.[99] A wide variety of medications may interfere with the accuracy of the mIBG scan, and if possible these should be discontinued before the study.[100] Image quality of ^{123}I-mIBG scans can be improved by using a medium-energy collimator.[101]

Accurate interpretation of mIBG scans requires familiarity with the normal physiologic uptake and accumulation of mIBG in the body. Normal uptake can be seen in the heart, liver, salivary and tear glands, lungs, and brown adipose tissue.[102,103] mIBG uptake in normal adrenal glands is not uncommon, especially after contralateral adrenalectomy. Excreted mIBG can be seen in the bowel and genitourinary system. Intense uptake also can be seen in the thyroid gland, although this may, in part, represent uptake of unincorporated free radioiodine in the administered radiopharmaceutical. Patients typically are pretreated with oral iodine to limit thyroid uptake.[104] This practice was started when ^{131}I-mIBG was in common use, but thyroid exposure is less of a concern with ^{123}I-mIBG and lower amounts of free radioiodine. However, pretreatment is still useful in limiting thyroid uptake that could interfere with image interpretation.

Hodgkin Disease

The most common sites of involvement by Hodgkin disease are mediastinal and other thoracic lymph nodes. Lung involvement is unusual at the time of diagnosis, but increases with disease progression and persistence.[105] In a patient with multiple sites of disease at the time of diagnosis, most sites of involvement are identified by imaging and are not confirmed by biopsy. However, sites that remain FDG-avid after completion of first-line therapy may not represent persistent disease and should be biopsied[106] before using high-risk therapy, such as bone marrow transplant. For the past few decades, the conventional imaging methods for evaluation of Hodgkin disease had been a CT scan of the neck and thorax and a whole-body gallium scan performed with ^{67}Ga–gallium citrate. Since its clinical introduction, FDG PET (**Fig. 10**) has supplanted the use of the gallium scanning for the evaluation of Hodgkin disease.[84,107] This trend is largely attributable to the perceived increased accuracy of FDG PET but also reflects the need to perform a gallium scan over a 3-day period. Similarly, there is little

indication to obtain a bone scan in addition to FDG PET.[108]

In children with Hodgkin disease, FDG PET identifies sites of lymph node disease that are not seen with conventional imaging such as CT and gallium scan. FDG PET also may help in identifying focal sites of bone marrow involvement. These additional sites of disease can increase the disease stage in up to one-fifth of all patients.[84,109,110] However, the effect of this upstaging on clinical outcome is not yet clear. It has not been determined whether upstaging has a beneficial effect on outcome, or if it leads only to more aggressive therapy with a commensurate increase in treatment morbidity and late effects.

FDG PET also is used for assessing the response of Hodgkin disease to chemotherapy. FDG avidity typically resolves before complete shrinkage of soft-tissue masses, and is highly predictive of disease remission.[110,111] The role of FDG PET for disease surveillance after completion of therapy is less clear, particularly in pediatric patients. Most Hodgkin disease recurrence is FDG-avid, but surveillance FDG PET can have a high false-positive rate,[112] and the relative utility

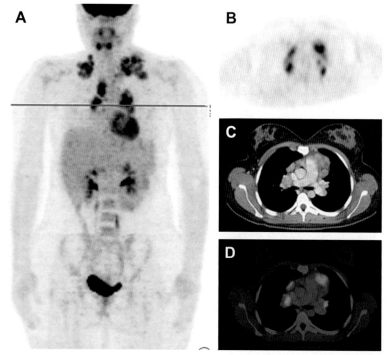

Fig. 10. FDG PET in an18-year-old girl with a new diagnosis of Hodgkin lymphoma. (*A*) The maximal intensity projection (MIP) of the FDG PET shows abnormal FDG uptake in both supraclavicular regions and mediastinum, but no abnormal uptake below the diaphragm. (*B*) In the transaxial plane, abnormal FDG uptake is seen bilaterally in the mediastinum. (*C*) CT demonstrates enlarged hilar and mediastinal lymph nodes lymph nodes. (*D*) Coregistration of PET and diagnostic CT images demonstrates FDG-avid disease in enlarged hilar and mediastinal lymph nodes, consistent with the diagnosis of Hodgkin lymphoma.

of FDG PET, CT, or clinical follow-up has not been defined for surveillance in pediatric Hodgkin disease patients.

Non-Hodgkin Lymphoma

Non-Hodgkin lymphoma includes a wide variety of subtypes, but in children the most common subtypes are Burkitt lymphoma, lymphoblastic lymphoma, large B-cell lymphoma, and anaplastic lymphoma.[83] These lymphomas are high-grade and, unlike Hodgkin disease, parenchymal lung involvement is seen in only a small number of patients with non-Hodgkin lymphoma.[113] Most cases of pediatric non-Hodgkin lymphoma demonstrate intense FDG avidity.[114] The use of FDG PET for pediatric non-Hodgkin lymphoma is based on experience with imaging non-Hodgkin lymphoma in adults,[115] but some studies have shown a role for FDG PET in pediatric patients.[110] By providing whole-body imaging, FDG PET can be helpful for staging by identifying remote sites of lymphoma not detected with conventional imaging. FDG PET may be particularly useful in identifying extranodal sites of disease, such as bone marrow, spleen, and soft tissue.[116] An early response to therapy for non-Hodgkin lymphoma identified by FDG PET may be predictive of a good long-term outcome.[110,115] This approach may be most useful for early identification of nonresponders who might benefit from a change in chemotherapy.

One special category of non-Hodgkin lymphoma includes the immunodeficiency lymphoproliferative disorders (**Fig. 11**). The most common are those occurring after solid organ transplant, but similar disease can be seen in patients with congenital immune disorders or acquired immunodeficiency, such as human immunodeficiency virus infection. FDG PET may have a role in staging and assessing the response to therapy for these tumors.[117]

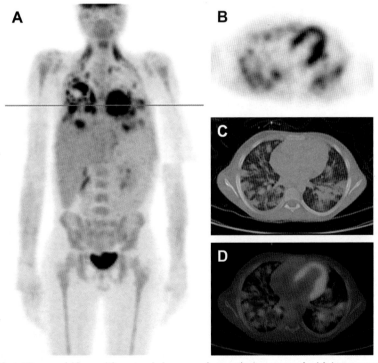

Fig. 11. FDG PET in a 15-year-old boy with systemic immune dysregulation treated with immunosuppression resulting in a B-cell lymphoproliferative disorder. (*A*) The MIP of the FDG PET shows widespread FDG-avid lung disease, hepatomegaly, and splenomegaly, but no other sites of FDG-avid lymphoproliferative disease. Diffuse bone marrow uptake was determined to not represent disease involvement and likely reflects physiologic marrow stimulation. Uptake in anterior neck muscles likely reflects an increased work of ventilation. (*B*) In the transaxial plane, numerous sites of abnormal FDG uptake are seen in both lungs. There is physiologic uptake in the myocardium. (*C*) CT demonstrates nodular parenchymal opacities throughout both lungs. (*D*) Coregistration of PET and diagnostic CT images of the lungs demonstrates that the parenchymal lung disease is FDG-avid, consistent with pulmonary involvement by the lymphoproliferative disorder.

Musculoskeletal Sarcomas in the Chest

Musculoskeletal sarcomas are not specific to the thorax, but many sites of primary or metastatic disease are within the chest. The most common of these tumors in children include osteosarcoma and Ewing sarcoma.[83] FDG PET may have a role in the clinical management of these tumors, including staging, assessing response to therapy, and evaluating for recurrence.[118] For these tumors, therapy includes a combination of systemic chemotherapy and some form of local control, which may be provided by either surgery or radiation therapy. Neoadjuvant chemotherapy may be used to treat disease before surgery and make possible limb-sparing surgery.[119] Successful disease management depends on disease stage, and FDG PET (**Fig. 12**) may have a special role in identifying all sites of disease. However, the utility of FDG PET has not been fully defined. In part, this likely reflects the tendency of published studies to combine different tumors within

one study, despite the likelihood that the clinical utility of FDG PET likely will be different for different sarcomas.

Osteosarcoma occurs primarily in the long bones of the extremities, but more than half of patients have metastases at or soon after diagnosis, with the skeleton and lungs the most common sites of metastases.[120] Most studies[121,122] have shown that whole-body bone scan is more effective than either FDG PET or whole-body magnetic resonance (MR) imaging for identifying skeletal metastases of osteosarcoma FDG PET. One recent study[123] suggested that the combination of whole-body bone scan and FDG PET may be the most sensitive approach. Lung metastases are best identified by CT, but sometimes can be identified on bone scan. Only occasionally are lung metastases large enough to be detected with FDG PET alone.

In patients with osteosarcoma, the histologic response to preoperative neoadjuvant chemotherapy predicts long-term outcome.[124] Early

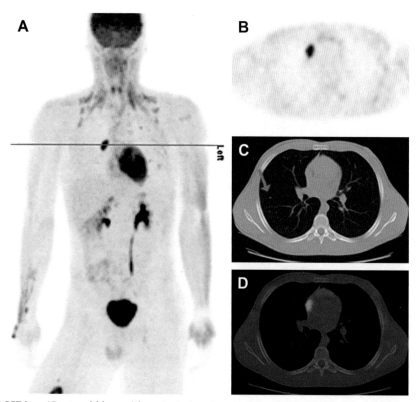

Fig. 12. FDG PET in a 15-year-old boy with metastatic osteosarcoma of the right femur. (*A*) The MIP of the FDG PET shows multiple FDG-avid metastases in the chest. The primary tumor in the distal right femur is seen at the edge of the torso field of view. (*B*) In the transaxial plane, abnormal FDG is seen adjacent to the right border of the mediastinum. (*C*) CT demonstrates a soft-tissue mass adjacent to the right border of the mediastinum and a small pulmonary nodule in the right lung (*arrow*). (*D*) Coregistration of PET and diagnostic CT images demonstrates intense uptake in a large metastasis adjacent to the mediastinum, while no abnormal uptake can be detected in smaller pulmonary nodule in the right lung.

studies showed that FDG PET performed better than bone scan in assessing the histologic response to chemotherapy,[125] probably reflecting a longer persistence of bone scan abnormalities. However, these studies have provided conflicting results regarding the overall clinical utility of FDG PET for preoperative assessment of osteosarcoma. Recent studies have shown that the maximum standardized uptake value (SUV_{max}) of the tumor is the best predictor of the histologic response to neoadjuvant chemotherapy,[126,127] but is limited at intermediate levels of FDG uptake. Another study[128] has suggested that the combination of decreased metabolic activity assessed by FDG and tumor shrinkage assessed by MR imaging provides the best prediction of the histologic response to preoperative chemotherapy. Therefore, in patients with osteosarcoma, there is not yet a definite role for imaging in the preoperative prediction of the histologic response to neoadjuvant chemotherapy.

The Ewing family of tumors encompasses a group of histologically distinct neoplasms that include sarcomas of bone, soft tissue, and the nerves, including primitive neuroectodermal

tumors. Metastatic disease is found in approximately one-quarter of patients at diagnosis,[129] with the lungs one of the most common sites of metastatic disease. Of patients without metastatic disease at diagnosis, up to one-third will present with metastatic relapse.[130] Anatomic imaging is most appropriate for imaging the primary site of disease, but FDG PET has a role in staging Ewing sarcoma (Fig. 13). FDG PET is more sensitive than either bone scan or whole-body MR imaging for finding metastases of Ewing sarcoma.[131] This aspect is important in Ewing sarcoma, as all sites of disease may receive local therapy.[132] However, chest CT is more sensitive than FDG PET for detecting lung metastases smaller than 8 mm,[123] and remains an important part of staging Ewing sarcoma. This staging may be acquired as part of a PET/CT or a separate diagnostic chest CT.

Although MR imaging is most commonly used to assess the response to therapy for Ewing sarcoma, preoperative FDG PET predicts the histologic response to neoadjuvant chemotherapy.[119] With nonmetastatic disease, an SUV_{max} of less than 2.5 after adjuvant chemotherapy predicts long-term progression-free survival.[132]

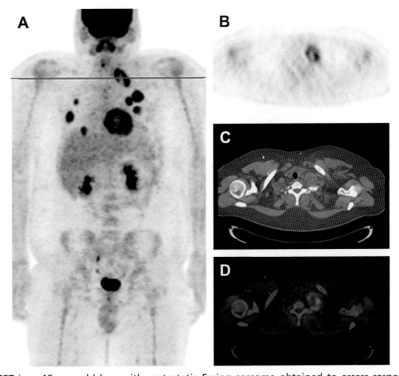

Fig. 13. FDG PET in a 15-year-old boy with metastatic Ewing sarcoma obtained to assess response to chemotherapy. (A) The MIP of the FDG PET shows multiple sites of abnormal uptake in the chest that are concerning for residual tumor. (B) In the transaxial plane, abnormal FDG uptake is seen in the left supraclavicular region. (C) Noncontrast CT demonstrates a left supraclavicular mass. (D) Coregistration of PET and diagnostic CT images demonstrates an FDG-avid supraclavicular mass consistent with a site of metastatic Ewing sarcoma.

The EURO-EWING 99 study[133] (European Ewing Tumour Working Initiatives of National Groups 1999) showed that FDG PET/CT combined with a diagnostic chest CT was more accurate than FDG PET alone. FDG PET/CT resulted in fewer equivocal skeletal lesions, but most of the improved performance reflected new lung metastases found with the diagnostic chest CT. There is little evidence to support replacing a diagnostic chest CT with a low-dose CT scan obtained as part of a PET/CT. FDG PET may have a role in finding recurrent Ewing sarcoma,[134] but the relative utility of FDG PET and bone scan has not been resolved.

Primary Lung Tumors

In children, primary malignant lung tumors are rare and pathologically diverse. Nearly all neoplastic lung lesions identified in this age group represent metastatic disease, while primary benign and malignant lung tumors each may account for less than 10% of all pulmonary tumors.[135] The most common primary malignant lung tumors in children are carcinoid tumor, inflammatory myofibroblastic

tumor, and pleuropulmonary blastoma.[136] The primary lung cancers of adulthood are very rarely reported in children.

Most reports regarding the use of FDG PET to evaluate primary lung tumors of children are case reports or small case series. Many primary malignant lung tumors of children have been demonstrated to be FDG-avid, including carcinoid tumors,[137] inflammatory fibroblastic tumors,[138,139] pleuropulmonary blastoma,[140] and mucoepidermoid tumors.[139,141] As in adults,[142] atypical carcinoid tumors are more likely than typical carcinoid tumors to be FDG-avid, but this difference is probably not sufficient to guide the diagnostic evaluation of a presumed bronchial carcinoid tumor.[137] Therefore, for most lung lesions in children FDG PET (**Figs. 14** and **15**) usually is not helpful for diagnostic evaluation, but can be useful for staging and posttherapy follow-up.[138,140]

FDG PET of the Thymus

Thymic FDG uptake can be normal in children (see **Fig. 9**), and should not be confused as a site of disease.[94] Even when there is intense FDG uptake

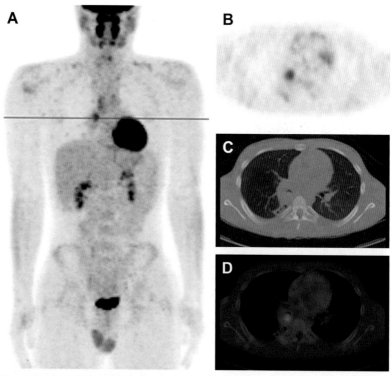

Fig. 14. FDG PET in a 15-year-old boy with a chronic cough obtained to assess an endobronchial lesion in the right lower bronchus seen on CT. (*A*) The MIP of the FDG PET shows a single focus of moderate uptake along the right side of the mediastinum. (*B*) In the transaxial plane, there is abnormal uptake adjacent to the right margin of the mediastinum, near the right hilum. (*C*) CT demonstrates an endobronchial lesion in the right lower bronchus. (*D*) Coregistration of PET and diagnostic CT images demonstrates a single FDG-avid endobronchial lesion in the right lower bronchus. Surgical resection demonstrated a typical carcinoid.

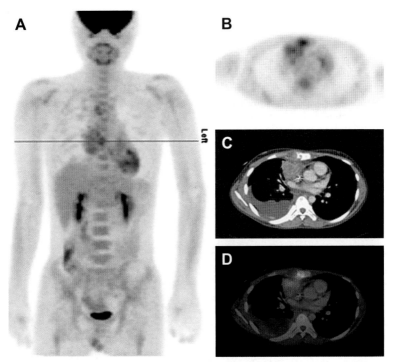

Fig. 15. FDG PET in a 14-year-old boy with carcinoma of the thymus. (A) The MIP of the FDG PET shows hetero-geneous FDG uptake in the mediastinum. (B) In the transaxial plane, there is a region of heterogeneous uptake in the anterior mediastinum. (C) CT of the chest shows a soft-tissue mass in the anterior mediastinum, in the ex-pected location of the thymus, that is eroding into the sternum. (D) Coregistration of PET and CT images confirms the presence of an FDG-avid anterior mediastinal mass. Surgical resection demonstrated carcinoma of the thymus.

in the thymus, a homogeneous pattern of uptake likely represents normal physiologic uptake in children. Similarly, after chemotherapy or radio-therapy to the chest, intense thymic uptake can be seen, particularly in children and young adults. Rather than being disease specific, this phe-nomenon of "thymic rebound" may reflect the combined use of a glucocorticoid-containing che-motherapy regimen and radiation therapy in these patients.[94]

Heterogeneous FDG uptake in the thymus, particularly if corresponding to structural lesions identified by CT, is much more concerning for a true disease process. Thymoma and thymic carcinoma are rare in children,[143] and abnormal findings in the thymus may represent involvement by lymphoma or metastatic disease. Overall, thy-moma and thymic carcinoma have substantially greater FDG uptake than thymic hyperplasia, but the level of FDG avidity cannot discriminate malig-nant pathology from a benign process.[144] Once a diagnosis of thymoma or thymic carcinoma has been made, FDG PET may be helpful for staging, assessing response to therapy, and follow-up.

Neuroblastoma

Neuroblastoma is the most common extracranial solid tumor in children,[83] and up to half of all cases may present with metastases. Although the most common site of disease is the abdomen, primary tumors and metastatic disease both occur in the chest.[145] Most posterior mediastinal masses in children are neurogenic tumors,[146] typically neuro-blastoma, ganglioneuroblastoma, and ganglioneu-roma. Whole-body scanning with radioiodinated mIBG has been the standard method for functional imaging of neuroblastoma.[147] In 2010 the Interna-tional Neuroblastoma Risk Group published a consensus guideline for the use of ^{123}I-mIBG scans in patients with neuroblastoma.[148] The guideline supports the use of ^{123}I-mIBG scans for initial staging at diagnosis, to assess response to therapy, and as posttherapy surveillance for relapse. The guideline also provides technical guidance for performing and interpreting ^{123}I-mIBG scans. ^{123}I-mIBG can have high accuracy for imaging neuroblastoma, but the performance of ^{123}I-mIBG depends on the quality of the scan im-ages, which is linked to imaging technique.[101,148]

Overall, ^{123}I-mIBG may have a sensitivity of greater than 95% for detecting neuroblastoma.[147] In a single recent prospective multicenter trial, Vik and colleagues[149] showed that ^{123}I-mIBG had a sensitivity of 93% and specificity of 92% among 87 patients with histologic confirmation of disease. This study also demonstrated that the addition of SPECT clarified the location of mIBG-avid disease in approximately half of the cases while providing additional diagnostic value in at least 30% of cases. After patients achieve remission, ^{123}I-mIBG is a sensitive method for surveillance of recurrent disease. Kushner and colleagues[150] found that ^{123}I-mIBG is more sensitive than bone scan, CT, or ^{131}I-mIBG scan for posttherapy surveillance. False-positive findings are rare with ^{123}I-mIBG, and usually are clarified by correlation with either CT or MR imaging.[151] Interpretation of

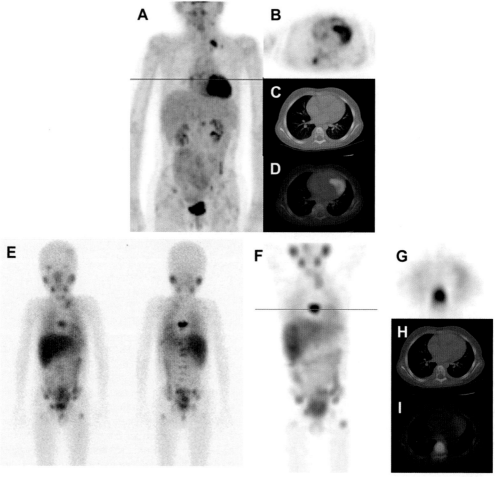

Fig. 16. Functional imaging of neuroblastoma. FDG PET identified fewer sites of disease than either whole-body or SPECT ^{123}I-mIBG scan in an 11-year-old boy with relapsed neuroblastoma. (A) The MIP of the FDG PET shows abnormal uptake in the neck, supraclavicular regions, and paravertebral region. Subtle abnormal focal uptake is also identified in the retroperitoneum and possibly in the pelvis. (B) In the chest, an image in the transaxial plane shows a single focus of abnormal mIBG uptake in the right paraspinal region. (C) On chest CT, there is a right paravertebral soft-tissue mass at the T7 level. (D) Coregistration of PET and CT images confirms an FDG-avid paravertebral soft tissue near vertebra T7. (E) Whole-body ^{123}I-mIBG scan (anterior and posterior) demonstrates numerous sites of abnormal uptake in neck, left supraclavicular region, in multiple vertebrae, numerous sites in the pelvis, and in both proximal femurs. (F) SPECT ^{123}I-mIBG scan confirms the sites of abnormal mIBG uptake, including intense uptake in the mid thorax. (G) A transaxial image from the SPECT shows intense uptake in the paravertebral region of the mid thorax. (H) Chest CT, also seen in (C), demonstrates the right paravertebral soft-tissue mass and sclerosis of the T7 vertebra. (I) Coregistration of mIBG and CT images demonstrates disease involvement of the T7 vertebral body that is not identified on the FDG PET as well as possible uptake in the paravertebral soft tissue. As this case demonstrates, FDG PET may be complementary to, but cannot replace ^{123}I-mIBG SPECT for the evaluation of neuroblastoma.

^{123}I-mIBG scans also requires familiarity with patterns of physiologic uptake in supraclavicular brown adipose tissue, salivary glands, liver, bowel, and the urinary collecting system.[152]

The role of FDG PET for the evaluation of neuroblastoma remains unclear (**Fig. 16**). Most (but not all) sympathochromaffin tumors are FDG-avid, but it is not clear that FDG PET offers a benefit over whole-body ^{123}I-mIBG scan. A recent report[153] suggested that ^{123}I-mIBG scans may be more useful in patients with low-stage disease, whereas FDG PET may be more useful for patients with stage III or stage IV disease, although this has not been confirmed by other investigators. In another study, Taggart and colleagues[154] showed that ^{123}I-mIBG scans outperformed FDG PET for evaluating the response to ^{131}I-mIBG therapy, with ^{123}I-mIBG scans more sensitive than FDG PET for identifying sites of diseases both before and after therapy. Because ^{123}I-mIBG and ^{18}F-FDG have different patterns of physiologic uptake that may hinder evaluation of a particular site of disease, either study might perform better in a specific patient. For example, FDG PET may not easily identify focal bone marrow disease in a patient that has received marrow-stimulating therapy.[155] In selected circumstances, such as following patients with known sites of mIBG-negative disease, FDG PET may serve as a complementary study to ^{123}I-mIBG scans.[156] However, current data does not support the routine replacement of ^{123}I-mIBG with ^{18}F-FDG for the evaluation of patients with neuroblastoma.

Other PET agents, including ^{18}F-dopamine and ^{18}F-DOPA, have been used successfully to image sympathochromaffin tumors, including neuroblastoma.[157] However, these agents are not widely available, and there is little evidence that they will perform better than either ^{123}I-mIBG whole-body scans or FDG PET in patients with neuroblastoma.

RADIATION EXPOSURE

Nuclear medicine studies typically expose children to low effective doses of radiation. For most studies, radiopharmaceutical doses are adjusted for patient size. However, there is variability among institutions in the administered doses of specific radiopharmaceuticals.[158] Some of this variability may be based on differences in technique or hardware, but may not reflect the improved performance of newer-generation cameras. Recent efforts in Europe[159] and North America[160] to standardize radiopharmaceutical doses offer opportunities to decrease radiation exposure that occurs with many nuclear medicine studies. Technical

advances, such as improved camera sensitivity and new methods of image processing,[161] have the potential for even further decreases in radiation exposure.

SUMMARY

In children, nuclear medicine is used to assess a wide range of disease processes and tumors in the chest. As in adults, nuclear medicine frequently provides functional information about tumors or other diseases that can complement anatomic imaging methods. Some indications for pediatric nuclear medicine studies, such as pulmonary embolism or gastroesophageal reflux, are similar to those seen in adults. However, other indications, such as congenital heart disease or cystic fibrosis, are more specific to children and young adults. In pediatric oncology imaging, FDG PET has a role in tumor staging, assessing response to therapy, and follow-up. For some tumors, such as lymphomas, the use of FDG PET can be guided by experience with similar diseases in adults. For more common pediatric tumors, such as neuroblastoma, clinical trials are available to help guide appropriate imaging in disease management. However, the lower incidence of pediatric cancers has made it more difficult to fully define the role of FDG PET for many less common tumors. Large, multi-institutional studies of the utility of ^{18}F-FDG, as well as other PET agents, are still needed. In the meantime, the use of FDG PET on a case-by-case basis can be helpful in the management of children with uncommon pediatric tumors. Nuclear medicine studies typically result in low radiation doses, but recent efforts to standardize radiopharmaceutical doses, the availability of improved cameras, and advances in image processing will lead to even lower radiation exposure for children undergoing nuclear medicine studies.

REFERENCES

1. Freeman LM, Stein EG, Sprayregen S, et al. The current and continuing important role of ventilation-perfusion scintigraphy in evaluating patients with suspected pulmonary embolism. Semin Nucl Med 2008;38:432–40.
2. Gelfand MJ, Gruppo RA, Nasser MP. Ventilation-perfusion scintigraphy in children and adolescents is associated with a low rate of indeterminate studies. Clin Nucl Med 2008;33:606–9.
3. Dae MW. Pediatric nuclear cardiology. Semin Nucl Med 2007;37:382–90.
4. Komori K, Kamagata S, Hirobe S, et al. Radionuclide imaging study of long-term pulmonary function after lobectomy in children with congenital

cystic lung disease. J Pediatr Surg 2009;44: 2096–100.

5. Johnson K. Ventilation and perfusion scanning in children. Paediatr Respir Rev 2000;1:347–53.

6. Navalkissoor S, Easty M, Biassoni L. Functional lung assessment with radionuclides in paediatric respiratory diseases: a useful, underutilized test in nuclear medicine? Nucl Med Commun 2010;31:896–902.

7. Ciofetta G, Piepsz A, Roca I, et al. Guidelines for lung scintigraphy in children. Eur J Nucl Med Mol Imaging 2007;34:1518–26.

8. Parker JA, Coleman RE, Hilson AJ, et al. Society of Nuclear Medicine procedure guideline for lung scintigraphy. Version 3.0, approved February 7, 2004. Available at: http://interactive.snm.org/LungScintigraphy_v3.0. Accessed June 2, 2011.

9. Darte L, Persson BR, Soderbom L. Quality control and testing of ^{99m}Tc-macroaggregated albumin. Nuklearmedizin 1976;15:80–5.

10. Heyman S. Toxicity and safety factors associated with lung perfusion studies with radiolabeled particles. J Nucl Med 1979;20:1098–9.

11. Treves ST, Packard AB. Lungs. In: Treves ST, editor. Pediatric nuclear medicine/PET. New York: Springer; 2006. p. 87–127.

12. Cao X, Treves ST. Automated software for analysis and reporting of Xenon-133 (Xe-133) pulmonary ventilation studies in children. J Nucl Med 2009; 50(Suppl 2):806.

13. Matthews JJ, Maurer AH, Steiner RM, et al. New ^{133}Xe gas trapping index for quantifying severe emphysema before partial lung volume reduction. J Nucl Med 2008;49:771–6.

14. Cabahug CG, McPeck M, Palmer LB, et al. Utility of technetium-99m-DTPA in determining regional ventilation. J Nucl Med 1996;37:239–44.

15. Trujillo NP, Pratt JP, Talusani S, et al. DTPA aerosol in ventilation/perfusion scintigraphy for diagnosing pulmonary embolism. J Nucl Med 1997;38:1781–3.

16. Jackson P, Mackey D, van der Wall H. Physical and chemical nature of Technegas. J Nucl Med 1998; 39:1646–9.

17. Pesavento R, de Conti G, Minotto I, et al. The value of 64-detector row computed tomography for the exclusion of pulmonary embolism. Thromb Haemost 2001;8:105.

18. Kristaneepaiboon S, Lee EY, Zurakowski D, et al. MDCT pulmonary angiography evaluation of pulmonary embolism in children. AJR Am J Roentgenol 2009;192(5):1246–52.

19. Lee EY, Kritsaneepaiboon S, Zurakowski D, et al. Beyond the pulmonary arteries: alternative diagnoses in children with MDCT pulmonary angiography negative for pulmonary embolism. AJR Am J Roentgenol 2009;193(3):888–94.

20. Lee EY, Zurakowski D, Diperna S, et al. Parenchymal and pleural abnormalities in children with and without pulmonary embolism at MDCT pulmonary angiography. Pediatr Radiol 2010;40(2):173–81.

21. Lee EY, Zurakowski D, Boiselle PM. Pulmonary embolism in pediatric patients: survey of CT pulmonary angiography practices and policies. Acad Radiol 2010;17(12):1543–9.

22. Prabhu SP, Mahmood S, Sena L, et al. MDCT evaluation of pulmonary embolism in children and young adults following a lateral tunnel Fontan procedure: optimizing contrast-enhancement techniques. Pediatr Radiol 2009;39(9):938–44.

23. Schembri GP, Miller AE, Smart R. Radiation dosimetry and safety issues in the investigation of pulmonary embolism. Semin Nucl Med 2010;40:442–54.

24. Pifarre P, Roca I, Irastorza I, et al. Lung ventilation-perfusion scintigraphy in children on long-term parenteral nutrition. Eur J Nucl Med Mol Imaging 2009;36:1005–8.

25. Bajc M, Neilly JB, Miniatti M, et al. EANM guidelines for ventilation/perfusion scintigraphy: part 2. Eur J Nucl Med Mol Imaging 2009;36:1528–38.

26. Bajc M, Jonson B. Ventilation/perfusion SPECT—an essential but underrated method for diagnosis of pulmonary embolism and other diseases. Eur J Nucl Med Mol Imaging 2009;36:875–8.

27. Miles S, Rogers KM, Thomas P, et al. A comparison of single-photon emission CT lung scintigraphy and CT pulmonary angiography for the diagnosis of pulmonary embolism. Chest 2009;136:1546–53.

28. Vettukattil JJ, Slavik Z, Lamb RK, et al. Intrapulmonary arteriovenous shunting may be a universal phenomenon in patients with the superior cavopulmonary anastomosis: a radionuclide study. Heart 2000;83:425–8.

29. Jeandot R, Lambert B, Brendel AJ, et al. Lung ventilation and perfusion scintigraphy in the follow up of repaired congenital diaphragmatic hernia. Eur J Nucl Med 1989;15:591–6.

30. Pal K, Gupta DK. Serial perfusion study depicts pulmonary vascular growth in the survivors of non-extracorporeal membrane oxygenation-treated congenital diaphragmatic hernia. Neonatology 2010;98:254–9.

31. Hayward MJ, Kharasch V, Sheils C, et al. Predicting inadequate long-term lung development in children with congenital diaphragmatic hernia: an analysis of longitudinal changes in ventilation and perfusion. J Pediatr Surg 2007;42:112–6.

32. Blickman JG, Rosen JG, Welch KJ, et al. Pectus excavatum in children: pulmonary scintigraphy before and after corrective surgery. Eur J Cardiothorac Surg 2006;30:637–43.

33. Pruckmayer M, Zacherl S, Ulrike SM, et al. Scintigraphic assessment of pulmonary and whole-body blood flow patterns after surgical intervention in congenital heart disease. J Nucl Med 1999;40: 1477–83.

34. Grimon G, Andre L, Bernard O, et al. Early radionuclide detection of intrapulmonary shunts in children with liver disease. J Nucl Med 1994;35:1328–32.

35. El-Shabrawi MH, Omran S, Wageeh S, et al. (99m) Technetium-macroaggregated albumin perfusion lung scan versus contrast enhanced echocardiography in the diagnosis of the hepatopulmonary syndrome in children with chronic liver disease. Eur J Gastroenterol Hepatol 2010;22:1006–12.

36. Orenstein SR. An overview of reflux-associated disorders in infants: apnea, laryngospasm, and aspiration. Am J Med 2001;111(Suppl 8A):60S–3S.

37. Heyman S, Kirkpatrick JA, Winter HS, et al. An improved radionuclide method for the diagnosis of gastroesophageal reflux and aspiration in children (milk scan). Radiology 1979;131:479–82.

38. Bar-Sever Z. Gastroesophageal reflux, gastric emptying, esophageal transit, and pulmonary aspiration. In: Treves ST, editor. Pediatric nuclear medicine/PET. New York: Springer; 2006. p. 162–91.

39. Baikie G, South MJ, Reddihough DS, et al. Agreement of aspiration tests using barium videofluoroscopy, salivagram, and milk scan in children with cerebral palsy. Dev Med Child Neurol 2005;47:86–93.

40. Bar-Sever Z, Connolly LP, Treves ST. The radionuclide salivagram in children with pulmonary disease and a high risk of aspiration. Pediatr Radiol 1995;25:S180–3.

41. Heyman S, Respondek M. Detection of pulmonary aspiration in children by radionuclide "salivagram". J Nucl Med 1989;30:697–9.

42. Baikie G, Reddihough DS, South M, et al. The salivagram in severe cerebral palsy and able-bodied adults. J Paediatr Child Health 2009;45:342–5.

43. Kaya M, Inan M, Bedel D. Detection of tracheoesophageal fistula caused by ingestion of a caustic substance by esophageal scintigraphy. Clin Nucl Med 2005;30:365–6.

44. Valenza V, Perotti G, DiGiuda D, et al. Scintigraphic evaluation of Zenker's diverticulum. Eur J Nucl Med Mol Imaging 2003;30:1657–64.

45. Heyman S. Volume-dependent pulmonary aspiration of a swallowed radionuclide bolus. J Nucl Med 1997;38:103–4.

46. Dodds WJ, Stewart ET, Logemann JA. Physiology and radiology of normal oral and pharyngeal phases of swallowing. Am J Roentgenol 1990; 154:953–63.

47. Warrington JC, Charron M. Pediatric gastrointestinal nuclear medicine. Semin Nucl Med 2007;37: 269–85.

48. Baulieu F, Boiron M, Bertrand P, et al. Evaluation of a solid bolus suitable for esophageal scintigraphy. Dysphagia 2007;22:281–9.

49. Odunsi S, Camilleri M. Selected interventions in nuclear medicine: gastrointestinal motor functions. Semin Nucl Med 2009;39:186–94.

50. Parkman HP, Maurer AH, Caroline DF, et al. Optimal evaluation of patients with nonobstructive esophageal dysphagia: manometry, scintigraphy, or videoesophagography? Dig Dis Sci 1996;41:1355–68.

51. Pasquili SK, Marino BS, McBride MG, et al. Coronary artery pattern and age impact exercise performance late after the arterial switch operation. J Thorac Cardiovasc Surg 2007;34:1207–12.

52. Chang RK, Gurvitz M, Rodriguwz S, et al. Current practice of exercise stress testing among pediatric cardiology and pulmonology centers in the United States. Pediatr Cardiol 2006;27:110–6.

53. Rhodes J, Tikkanen AU, Jenkins KJ. Exercise testing and training in children with congenital heart disease. Circulation 2010;122:1957–67.

54. Chatriwalla AK, Prieto LR, Brunken RC, et al. Preliminary data on the diagnostic accuracy of rubidium-82 cardiac PET imaging for the evaluation of ischemia in a pediatric population. Pediatr Cardiol 2008;29:732–8.

55. Khorsand A, Graf S, Pirich C, et al. Assessment of myocardial perfusion by dynamic N-13 ammonia PET imaging: comparison of 2 tracer kinetic models. J Nucl Cardiol 2005;12:410–7.

56. Silverstein J, Haller M. Coronary artery disease in youth: present markers, future hope? J Pediatr 2010;157:523–4.

57. Newberger JW, Fulton DR. Coronary revascularization in patients with Kawasaki disease. J Pediatr 2010;157:8–10.

58. Muta H, Ishii M. Percutaneous coronary intervention versus coronary artery bypass grafting for stenotic lesions after Kawasaki disease. J Pediatr 2010;157:120–6.

59. Tsuda E, Abe T, Tamaki W. Acute coronary syndrome in adult patients with coronary artery lesions caused by Kawasaki disease: review of case reports. Cardiol Young 2011;21:74–82.

60. Zanon G, Zucchetta P, Varnier M, et al. Do Kawasaki disease patients without coronary artery abnormalities need a long-term follow-up? A myocardial single-photon emission computed tomography study. J Paediatr Child Health 2009;45:419–24.

61. Gazarian M, Feldman BM, Benson LN, et al. Assessment of myocardial perfusion and function in childhood systemic lupus erythematosus. J Pediatr 1998;132:109–16.

62. Espinola-Zavaleta N, Alexanderson-Rosas E, Granados N, et al. Myocardial perfusion defects in patients with autoimmune diseases: a prospective study. Analysis of two diagnostic tests. Lupus 2006;15:38–43.

63. Frommell PC. Congenital coronary artery abnormalities predisposing to sudden cardiac death. Pacing Clin Electrophysiol 2009;32(Suppl 2):S63–6.

64. Kane DA, Fulton DR, Saleeb S, et al. Needles in hay: chest pain as the presenting symptom in

children with serious underlying cardiac pathology. Congenit Heart Dis 2010;5:366–73.

65. Hauser M, Bengel FM, Kuhn A, et al. Myocardial blood flow and flow reserve after coronary reimplantation in patients after arterial switch and Ross operation. Circulation 2001;103:1875–80.

66. Hutter PA, Bennink GB, Ay L, et al. Influence of coronary anatomy and reimplantation on the long-term outcome of the arterial switch. Eur J Cardiothorac Surg 2000;18(2):207–13.

67. Raisky O, Bergoend E, Agnoletti G, et al. Late coronary artery lesions after neonatal arterial switch operation. Results of surgical coronary revascularization. Eur J Cardiothorac Surg 2007;31:894–8.

68. Espinola-Zavaleta N, Alexanderson E, Attie F, et al. Right ventricular function and ventricular perfusion defects in adults with congenitally corrected transposition: correlation of echocardiography and nuclear medicine. Cardiol Young 2004;14:174–81.

69. Zuppan CW, Wells LM, Kerstetter JC, et al. Cause of death in pediatric and infant heart transplant recipients: review of a 20-year, single-institution cohort. J Heart Lung Transplant 2009;28:579–84.

70. Maiers J, Jurwitz R. Identification of coronary artery disease in the pediatric cardiac transplant patient. Pediatr Cardiol 2008;29:19–23.

71. Dandel M, Hetzer R. Impact of immunosuppressive drugs on the development of cardiac allograft vasculopathy. Curr Vasc Pharmacol 2010;8:706–19.

72. Nagji AS, Hranjec T, Swenson BR, et al. Donor age is associated with chronic allograft vasculopathy after adult heart transplantation: implications for donor allocation. Ann Thorac Surg 2010;90:168–75.

73. Treves ST, Blume ED, Armsby L, et al. Cardiovascular system. In: Treves ST, editor. Pediatric nuclear medicine/PET. New York: Springer; 2006. p. 128–61.

74. Hor G. What is the current status of quantification and nuclear medicine in cardiology? Eur J Nucl Med 1996;23:815–51.

75. Massardo T, Jaimovich R, Lavados H, et al. Comparison of radionuclide ventriculography using SPECT and planar techniques in different cardiac conditions. Eur J Nucl Med Mol Imaging 2007;34:1735–46.

76. Gedik GK, Caglar M, Unal S, et al. Evaluation of cardiovascular complications with ^{99m}Tc tetrofosmin gated myocardial perfusion scintigraphy in patients with thalassemia major. Rev Esp Med Nucl 2008;27:191–8.

77. Kiratli PO, Tuncei M, Oskutlu S, et al. Gated myocardial perfusion scintigraphy in children with myocarditis: can it be considered as an indicator of clinical outcome. Nucl Med Commun 2008;29:907–14.

78. Szuba A, Shin WS, Strauss HW, et al. The third circulation: radionuclide lymphoscintigraphy in the evaluation of lymphedema. J Nucl Med 2003;44:43–57.

79. Bellini C, Boccardo F, Campisi C, et al. Congenital pulmonary lymphangiectasis. Orphanet J Rare Dis 2006;1:43.

80. Biewer ES, Zurn C, Arnold R, et al. Chylothorax after surgery on congenital heart disease in newborns and infants—risk factors and efficacy of MCT-diet. J Cardiothorac Surg 2010;13:127.

81. Siu SL, Yang JY, Hui JP, et al. Chylothorax secondary to catheter related thrombosis successfully treated with heparin. J Paediatr Child Health 2011. [Epub ahead of print]. DOI:10.1111/j.1440-1754.2010.01936.x.

82. Peterss S, Gratz KF, Khaladj N, et al. Lymphoscintigraphic localization of a high-output chylous leak after bilateral lung transplantation. J Heart Lung Transplant 2011;30(4):481–3.

83. Ries LA. Childhood cancer mortality. In: Ries LA, Smith MA, Gurney JG, et al, editors. Cancer incidence and survival among children and adolescents: United States SEER Program 1975-1995. Bethesda (MD): National Cancer Institute; 1999. SEER Program. NIH Pub. No. 99–4649. p. 165–9.

84. Mody RJ, Bui C, Hutchinson RJ, et al. Comparison of (18)F fluorodeoxyglucose PET with Ga-67 scintigraphy and conventional imaging modalities in pediatric lymphoma. Leuk Lymphoma 2007;48:699–707.

85. Chen K, Chen X. Positron emission tomography imaging of cancer biology: current status and future prospects. Semin Oncol 2011;38:70–86.

86. Rohren EM, Turkington TG, Coleman RE. Clinical applications of PET in oncology. Radiology 2004; 231:305–32.

87. McQuattie S. Pediatric PET/CT imaging: tips and techniques. J Nucl Med Technol 2008;36:171–8.

88. Nadel HR, Shulkin B. Pediatric positron emission tomography-computed tomography protocol considerations. Semin Ultrasound CT MR 2008;29:271–6.

89. Zukotynski KA, Fahey FH, Laffin S, et al. Constant ambient temperature of 24 degrees C significantly reduces FDG uptake by brown adipose tissue in children scanned during the winter. Eur J Nucl Med Mol Imaging 2009;36:602–6.

90. Parysow O, Mollerach AM, Jager V, et al. Low-dose oral propranolol could reduce brown adipose tissue F-18 FDG uptake in patients undergoing PET scans. Clin Nucl Med 2007;32:351–7.

91. Gelfand MJ, O'Hara SM, Curtwright LA, et al. Premedication to block [^{18}F] FDG uptake in brown adipose tissue of pediatric and adolescent patients. Pediatr Radiol 2005;35:984–90.

92. Williams G, Kolodny GM. Method for decreasing uptake of ^{18}F-FDG by hypermetabolic brown adipose tissue on PET. AJR Am J Roentgenol 2008;190:1406–9.

93. Shammas A, Lim R, Charron M. Pediatric FDG PET/CT: physiologic uptake, normal variants, and benign conditions. Radiographics 2009;29:1467–86.

94. Jerushalmi J, Frenkel A, Bar-Shalom R, et al. Physiologic thymic uptake of ^{18}F-FDG in children and young adults: a PET/CT evaluation of incidence, patterns, and relationship to treatment. J Nucl Med 2009;50:849–53.

95. Williams G, Kolodny GM. Suppression of myocardial ^{18}F-FDG uptake by preparing patients with a high-fat, low-carbohydrate diet. AJR Am J Roentgenol 2008;190:W151–6.

96. Sisson JC, Frager MS, Valk TW, et al. Scintigraphic localization of pheochromocytoma. N Engl J Med 1981;305:12–7.

97. Kimmig B, Brandeis WE, Eisenhut M, et al. Scintigraphy of a neuroblastoma with I-131 meta-iodobenzylguanidine. J Nucl Med 1984;25:773–5.

98. Paltiel HJ, Gelfand MJ, Elgazzar AH, et al. Neural crest tumors: I-123 imaging in children. Radiology 1994;190:117–21.

99. Sharp SE, Gelfand MJ, Shulkin BL. Pediatrics: diagnosis of neuroblastoma. Semin Nucl Med 2011;41: 345–53.

100. Bombardieri E, Giammarile F, Aktolun C, et al. [131]I/^{123}I-metaiodobenzylguanidine (mIBG) scintigraphy: procedure guidelines for tumor imaging. Eur J Nucl Med Mol Imaging 2010;37:2436–46.

101. Snay ER, Treves ST, Fahey FH. Improved quality of pediatric ^{123}I-MIBG images with medium-energy collimators. J Nucl Med Technol 2011;39:100–4.

102. Bonnin F, Lumbrusco J, Tenenbaum F, et al. Refining interpretation of MIBG scans in children. J Nucl Med 1994;35:803–10.

103. Okuyama C, Ushijima Y, Kubota T, et al. ^{123}I-metaiodobenzylguanidine uptake in the nape of the neck of children: likely visualization of brown adipose tissue. J Nucl Med 2003;44:1421–5.

104. van Santen HM, de Kraker J, van Eck BL, et al. Improved radiation protection of the thyroid gland with thyroxine, methimazole, and potassium iodide during diagnostic and therapeutic use of radiolabeled metaiodobenzylguanidine in children with neuroblastoma. Cancer 2003;98:389–96.

105. Leone G, Castellana M, Rabitti C, et al. Escavative pulmonary Hodgkin's lymphoma: diagnosis by cutting needle. Eur J Haematol 1990;44:139–41.

106. Schaefer HG, Taverna C, Strobel K, et al. Hodgkin disease: diagnostic value of FDG PET/CT after first-line therapy—is biopsy of FDG-avid lesions still needed? Radiology 2007;244:257–62.

107. Hudson MM, Krasin MJ, Kaste SC. PET imaging in pediatric Hodgkin's lymphoma. Pediatr Radiol 2004;34:190–8.

108. Shulkin BL, Goddin GS, McCarville MB, et al. Bone and [18F]fluorodeoxyglucose positron-emission tomography/computed tomography scanning for the assessment of osseous involvement in Hodgkin lymphoma in children and young adults. Leuk Lymphoma 2009;11:1794–802.

109. Kabickova E, Sumerauer D, Cumlivska E, et al. Comparison of ^{18}F-FDG-PET and standard procedures for the pretreatment staging of children and adolescents with Hodgkin's disease. Eur J Nucl Med Mol Imaging 2006;33:1025–31.

110. Miller E, Metser U, Avrahami G, et al. Role of ^{18}F-FDG PET/CT in staging and follow-up of lymphoma in pediatric and young adult patients. J Comput Assist Tomogr 2006;30:689–94.

111. Hutchings M, Loft A, Hansen M, et al. FDG-PET after two cycles of chemotherapy predicts treatment failure and progression-free survival in Hodgkin lymphoma. Blood 2006;107:52–9.

112. Crocciolo R, Fallanca F, Giovacchini G, et al. Role of [18]FDG-PET/CT in detecting relapse during follow-up of patients with Hodgkin's lymphoma. Ann Hematol 2009;88:1229–36.

113. Au V, Leung AN. Radiologic manifestations of lymphoma in the thorax. AJR Am J Roentgenol 1997;168:93–8.

114. Weiler-Sagie M, Bushelev O, Epelbaum R, et al. ^{18}F-FDG avidity in lymphoma readdressed: a study of 766 patients. J Nucl Med 2010;51:25–30.

115. Castellucci P, Zinzani P, Pourdehnad M, et al. ^{18}F-FDG PET in malignant lymphoma: significance of positive findings. Eur J Nucl Med Mol Imaging 2005;32:749–56.

116. Even-Sapir E, Lievshitz G, Perry C, et al. Fluorine-18 fluorodeoxyglucose PET/CT patterns of extranodal involvement in patients with non-Hodgkin lymphoma and Hodgkin's disease. Radiol Clin North Am 2007;45:697–709.

117. Von Falck C, Maecker B, Schirg E, et al. Post-transplant lymphoproliferative disease in pediatric solid organ transplant patients: a possible role for [^{18}F]-FDG-PET/CT in initial staging and therapy monitoring. Eur J Radiol 2007;63:427–35.

118. Grant FD, Drubach LA, Treves ST. ^{18}F-Fluorodeoxyglucose PET and PET/CT in pediatric musculoskeletal malignancies. PET Clin 2010;5:349–61.

119. Hawkins DS, Rajendren JG, Conrad EU, et al. Evaluation of chemotherapy response in pediatric bone sarcomas by [F-18]-fluorodeoxy-D-glucose positron emission tomography. Cancer 2002;94: 3277–84.

120. Brenner W, Bohuslavizki KH, Eary JF. PET imaging of osteosarcoma. J Nucl Med 2003;44:930–42.

121. Franzius C, Sciuk J, Daldrup-Link HE, et al. FDG-PET for detection of osseous metastases from malignant primary bone tumors: comparison with bone scintigraphy. Eur J Nucl Med 2000;27: 1305–11.

122. Daldrup-Link HE, Franzius C, Link TM, et al. Whole-body MR imaging for detection of bone metastases in children and young adults: comparison with skeletal scintigraphy and FDG PET. AJR Am J Roentgenol 2001;177:229–36.

123. Volker T, Denecke T, Steffen I, et al. Positron emission tomography for staging of pediatric sarcoma patients: results of a prospective multicenter trial. J Clin Oncol 2007;25:5435–41.

124. Schulte M, Brecht-Krauss D, Werner M, et al. Evaluation of neoadjuvant therapy response of osteogenic sarcoma using FDG PET. J Nucl Med 1999; 40:1637–43.

125. Bielack SS, Kempf-Bielack B, Delling G, et al. Prognostic factors in high-grade osteosarcoma of the extremities or trunk: an analysis of 1,702 patients treated on neoadjuvant cooperative osteosarcoma study group protocols. J Clin Oncol 2002; 20:776–90.

126. Ye Z, Zhu J, Tian M, et al. Response of osteogenic sarcoma to neoadjuvant therapy: evaluated by ^{18}F-FDG-PET. Ann Nucl Med 2008;22:475–80.

127. Hawkins DS, Conrad EU III, Butrynski JE, et al. [F-18]-Fluorodeoxy-D-glucose positron emission tomography response is associated with outcome for extremity osteosarcoma in children and young adults. Cancer 2009;115(35):19–25.

128. Cheon GJ, Klim MS, Lee JA, et al. Prediction model of chemotherapy response in osteosarcoma by ^{18}F-FDG PET and MRI. J Nucl Med 2009;50: 1435–40.

129. Marec-Berard P, Philip T. Ewing sarcoma: the pediatrician's point of view. Pediatr Blood Cancer 2004; 42:477–80.

130. Paulussen M, Ahrens S, Dunst J, et al. Localized Ewing tumor of the bone: final results of the cooperative Ewing's sarcoma study CESS 86. J Clin Oncol 2001;19:1818–29.

131. Furth C, Amthauer H, Deneke T, et al. Impact of whole-body MRI and FDG-PET on staging and assessment of therapy response in a patient with Ewing sarcoma. Pediatr Blood Cancer 2006;47: 607–11.

132. Barker LM, Pendergrass TW, Sander JE, et al. Survival after recurrence of Ewing's sarcoma family of tumors. J Clin Oncol 2005;23:4354–62.

133. Gerth HU, Juergens KU, Dirksen U, et al. Significant benefit of multimodal imaging: PET/CT compared with PET alone in staging and follow-up of patients with Ewing tumors. J Nucl Med 2007;48:1932–9.

134. Weyl Ben AM, Israel O, Postovsky S, et al. Positron emission tomography/computed tomography with [18]Fluor-deoxyglucose in the detection of local recurrence and distant metastasis of pediatric sarcoma. Pediatr Blood Cancer 2007;49:901–5.

135. Dishop MK, Kuruvilla S. Primary and metastatic lung tumors in the pediatric population: a review and 26-year experience at a large children's hospital. Arch Pathol Lab Med 2008;132(7):1079–103.

136. Yu DC, Grabowski MJ, Kozakewich HP, et al. Primary lung tumors in children and adolescents:

137. a 90-year experience. J Pediatr Surg 2010;45: 1090–5.

137. Suemitsu R, Maruyama R, Nishiyama K, et al. Pulmonary typical carcinoid tumor and liver metastasis with hypermetabolism on 18-fluorodeoxyglucose PET: a case report. Ann Thorac Cardiovasc Surg 2008;14:109–11.

138. Howman-Giles R, London K, McCowage G, et al. Pulmonary inflammatory myofibroblastic tumor after Hodgkin's lymphoma and application of PET imaging. Pediatr Surg Int 2008;24:947–51.

139. Kumar A, Jindal T, Dutta R, et al. Functional imaging in differentiating bronchial masses: an initial experience with a combination of (18)F-FDG-PET-CT scan and (68)Ga DOTA-TOC PET-CT scan. Ann Nucl Med 2009;23:745–51.

140. Geiger J, Walter K, Uhl M, et al. Imaging findings in a 3-year old girl with type III pleuropulmonary blastoma. In Vivo 2007;21:1119–22.

141. Lee EY, Vargas SO, Sawicki GS, et al. Mucoepidermoid carcinoma of bronchus in a pediatric patient: (18)F-FDG PET findings. Pediatr Radiol 2007;37: 1278–82.

142. Daniels CE, Lowe VJ, Aubry MC, et al. The utility of fluorodeoxyglucose positron emission tomography in the evaluation of carcinoid tumors presenting as pulmonary nodules. Chest 2007;131: 255–60.

143. Rothstein DH, Voss SD, Isakoff M, et al. Thymoma in a child: case report and review of the literature. Pediatr Surg Int 2005;21:548–51.

144. Kumar A, Regmi SK, Dutta R, et al. Characterization of thymic masses using (18)F-FDG PET-CT. Ann Nucl Med 2009;23:569–77.

145. Kushner BH. Neuroblastoma: a disease requiring a multitude of imaging studies. J Nucl Med 2004; 45:1172–88.

146. Massie RJ, Van Asperen PP, Mellis CM. A review of open biopsy for mediastinal masses. J Paediatr Child Health 1997;33:230–3.

147. Jacobson AF, Deng H, Lombard J, et al. ^{123}I-meta-iodobenzylguanidine scintigraphy for the detection of neuroblastoma and pheochromocytoma: results of a meta-analysis. J Clin Endocrinol Metab 2010; 95:2596–606.

148. Matthay KK, Shulkin B, Ladenstein R, et al. Criteria for evaluation of disease extent by ^{123}I-metaiodobenzylguanidine scans in neuroblastoma: a report for the International Neuroblastoma Risk Group (INRG) task force. Br J Cancer 2010; 102:1319–26.

149. Vik TA, Pfluger T, Kadota R, et al. ^{123}I-mIBG scintigraphy in patients with known or suspected neuroblastoma: results from a prospective multicenter trial. Pediatr Blood Cancer 2009;52:784–90.

150. Kushner BH, Kramer K, Modak S, et al. Sensitivity of surveillance studies for detecting asymptomatic

and unsuspected relapse of high-risk neuroblastoma. J Clin Oncol 2009;27:1041–6.

151. Kushner BH, Kramer K, Modak S, et al. Reply to K. Satharasinghe et al. J Clin Oncol 2009;27:e235.

152. Pfluger T, Schmied C, Porn U, et al. Integrated imaging using MRI and ¹²³I metaiodobenzylguanidine scintigraphy to improve sensitivity and specificity in the diagnosis of pediatric neuroblastoma. AJR Am J Roentgenol 2003;181:1115–24.

153. Sharp SE, Shulkin BL, Gelfand MJ, et al. ¹²³I-MIBG scintigraphy and ¹⁸F-FDG PET in neuroblastoma. J Nucl Med 2009;50:1237–43.

154. Taggart DR, Han MM, Quach A, et al. Comparison of iodine-123 metaiodobenzylguanidine (MIBG) scan and [¹⁸F] fluorodeoxyglucose positron emission tomography to evaluate response after iodine-131 MIBG therapy for relapsed neuroblastoma. J Clin Oncol 2009;27:5343–9.

155. Sharp SE, Shulkin BL, Gelfand MJ, et al. Reply to: letter to the editor. J Nucl Med 2010;51:331.

156. Colavolpe C, Guedj E, Cammilleri S, et al. Utility of FDG-PET/CT in the follow-up of neuroblastoma which became MIBG-negative. Pediatr Blood Cancer 2008;51:828–31.

157. Rufini V, Calcagni ML, Baum RP. Imaging of neuroendocrine tumors. Semin Nucl Med 2006;36:228–47.

158. Treves ST, Davis RT, Fahey FH. Administered radiopharmaceutical doses in children: a survey of 13 pediatric hospitals in North America. J Nucl Med 2008;49:1024–7.

159. Lassman M, Biassoni L, Monsieurs M, et al, EANM Dosimetry and Paediatrics Committees. The new EANM paediatric dosage card. Eur J Nucl Med Mol Imaging 2007;34:796–8.

160. Gelfand MJ, Parisi MT, Treves ST. Pediatric radiopharmaceutical administered doses: 2010 North American consensus guidelines. J Nucl Med 2010;52:318–22.

161. Stansfield EC, Sheehy N, Zurakowski D, et al. Pediatric 99mTc-MDP bone SPECT with ordered subset expectation maximization iterative reconstruction with isotropic 3D resolution recovery. Radiology 2010;257:793–801.

Radiation, Thoracic Imaging, and Children: Radiation Safety

Donald P. Frush, MD

KEYWORDS
- Computed tomography • Infants and children
- Radiation dose • Radiation risk

The chest is the most frequently evaluated region of the body in children.[1] In this issue of *Radiologic Clinics* the various applications and benefits of chest imaging are detailed. The majority of thoracic diagnostic imaging involves modalities that depend on ionizing radiation, consisting of "conventional" radiography (film screen, computed radiography [CR], and direct/digital radiography [DR]), fluoroscopy, angiography, multidetector computed tomography (MDCT), and nuclear imaging. While radiography has been a mainstay for chest imaging across the pediatric population, computed tomography (CT) is the second most commonly used modality, with an established record for improving care for both diagnosis and management strategies.[1–3] In particular, with the availability of isotropic datasets with thin detector array technology combined with high-quality 2-dimensional and 3-dimensional reconstruction MDCT images, evaluation of the cardiovascular system and airway has been a particular advantage in children.[4,5] CT angiography, including electrocardiogram gating CT angiography, has been especially helpful in evaluation, reducing the risks associated with conventional catheter-based angiography.[5,6] Paralleling these broadening applications are advancements in radiation protection through technical advancements as well as improved protocols. For CT, these technical advances include automatic tube current modulation and, more recently,

iterative reconstruction as well as in-plane breast shielding. For fluoroscopic evaluation, pulsed fluoroscopy substantially decreases radiation exposure in children. CR and DR, when used appropriately, also have the potential for dose reduction in pediatric imaging. These improvements in reducing radiation exposure risk, when matched with appropriate use strategies,[7–9] are essential for safe and effective health care in thoracic imaging in children.

Ionizing radiation is fundamental in the overwhelming majority of thoracic imaging in children, and radiation exposure is the most common risk. Physician imaging experts, especially radiologists, have the most extensive training and experience with the combination of radiation bioeffects, medical physics, epidemiology, and risk-reduction strategies. But there must also be a dynamic partnership with technologists, medical and health physicists, epidemiologists, regulators and policy experts, educators, nurses, other investigators in allied imaging health fields, and industry representatives. It is incumbent on this community to maximize the yield and minimize both the real and potential radiation risks of diagnostic imaging.

Mistakes, oversights, and inattention to radiation exposure continue to be an extremely visible issue for radiology in the public eye.[10,11] Radiation exposure has a long history in diagnostic imaging, especially pediatric radiology where John Caffey,

Disclosure: The author is a principal investigator for CT research in children from GE Healthcare. No salary support.
Pediatric Radiology, Department of Radiology, 1905 Children's Health Center, Duke University Medical Center, Box 3808 DUMC, Durham, NC 27710, USA
E-mail address: frush943@mc.duke.edu

Radiol Clin N Am 49 (2011) 1053–1069
doi:10.1016/j.rcl.2011.06.003

an outspoken critic of thymic radiation for treatment of what is now recognized as normal thymus in children, was reported to emphasize that "destroying the thymus myth" was one of pediatric radiology's most significant contributions to medicine.[12] Even recently, risks of breast and thyroid cancer were reported with thymic radiation during childhood.[13,14] In addition, the introduction section of Consumer Reports, 50 years ago, included the statement "…2 serious abuses…are frequently met with today—the improper use of x-rays and the use of unnecessarily large doses." This introduction ended with a still timely though potentially underappreciated admonishment that "…a patient who refuses to be x-rayed because of fear of radiation will not be protecting his health but jeopardizing it."[15] Up until 10 years ago, radiation dose and attendant risks from CT were often frankly ignored and often unrecognized in children[16,17] by those professionally responsible for their welfare. At present, radiation risks from diagnostic imaging are still recognized in industry journals. In the Top Ten Technical Hazards for 2011 from the ECRI Institute, the radiation dose from CT scans was listed as fourth in priority, and superseded information technology, complications, patient-controlled analgesia overdoses (ironically, another "dosing" problem), as well as needle sticks all more traditionally recognized as "dangers" in medical care.[18] Recently, state legislation in California mandated dose index recording from CT examinations on radiology reports.[19] It is not difficult to see that there is a long-standing and increasingly compelling need to address radiation safety from a myriad of sectors, across all ages, and inclusive of thoracic imaging.

To these ends, this article reviews practice patterns, dose measures and modality doses, radiation biology and risks, and risk-reduction strategies for thoracic imaging in children. Although the real and potential risks cannot be entirely eliminated, improvements in radiation protection can be achieved while maintaining diagnostic capabilities. Because radiography and CT examinations are most commonly used for thoracic imaging in children,[1] most of the discussion focuses on these two modalities.

PRACTICE PATTERNS

Medical imaging now accounts for nearly 50% of the radiation exposure to the United States population as opposed to 15% 30 years ago (Fig. 1).[20] At present, CT scanning is responsible for about half of all medical imaging exposure, and nearly 25% of all radiation exposure to the United States population.[20] As many as 2 to 7 million children per

year undergo CT examinations.[1,21] While there have been indications of increasing use of CT over the past two decades, new data suggest that the performance may be decreasing, at least in children's hospitals.[22] In the 2008 survey of the Society of Chairpersons of Radiology at Children's Hospitals (SCORCH) membership, including institutional data from 2003 to 2007, there was an overall decrease in the percentage of pediatric CT examinations as a function of the total number of cross-sectional imaging (CT, magnetic resonance (MR), and sonography examinations) from about 41% in 2003 to 35% in 2007. At present, a survey to assess pediatric CT usage in institutions and practices that image children but are not centers for pediatric imaging is being performed (Michael Callahan, MD, Boston, MA, personal communication, December 2010).

Recent extensive data by Dorfman and colleagues[1] provide some interesting perspectives on imaging in children. This investigation looked at about 350,000 children in 5 health care markets across the country and included fairly detailed age-, gender-, modality-, and indication-specific data. As many as 42% of children younger than 18 years underwent medical imaging involving ionizing radiation, with higher rates of use in children older than 10 years and younger than 2 years. CT examinations were performed in 7.9%, with more than one examination in 3.5% of the population. Fluoroscopy and angiography were relatively infrequent, accounting for 2% of the total, with only 0.7% receiving nuclear imaging examinations. Chest radiography was nearly double the relative percentage of the next closest radiographic procedure or region. Chest CT was performed about 15% of the time compared with brain CT. Abdomen/pelvis CT, maxillofacial CT, and spine CT were performed more often than chest CT in children. Investigators extrapolated that about 1.9 million children per year underwent CT examination, with 0.9 million having 2 or more examinations. For fluoroscopic evaluation, the upper gastrointestinal examination (obviously involving some thoracic radiation exposure) was the most frequent examination performed, with dedicated evaluation of the pharynx or esophagus as the third most frequently performed examination. These data show that when fluoroscopy is performed in children, the chest is often involved. While the frequency of CT examination in pediatric specialty centers such as children's hospitals may be decreasing, Broder and colleagues[23] noted that in a 6-year period from 2000 to 2006 the frequency of chest CT imaging rose by 435%, despite increases in visit frequency of 2%. More recently, in two separate articles by Larson and

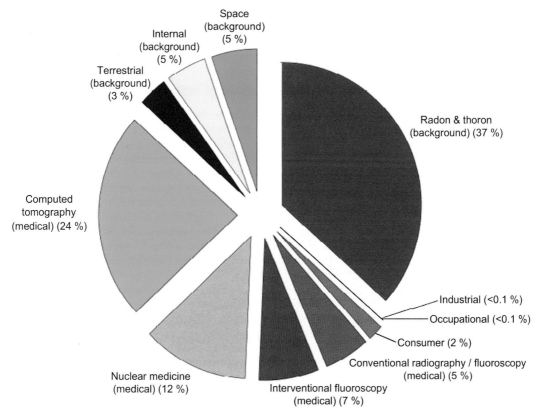

Fig. 1. All exposure categories: collective effective dose (percent), 2006. (*From* National Council on Radiation Protection and Measurements. Ionizing radiation exposure of the population of the United States. National Council on Radiation Protection and Measurements Report No. 160. Bethesda, MD: National Council on Radiation Protection and Measurements, 2009; with permission.)

colleagues[24,25] also noted that the frequency of imaging of children in the emergency department was increasing. First,[24] there has been a fivefold increase (0.33 million to 1.6 million) in the number of pediatric CT examinations performed in the emergency department from 1995 to 2008. Larson and colleagues[25] also observed in another investigation that "the compound annual growth rates in the percentage of ED visits in which CT was performed in children, young adults, middle-aged adults… were 12.7%, 15.2%, 14.4%…," also noting a brief inflection point in 2005 to 2006 that suggested (but was not conclusive) that the growth rate was near zero for this period. Therefore, while there may be some overall trends in children's hospitals, it is not yet clear that CT use in children for all indications and across all practice environments is substantially decreasing.

RADIATION DOSE

A recent review by Huda[26] and an educational module of the International Atomic Energy Agency (IAEA)[27] are excellent resources for radiation units,

especially in CT. The more common dose units are summarized here. Most metrics will be incidental radiation, or exposure (air kerma, kerma area product), or absorbed radiation (eg, absorbed dose to an organ) and effective dose. Air kerma (kinetic energy released per unit mass) is measured in Gray (Gy). The dose area product (DAP, also called kerma air product or KAP) is measured in $Gy \cdot cm^2$ (or more appropriately for medical imaging as $mGy \cdot cm^2$), the area factor representing a plane perpendicular to the beam. Because of the relationship with increasing area the further from the source of radiation, as well as the inverse square law with distance, the KAP in the balance does not change based on where it is measured in the primary beam. In angiography and potentially fluoroscopy, cumulative dose relative to the International Reference Point (usually 15 cm from the gantry source) can be used in addition to KAP. Fluoroscopic time is an insensitive indicator of radiation exposure given the high rate of variable influence on radiation from parameters such as magnification, source to patient distance, and collimation,[9] although it may often be part of the archived and potentially formal dictated patient report. Cine runs and number of images are also only crude indicators of dose and are not recommended as measures of radiation exposure in medical imaging. In radiography, there have been several dose descriptors, most being distilled down to an exposure index. At present, vendors are moving toward more consensus measures of exposure index for CR and DR.

Conversion from these various dose amounts to effective dose for all imaging modalities is beyond the aim of this article. However, it is worthwhile to understand this conversion for CT because it is often reported, and CT dose estimation does have some limitations, especially in children. For CT examinations this can be calculated by multiplying the CT dose index (CTDI) available on CT equipment by the scan length product to obtain the dose length product (DLP). Multiplication of the DLP with various age-based and region-based conversion (K coefficient) factors can provide an estimate of effective dose, as recently reviewed by Thomas and Wang.[28] The DLP method in children is problematic, because measures are performed in a body (32 cm) and head (16 cm, the default "pediatric size" for small children) acrylic cylindrical phantoms. At present, collaborative groups within the American Association of Physicists in Medicine (Keith Strauss, MS, Boston, MA, personal communication, February 2011; Report of AAPM Task Group 204) are working on more appropriate pediatric dose estimations for CT examinations. Other ways to convert estimated effective dose for CT include published tables,[28,29] Monte Carlo simulations, and phantom dosimetry. In addition, in 2007 Martin[30] published a set of recommendations providing an indication of how much reliance can be placed on effective dose as an indicator of risk for patients.

DOSE ESTIMATIONS FOR THORACIC IMAGING IN CHILDREN

Radiographic doses in general are low compared with other modalities using ionizing radiation. Chest radiographic examinations can be more than 2 orders of magnitude lower than a CT examination, as shown in **Table 1** (data provided by Steve Don from St Louis Children's Hospital).[31]

Dose estimations from fluoroscopic and angiographic evaluation are highly variable, dependent to a large extent on the nature of the procedure, ranging from effective doses of less than 1 mSv to doses which for interventional therapeutic procedures may rarely exceed deterministic thresholds. For CT examinations, doses for chest imaging can range from less than 1 mSv to the

doses at or above 10 times this dose, especially for cardiac-gated examinations.[32] Whereas reference levels for chest examinations are not available in the United States, they are more developed in Europe. The National Council on Radiation Protection and Measurement (NCRP) is currently finalizing a report on diagnostic reference levels in medical imaging and dentistry (David Schauer, NCRP, personal communication, 2011).

Effective dose estimations from CT examinations in children can be variable. One recent article from Switzerland[33] provided dose-length product numbers from several institutions and demonstrated effective dose for chest CT (using the K coefficient) in children of 2.1 to 3.3 mSv (<1 year old), 2.9 to 4.2 mSv (1–5 years old), 2.3 to 3.2 mSv (5–10 years old), and 4.8 to 5.1 mSv (10–15 years old).[33] Of note, investigators also reported a tenfold variation in children younger than 1 year, a 20-fold variation in doses in children from 1 to 5 years old, with as high as a 40-fold variation in the teenage years. In addition, Muhogora and colleagues,[34] surveying the CT techniques in developing countries, have noted a wide variation in doses in children. In the United States, Thomas and Wang[28] provided a very thorough survey of their techniques, noting effective doses of 2.8 mSv at 0 years old, 3.4 mSv at 1 year of age, 3.7 mSv at 5 years of age, 4.1 mSv at 10 years of age, and 2.8 mSv at 15 years of age. A survey of Australian practices noted a 12-fold variation in the child and 24-fold variation in a baby for chest CT examinations, and resultant potential for large dose reductions in chest imaging.[35] Finally, unpublished data from a recent literature review performed by the author's group at Duke Medical Center demonstrated that chest CT doses across all ages range between 4.5 and 5.5 mSv, with higher dose estimations at younger ages. Together, these investigations demonstrate a wide range of chest CT doses that are not necessarily reflective of age or indication. This finding underscores the need to define reference levels more clearly. Current work through the American College of Radiology and 6 institutions (Children's Hospital of Boston, Children's Hospital Philadelphia, Cincinnati Children's Hospital, Massachusetts General Hospital, Duke Medical Center, Primary Children's Salt Lake City) is aimed at establishing preliminary reference levels for pediatric CT.

Of note, current MDCT technology can provide relatively high doses to children. For example, past work in the author's laboratory on a 64-slice scanner using metal oxide semiconductor field effect transistors (MOSFET), with all selectable CT parameters that effect radiation dose such as tube current, peak kilovoltage, and pitch, maximized for highest dose, demonstrated that chest

Table 1
Typical exposure received from common examinations at St Louis Children's Hospital

Examination	Preterm Weight or Age	No. of Images	kVp	mAs	Entrance Skin Exposure, mGy[a]	Bone Marrow, mGy	Effective Dose, mSv[b]
Portable chest	1000 g	1	64	1.6	0.072	0.008	0.009
Portable abdomen	1000 g	1	64	1.6	0.072	0.009	0.010
Portable chest	2000 g	1	70	2.5	0.15	0.017	0.020
Portable abdomen	2000 g	1	70	2.5	0.15	0.021	0.021
Chest PA	5 y	1	96	5	0.55	0.11	0.06
Chest Lat	5 y	1	96	7	0.77	0.11	0.09
Abdomen AP	5 y	1	66	10	0.45	0.037	0.040
Abdomen decubitus	5 y	1	66	12.5	0.56	0.070	0.078
Wrist AP	5 y	1	60	3.5	0.20	0.008	0.001
Wrist oblique	5 y	1	60	3.5	0.20	0.008	0.001
Wrist Lat	5 y	1	60	4	0.23	0.01	0.0012
Pelvis AP	5 y	1	66	10	0.45	0.032	0.041
Pelvis Frog	5 y	1	66	10	0.45	0.032	0.041
Scoliosis AP	11 y		68	20	1	0.054	0.130
Scoliosis Lat	11 y		68	40	2	0.100	0.095
Head CT	5 y	30	120	250		3.70	5.8
Abdomen/Pelvic CT	5 y	90	120	85		4.10	7.3
Fluoroscopy 3 min continuous	5 y	18			18	1.5	1.2
Fluoroscopy 3 min 8-pulse	5 y	18			4.8	0.4	0.32

Abbreviations: AP, anteroposterior; Lat, lateral; PA, posteroanterior.
[a] mGray.
[b] mSievert.
From Don S. Radiosensitivity of children: potential for overexposure in CR and DR and magnitude of doses in ordinary radiographic examinations. Pediatr Radiol 2004;34(3):S167–72; with permission.

CT effective dose could exceed 43 mSv in a 5-year-old anthropomorphic phantom. This scan was able to be completed without any sort of alert for the relatively high dose. Recently, both the Food and Drug Administration[36] and the National Electrical Manufacturers Association[37] have called for and developed recommendations for dose alerts on CT scanners.

RISK ESTIMATIONS

X-rays consist of high-energy photons that can transfer this energy into tissues and organs through which they pass. The energy transfer results in ionizations with either a direct effect of electrons on adjacent molecules, such as DNA, or production of free radicals when there is an interaction with water also affecting adjacent molecules such as DNA. Disruption in DNA may lead to poor repair and cell death but also may lead to altered function. Free electron or free radical effects on DNA can cause either single-stranded or double-stranded disruptions. Single-stranded breaks are often repaired. However, some double-stranded breaks, especially those separated some distance through several base pairs, cannot be adequately repaired and cell death or nonlethal chromosomal aberrations can occur, ultimately leading to potential dysregulation of normal growth and development, responsible for genetic defects and carcinogenesis. An excellent review of radiobiology for imagers was recently provided by Hall.[38]

Based on International Commission on Radiological Protection 103, the most radiosensitive tissues affected in thoracic imaging with ionizing radiation are the breast, red marrow, and lung, followed by the thyroid and esophagus.[39]

Children are more sensitive than adults to radiation by as much as a factor of 15, depending on age and gender.[40] However, it is important to realize that induction of fatal cancer by low-level radiation is uncertain; therefore, cautious interpretation of risks during medical imaging is warranted, particularly in discussions with individual patients, families, and caregivers.

In general, low-level radiation exposure is under 100 to 150 mSv. Risks above this level are not debated; however, there is disagreement regarding possible risk below this level. There are a great many variables that come into play, including gender, age, area of exposure, genetic susceptibility, and acute versus protracted exposure. In addition, one must recognize that a 1.0-mSv chest exposure in a 5-year-old girl carries a greater risk of breast cancer than a 10-mSv pelvic MDCT examination, despite an effective dose for the chest CT of one order of magnitude lower. This is due to the limited exposure to the breasts (scatter only) from the pelvic scan. The linear no-threshold model (LNT) is considered by many organizations to be the most conservative and reasonable model, although this has been recently debated.[41,42] In general, the teaching has been that there is a 5% risk of developing fatal cancer for every 1.0 mSv of exposure. Therefore, an effective dose of 100 mSv would result in a 0.5% (or 1 in 200) risk of cancer, and 10 mSv exposure would lead to a 0.05% (or 1 in 2000) risk of cancer. Again, this effective dose determination does not take into account age differences, and it may be that risk should be adjusted to as high as, say, 15% for younger children.

Epidemiologic studies for cancer risks in children provide important perspectives on what we know as well as uncertainties in radiation-related cancer from low levels of radiation exposure. Linet and colleagues[43] recently provided a comprehensive and excellent review of epidemiologic studies, which included low-level radiation in children (Table 2). There are several sources cited in the imaging literature suggesting a significant risk of cancer for exposure under 50 mSv that are familiar to pediatric radiologists. For example, Brenner and colleagues have noted that "the epidemiologic data suggest good evidence of increased cancer risks for 10–50 mSv for acute exposure and 50–100 mSv for protracted exposure."[44] In addition, they note that "…there is reasonable, though not definitive, epidemiologic evidence that organ doses in the range from 5–125 mSv result in very small but statistically significant increase in cancer risk."[2] Chodick and colleagues[45] reviewed pediatric CT examinations in Israel, concluding, "…17,686 pediatric scans were conducted annually in Israel during 1999–2003. We projected 9.5 lifetime deaths would be associated with one year of pediatric CT scanning. This number represents an excess of 0.29% over the total number of patients who are eventually estimated to die from cancer in their lifetime." One relatively extreme example of low-level radiation exposure and cancer risks in children from chest imaging was recently reported in the *International Journal of Epidemiology* by Bartley and colleagues,[46] who concluded "…the risk of ALL was elevated in children exposed to 3 or more postnatal x-rays." Citing Little in their review of cancer risks in children, Linet and colleagues[43] state that "…no consistent association has been observed for diagnostic radiation exposure and risk of childhood lymphoma, osteosarcoma, Ewing sarcoma, soft tissue sarcoma, or neuroblastoma."

STRATEGIES FOR RADIATION PROTECTION

The fundamental principles for radiation protection in pediatric imaging include justification and optimization. Justification, which implies "appropriate imaging," is an extremely complicated topic. The term "appropriate" is difficult to adjudicate, and examinations can be performed for a variety of arguably supportable reasons, including evidence-based data, experience (including anecdotal evidence), inexperience, self-referral, legal pressures (ie, defensive medicine), variations in resources, pressures by lay press, influence by third-party payers (reimbursement), and influences by parents or other caregivers. Recently the American Board of Radiology Foundation sponsored a symposium in Bethesda, Maryland, addressing issues of justification. Summary recommendations included: development of evidence-based appropriateness criteria; greater use of practice guidelines; decision support at the point of care; education of referring physicians, patients, and the public; accreditation of imaging facilities; management of self-referral and defensive medicine; and payment reform.[7] A recent example of how decision support can influence imaging was reported by Sistrom and colleagues[8] wherein American College of Radiology appropriateness criteria were embedded in a physician order entry system. Sistrom and colleagues demonstrated a decrease in the quarterly compound growth rate of outpatient CT from 3.0% to 0.25% coincident with the integration of the decision support system with computerized order entry. The use of imaging will clearly be furthered by investment in evidence-based medicine. At this point in time, appropriateness criteria and guidelines are useful but are all far from comprehensive. One often underemphasized aspect of controlling justification or appropriateness is the understanding that other imaging strategies that do not use ionizing radiation should be considered, especially sonography for evaluation of pleural processes and mediastinal abnormalities, particularly in younger children. MR imaging for chest wall and mediastinal and cardiovascular evaluation should also be considered.

A second principle of radiation protection is optimization. That is, when an examination is deemed appropriate, what measures can be taken to optimize the balance between radiation exposure and diagnostic yield?

For all imaging modalities, patient preparation is important. Children should be appropriately immobilized in the case of radiography, fluoroscopy, CT, and nuclear imaging, and sedation used only when necessary. For complex CT examinations such as CT angiography, understanding the clinical questions will help to design the examinations. Poor contrast enhancement may result in limited diagnostic yield and wasteful radiation exposure. During fluoroscopy, constant communication between radiologists and technologists with respect to positioning, and timing and amount of contrast for esophagography will help to minimize unnecessary fluoroscopic time. It is also important to have modality-credentialed staff. Incorrect settings for CR and DR examinations and fluoroscopy and angiography, as well as CT examination, can result in excess radiation exposure. With all modalities, a team approach among radiologists, technologists, and medical physicists will assure proper equipment function and use.

At the 2004 ALARA (As Low As Reasonably Achievable) symposium for CR and DR, experts emphasized the need for appropriate collimation, shielding, judicious use of grids, appropriate exposure factors, adequate preparation (immobilization and inspiratory effort), and post processing.[47,48] In addition, quality assessment and improvement programs were deemed critical, especially as modifications in existing radiography equipment occur or new equipment is installed. CR and DR have broad technical demands in pediatric imaging, due to the wide range of patient sizes. Establishment of appropriate settings and postprocessing protocols must be performed with as much expertise as possible by application specialists, technologists, and radiologists.

General strategies for radiation protection in radiography for screen film systems as well as CR and DR can be found in the IAEA educational material on radioprotection in children released in 2010.[26] Points emphasized included appropriate use of grids (minimizing use in very small children), use of posteroanterior versus anteroposterior projections in spine and chest radiography, assuring that the appropriate filtration is used,

minimizing exposure times to reduce motion artifacts, consideration of relatively higher kVp (with reduced mAs) examination techniques, attending to appropriate source to film distances, and minimizing patient to film distance. Shielding during radiography may reduce the minimal amount of external radiation but does not affect internal scatter. However, the use of shielding should not be discouraged because it is an overt acknowledgment to the child, parents, or other caregivers that every attention to minimizing exposure has been addressed. Appropriate collimation must be performed. For example, a review by Datz and colleagues[49] indicated that poor collimation resulted in increased exposure by a factor of 2 for chest imaging and neonatal nurseries.

Tomosynthesis has the potential to provide additional anatomic information compared with conventional radiography, and at lower doses compared with CT. The technique has recently been reviewed,[50] and increasing pediatric investigations and applications are anticipated.

Fluoroscopy and angiography, as already noted, are relatively infrequently used for thoracic imaging in children compared with radiography and CT.[1] As with radiography, the IAEA summary of measures to reduce fluoroscopic and angiographic radiation exposure in children is instructive.[26] Strategies outlined include avoiding field overlap with different series, excluding radiosensitive tissues when possible, minimizing the use of electronic magnification, judicious use of grids in young children, proper positioning of the image intensifier receptor before engaging fluoroscopy, optimizing collimation, using imaging hold rather than continuous fluoroscopy, copper filtration, use of pulsed fluoroscopy (including grid control fluoroscopy), use of last image store capabilities, appropriate alerts during procedures, and recording of appropriate measures (such as DAP or cumulative dose). Also, video recording during studies can provide for review without using additional fluoroscopy. Recently, the Alliance for Radiation Safety in Pediatric Imaging, through the Step Lightly campaign, reinforced these measures for radiation reduction in children (**Fig. 2**).[51]

Strategies for radiation dose reduction in CT consist of adjustment in technical parameters, appropriate protocol optimization (especially related to clinical indication), and use of some newer strategies for dose reduction. Many of these strategies were recently reviewed by Nievelstein and colleagues[52] in *Pediatric Radiology*.

CT examination techniques should be based on indication. For example, evaluation of osseous abnormalities, such as for pectus excavatum, can be performed at relatively low tube current.

Table 2
Risk of specific and total childhood cancers associated with early-life postnatal medical radiation exposure

Authors, Year, Published Location, Study Duration	Upper Age Limit	No. Cases/No. Controls	Type of Cases	Type of Controls	Method of Exposure Assessment	Type of Exposure	Exposure Prevalence in Controls	Estimated Relative Risk
Leukemia								
Stewart et al, 1958, Great Britain, 1953–1955	10	619/619	Deceased	Population	Interview, medical records	Diagnostic / Therapeutic	12.9 / 0.2	1.2 / 5.0
Polhemus and Koch, 1959, USA. Los Angeles, 1950–1957	n/s	251/251	Incident	Hospital	Questionnaire	Diagnostic / Fluoroscopy / Therapeutic	41.4 / 3.2 / 3.6	2.1* / 3.5* / 3.7*
Ager et al, 1965, USA, Minnesota, 1953–1957	4	109/102 (siblings) 110 (neighborhood)	Deceased	Siblings Neighborhood	Interview, medical records	Any	16.7 / 18.2	1.3 / 1.1
Graham et al, 1966, USA, New York State, Baltimore and Minneapolis-St Paul, 1959–1962	14	319/884	Incident	Population	Medical records	Any / >1 site	36.0 / 7.6	1.2 / 2.1
Shu et al, 1988, China, Shanghai, 1974–1986	14	309/618	Incident, prevalent	Population	Interview	Any	27.3	0.9
Fajardo-Gutierrez et al, 1993, Mexico, Mexico City	14	79/148	Incident, prevalent	Population, Hospital	Interview	Any	27.0	1.1
Acute Lymphoblastic Leukemia								
Shu, 1988, China, Shanghai, 1974–1986	14	172/618	Incident, prevalent	Population	Interview	Any	27.3	0.9
Magnani et al, 1990, Italy, Turin, 1981–1984	n/s	142/307	Incident, prevalent	Hospital	Interview	Diagnostic	45.9	0.7
Shu et al, 1994, China, Shanghai, 1986–1991	14	166/166	Incident	Population	Interview	Any	—	1.6
Shu. 2002, USA, 1989–1993	15	1842/1986	Incident	Population	Interview	Diagnostic	39	1.1
Infantc-Rivard, 2003, Canada, Quebec, 1980–1998	14	701/701	Incident	Population	Interview	Diagnostic 1 / 2 or more	19.1 / 18.8	1.1 / 1.5*

Study						Exposure		
Acute Myeloid Leukemia								
Shu et al, 1988, China, Shanghai, 1974–1986	14	92/618	Incident, prevalent	Population	Interview	Any	27.3	1.0
Lymphoma								
Shu et al, 1994, China, Shanghai, 1981–1991	14	87/166	Incident	Population	Interview	Any	—	1.6*
Brain Tumors								
Howe et al, 1989, Canada, Toronto, 1977–1983	19	74/138	Incident	Population	Interview	Chest diagnostic Skull diagnostic	8.0 4.3	2.1 6.7*
McCredie et al, 1994, Australia, NSW, 1985–1989	14	82/164	Incident	Population	Interview	Dental, Skull diagnostic	9.1	0.4
Shu et al, 1994, China, Shanghai, 1981–1991	14	107/107	Incident	Population	Interview	Any	—	1.5
Schuz et al, 2001, Germany, 1993–1997	15	466/2458	Incident	Population	Interview	Any	4.3	0.8
Astrocytoma								
Kuijten et al, 1990, USA, PA, NJ, DE, 1980–1986	14	163/163	Incident	RDD	Interview	Head or neck Dental	n/s n/s	1.0 0.9
Bunin et al, 1994, USA, Canada, 1986–1989	5	155/155	Incident	RDD	Interview	Head, neck or dental Dental Head	13.5 9.0 3.2	1.2 1.0 1.1
PNET								
Bunin et al, 1994, USA, Canada, 1986–1989	5	166/166	Incident	RDD	Interview	Head, neck or dental Dental Head	12.0 8.4 4.2	1.1 0.5 0.9
Neuroblastoma								
Greenberg et al, 1983, USA, North Carolina, 1972–1981	14	104/208 (hospital) 105 (Wilm)	Incident	Hospital Wilm	Medical records	Chest Cranial Abdominal 	33.2 11.7 6.2 1.3 6.7 3.9	0.3* 2.0 0.3 1.6 0.4 0.8

(continued on next page)

Table 2
(continued)

Authors, Year, Published Location, Study Duration	Upper Age Limit	No. Cases/No. Controls	Type of Cases	Type of Controls	Method of Exposure Assessment	Type of Exposure	Exposure Prevalence in Controls	Estimated Relative Risk
Osteosarcoma								
Gelberg et al, 1997, USA, New York	24	130/130	Incident	Population	Interview	Medical	n/s	1.0
Ewing Sarcoma								
Daigle et al, 1987, USA, Minnesota, 1975–1981	20	98/98 95/95	Incident, prevalent	RDD Siblings	Interview	Any	n/s n/s	1.0 1.0
Winn et al, 1992, USA, multicenter, 1983–1985	22	204/204 191/191	Incident	RDD Siblings	Interview	Diagnostic Dental Diagnostic Dental	37.7 50.0 39.8 53.9	1.6* 1.2 1.6 0.9
All Sites								
Stewart et al, 1958, Great Britain, 1953–1955	10	1299/1299	Deceased	Population	Interview, medical records	Diagnostic Therapeutic	13.6 0.2	1.0 2.7
Hartley et al, 1988, UK, North West, West Midlands, Yorkshire, 1980–1983	14	535/1068 465/928	Incident	General practitioner, hospital	Interview, medical records	Neonatal diagnostic	0.3 1.0	2.0 1.1
Shu et al, 1994, China, Shanghai	14	642/642	Incident	Population	Interview	Any	—	1.3*

* Statistically significant.

Abbreviations: n/s, not stated; PNET, primitive neuroectodermal tumor; RDD, Random digit dialing.

From Linet M, Kim K, Rajaraman P. Children's exposure to diagnostic medical radiation and cancer risk: epidemiologic and dosimetric considerations. Pediatr Radiol 2009;39(1): S4–26; with permission.

Patient's Name _____ MR# _____ Date of exam _____

image gently℠

Step Lightly Checklist

Review steps below before starting the procedure.

Safety is a team effort: don't be afraid to ask the necessary questions to ensure you are working as a team to keep radiation dose to patients and staff as low as possible.

Reducing radiation dose must be balanced with safe, accurate and effective completion of the procedure. Not all the steps below may be possible in each case, depending on patient size, technical challenge and critical nature of the procedure. Overall patient safety is most important. The goal is to minimize the dose to the patient while providing important and necessary medical care.

- ❏ Ask patient or family about previous radiation (record card downloadable at this link). Answer questions about radiation safety (parent/patient brochure downloadable here)
- ❏ Use ultrasound when possible
- ❏ Position hanging table shields and overhead lead shields prior to procedure with reminders during the case as needed
- ❏ Operators and personnel wear well fitted lead aprons, thyroid shield and leaded eye wear
- ❏ Use pulse rather than continuous fluoroscopy when possible, and with as low a pulse as possible
- ❏ Position and collimate with fluoroscopy off, tapping on the pedal to check position
- ❏ Collimate tightly. Exclude eyes, thyroid, breast, gonads when possible
- ❏ Operator and personnel hands out of beam
- ❏ Step lightly: tap on pedal and review anatomy on last image hold rather than with live fluoroscopy when possible; minimize live fluoroscopy time
- ❏ Minimize use of electronic magnification; use digital zoom whenever possible
- ❏ Acknowledge fluoroscopy timing alerts during procedure
- ❏ Use last image hold whenever possible instead of exposures
- ❏ Adjust acquisition parameters to achieve lowest dose necessary to accomplish procedure: use lowest dose protocol possible for patient size, lower frame rate, minimize magnification, reduce length of run
- ❏ Plan and communicate number and timing of acquisitions, contrast parameters, patient positioning and suspension of respiration with radiology and sedation team in advance to minimize improper or unneeded runs
- ❏ Move table away from X-ray tube in both planes. Move patient as close to detector in both planes
- ❏ Use a power injector, or extension tubing if injected by hand
- ❏ Move personnel away from table or behind protective shields during acquisitions
- ❏ Minimize overlap of fields on subsequent acquisitions
- ❏ After procedure: record and review dose

Fig. 2. Radiation protection check list from Step Lightly Campaign for pediatric interventional radiology. (*From* Sidhu M, Goske MJ, Connolly B, et al. Image gently, step lightly: promoting radiation safety in pediatric interventional radiology. AJR Am J Roentgenol 2010;195:299–301; with permission from Alliance for Radiation Safety in Pediatric Imaging.)

CT angiography is amenable to lower kVp because of the relatively high contrast enhancement. Recently, Singh and colleagues[53] provided a review of dose-reduction strategies for pediatric CT based on clinical indication, as well as patient size, and prior CT examinations. Routine chest evaluation can be performed at lower peak kilovoltage and tube current than abdominal examinations. Protocols for chest MDCT are available.[52,54] In general, 80 kVp for the youngest (smallest) children, increasing to 100 kVp in school-age children, with a maximum of 120 kVp is generally recommended for general chest MDCT. Kim and Newman[55] have reported on the benefits of lower kVp in chest CT in children and have found that reductions of 40% to 50% in dose were possible. Because of the relatively high contrast resolution of lung tissue, lower tube currents are also useful in chest imaging. For example, Li and colleagues,[56] in a lung nodule study, demonstrated that tube current could be as low as 17.5 mA for nodule detection in a model of digital nodule insertion and simulated tube current reduction. The use of tube current modulation in children has also been helpful in reducing dose.[57–59] Recently, Peng and colleagues[60] reported decreases of about 65% in $CTDI_{vol}$ compared with a fixed tube current while maintaining acceptable image quality. Pitch is

Table 3
Published dosimetry: investigations of bismuth shield techniques

Investigation	Region Scanned (No. of Patients)	Organ Assessed (Shield Layers)	Patient Type (No. of Patients)	Dose Reduction	Comments on Image Quality
Mukundan et al	Head	Eye (2)	5-y-old pediatric phantom	42%	Shield artifact fell outside the diagnostic area of interest
Fricke et al	Chest (29), Abdomen (21)	Breast (2)	2-mo to 18-y-old pediatric patients, neonatal phantom	29%	No statically significant difference in noise between the shielded and nonshielded lung regions of interest
Coursey et al	Chest	Breast (2)	5-y-old pediatric phantom	26% (Bi only) 52% (Bi + ATCM)	Image noise increased but remained close to the target noise index (12 HU)
Melaughlin et al	Brain (20) Chest (20)	Eye, thyroid (4)	20 controlled group, 20 uncontrolled group	18% (eye), 56% (thyroid)	Image artifacts are a problem if the shield is placed in inappropriate way
Hopper et al	Chest (45), head, neck, pelvis	Breast, thyroid, eye testes (4)	Female patients (chest), Phantom (thyroid, eye, testes)	57% (breast), 60% (thyroid) 40% (eye), 51% (testes)	Shield did not affect the diagnostic CT image but reduced the amount of radiation to radiosensitive structures
Hopper et al	Head (30)	Eye (4)	Phantom, patients	49% (phantom), 40% (patients)	No significant artifact caused by the eye shielding
Kalra et al	Chest	Breast (4)	Phantom	40%	In-plane shields are associated with greater image noise, artificially increased attenuation values, and streak artifacts
Yilmaz et al	Chest (50)	Breast	Adult female patients	41%	No qualitative changes in image quality
Hohl et al	Nock, chest	Thyroid, breast	Phantom	47% (thyroid), 32% (breast)	No deterioration in image quality